The Sjögren's Book

The Sjögren's Book

FOURTH EDITION

Edited by Daniel J. Wallace, MD

Associate Editors:

Steven E. Carsons, MD
Elaine Alexander, MD, PhD
Frederick B. Vivino, MD
Katherine Morland Hammitt, MA
Steven Taylor, SSF CEO

Assistant Editor:

Patricia Spolyar, RN

A publication of the Sjögren's Syndrome Foundation

and

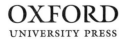

OXFORD
UNIVERSITY PRESS

OXFORD
UNIVERSITY PRESS

Oxford University Press, Inc., publishes works that further
Oxford University's objective of excellence
in research, scholarship, and education.

Oxford   New York
Auckland   Cape Town   Dar es Salaam   Hong Kong   Karachi
Kuala Lumpur   Madrid   Melbourne   Mexico City   Nairobi
New Delhi   Shanghai   Taipei   Toronto

With offices in
Argentina   Austria   Brazil   Chile   Czech Republic   France   Greece
Guatemala   Hungary   Italy   Japan   Poland   Portugal   Singapore
South Korea   Switzerland   Thailand   Turkey   Ukraine   Vietnam

Published by Oxford University Press, Inc.
198 Madison Avenue, New York, New York 10016
www.oup.com

Oxford is a registered trademark of Oxford University Press

Library of Congress Cataloging-in-Publication Data

The Sjogren's book / edited by Daniel J. Wallace.—4th ed.
p. cm.
Rev. ed. of: New Sjogren's syndrome handbook editor, Daniel J. Wallace;
associate editors, Evelyn J. Bromet ... [et al.].
Includes bibliographical references and index.
ISBN 978-0-19-973722-2
1. Sjogren's syndrome—Popular works. I. Wallace, Daniel J. (Daniel Jeffrey),
1949- II. New Sjogren's syndrome handbook.
RC647.5.S5N49 2011
616.7'75—dc23   2011022192

9 8 7 6 5 4 3 2
Printed in USA
on acid-free paper

CONTENTS

CONTRIBUTORS

Soo Kim Abboud, MD Assistant Professor, Department of Otolaryngology–
Head and Neck Surgery, University of Pennsylvania School of Medicine;
Chief of Otolaryngology, Penn Presbyterian Medical Center, Philadelphia,
Pennsylvania

Elaine Alexander, MD, PhD Biomedical Consultant, San Diego, California

Thomas R. Allan, MD Department of Obstetrics and Gynecology, Hartford
Hospital, Hartford, Connecticut. Assistant Clinical Professor, University of
Connecticut, Farmington, Connecticut

Eva Baecklund, MD, PhD Senior Consultant, Unit of Rheumatology,
Department of Medical Sciences, Uppsala University, Uppsala, Sweden

Alan N. Baer, MD Associate Professor of Medicine and Director,
Jerome L. Greene Sjögren's Syndrome Clinic, Division of Rheumatology,
Johns Hopkins University School of Medicine, and Chief of Rheumatology,
Good Samaritan Hospital, Baltimore, Maryland

Margaret Baim, MS, NP Clinical Director for Training, Benson Henry
Institute for Mind Body Medicine, Massachusetts General Hospital, Boston,
Massachusetts

Richard D. Brasington, Jr., MD Professor of Medicine, Director of
Clinical Rheumatology, Washington University School of Medicine,
St. Louis, Missouri

Anne E. Burke, MD, MPH Assistant Professor of Gynecology and Obstetrics,
Johns Hopkins University School of Medicine, Bayview Medical Center,
Baltimore, Maryland

Steven E. Carsons, MD Chief, Division of Rheumatology, Allergy and
Immunology, Winthrop University Hospital, and Professor of Medicine,
SUNY, Stony Brook, Mineola, New York

Lan Chen, MD, PhD Clinical Associate of Medicine and Attending
Rheumatologist, Division of Rheumatology, Penn Presbyterian Medical
Center; Penn Sjögren's Center, University of Pennsylvania School of
Medicine, Philadelphia, Pennsylvania

Janine Austin Clayton, MD Deputy Director, Office of Research on Women's Health, National Institutes of Health, Bethesda, Maryland

Philip L. Cohen, MD Professor of Medicine, Chief of Rheumatology Section, Temple University School of Medicine, Philadelphia, Pennsylvania

Reza Dana, MD, MPH, M.Sc. Professor of Ophthalmology, Director of Cornea Service, Massachusetts Eye and Ear Infirmary, Harvard Medical School, Boston, Massachusetts

Troy E. Daniels, DDS, MS Professor of Oral Medicine and Pathology, Schools of Dentistry and Medicine, University of California, San Francisco, San Francisco, California

Lynn C. Epstein, MD, DLFAPA, FAACAP Clinical Professor of Psychiatry, Tufts University School of Medicine, Boston, Massachusetts

John R. Fenyk, Jr., MD Professor, Department of Dermatology, University of Minnesota, Minneapolis, Minnesota

H. Kenneth Fisher, MD, FACP, FCCP Professor of Clinical Medicine, University of California, Los Angeles, California, and Consultant in Pulmonary and Sleep Medicine, Wyoming Cardiopulmonary Services, Casper, Wyoming

S. Lance Forstot, MD, FACS Clinical Professor of Ophthalmology, University of Colorado Medical School, Denver, Colorado

Gary N. Foulks, MD, FACS Emeritus Professor of Ophthalmology, University of Louisville School of Medicine, Louisville, Kentucky

Robert I. Fox, MD, PhD Chief of Rheumatology, Scripps Memorial Hospital and Research Foundation, La Jolla, California

Philip C. Fox, DDS Visiting Scientist, Carolinas Medical Center, Charlotte, North Carolina

Arthur I. Grayzel, MD, MACR Past Medical Director, Arthritis Foundation, and Past President, Sjögren's Syndrome Foundation, New York, New York

Abha Gulati, MD Early Clinical Development Specialist, Merck Pharmaceuticals, Rahway, New Jersey

Katherine Morland Hammitt, MA Vice President of Research, Sjögren's Syndrome Foundation, Bethesda, Maryland

Paul F. Howard, MD, FACR, FACP Director, Arthritis Health, Scottsdale, Arizona, Clinical Lecturer, University of Arizona, Affiliate Assistant Professor, Midwestern University, Phoenix, Arizona

John A. Ice, MD Research Associate, Arthritis and Clinical Immunology Research Program, Oklahoma Medical Research Foundation, Oklahoma City, Oklahoma

Stuart S. Kassan, MD, FACP, FACR Clinical Professor of Medicine, University of Colorado Health Sciences Center, Denver, Colorado

Robert S. Lebovics, MD, FACS Head and Neck Surgical Group, and Surgical Consultant, New York, New York

Young H. Lee, BA, E. Medical Student (MSIII), Temple University School of Medicine, Philadelphia, Pennsylvania

Christopher J. Lessard, PhD Associate Research Scientist, Arthritis and Clinical Immunology Research Program, Oklahoma Medical Research Foundation, Oklahoma City, Oklahoma

Carla LoPinto-Khoury, MD Neurology Resident, Thomas Jefferson University, Jefferson Medical College, Philadelphia, Pennsylvania

Ian R. Mackay, MD, FRCP, FRACP, FRCPA, FAA Honorary Professor, Department of Biochemistry and Molecular Biology, Monash University, Melbourne, Australia

Steven Mandel, MD Professor of Neurology and Anesthesiology, Thomas Jefferson University, Jefferson Medical College, Philadelphia, Pennsylvania Adjunct Professor of Neurology, Temple University School of Podiatric Medicine. Adjunct Professor of Psychology, Widener University

Ramon Manon-Espaillat, MD, MA Clinical Professor of Neurology, Thomas Jefferson University, Jefferson Medical College, Philadelphia, Pennsylvania

Richa Mishra, MD Rheumatology Fellow, University of Pennsylvania, Philadelphia, Pennsylvania

Serena Morrison, MD Faculty Member, West Virginia University, Morgantown, West Virginia

Kathy L. Moser, PhD Director, Sjögren's Research Clinic, and Associate Member, Arthritis and Immunology Research Program, Oklahoma Medical Research Foundation, Oklahoma City, Oklahoma

Haralampos M. Moutsopoulos, MD, FACP, FRCP Professor and Director, Department of Pathophysiology, School of Medicine, National University of Athens, Athens, Greece

William Neil, MD Neurology Resident, Thomas Jefferson University, Jefferson Medical College, Philadelphia, Pennsylvania

Matthew Nichols, MD Assistant Clinical Professor, Department of Medicine, University of Colorado, School of Medicine; South Denver Gastroenterology, PC, Denver, Colorado

Athena S. Papas, DMD, PhD Head, Division of Public Health Research and Oral Medicine; Johansen Professor of Dental Research, Tufts University School of Dental Medicine, Boston, Massachusetts

Ann Parke, MD Professor of Medicine, University of Connecticut Health Center at St Francis Hospital, Hartford, Connecticut

Scott Pello, MD Neurology Resident, Thomas Jefferson University, Jefferson Medical College, Philadelphia, Pennsylvania

Lynn M. Petruzzi, RN, MSN Chair, Sjögren's Syndrome Foundation Board of Directors, and Chair, SSF Nursing & Allied Health Professional Awareness, Harrisburg, Pennsylvania

Theresa L. Ray, MD Medical Resident, Department of Dermatology, University of Minnesota, Minneapolis, Minnesota

David A. Roshal, DO Neurology Resident, Thomas Jefferson University, Jefferson Medical College, Philadelphia, Pennsylvania

Teri P. Rumpf, PhD Psychologist, Newton Highlands, Massachusetts

Barbara M. Segal, MD Associate Professor, Department of Medicine, University of Minnesota Medical School, Minneapolis, Minnesota

Katy M. Setoodeh, MD, Attending Rheumatologist, Department of Rheumatology, Cedars-Sinai Medical Center, Los Angeles, California

Mabi L. Singh, DMD, MS Associate Professor, Tufts University School of Dental Medicine, Boston, Massachusetts

Daniel Small, MD, M.M.Sc., F.A.C.P., F.A.C.R., Rheumatologist Director, Sjögren's Center of Florida, Sarasota, Florida

Meredith Snapp, MD Neurology Resident, Thomas Jefferson University, Jefferson Medical College, Philadelphia, Pennsylvania

Fotini C. Soliotis, MD, MRCP Rheumatologist, Euroclinic, Athens, Greece

Nehad R. Solomon, MD, FACR Rheumatologist, Valley Arthritis Care, Peoria, Arizona

Robert F. Spiera, MD Associate Professor of Clinical Medicine, Weill Medical College of Cornell University, New York, New York

Harry Spiera, MD Clinical Professor of Medicine, Mount Sinai School of Medicine, New York, New York

E. William St. Clair, MD Professor of Medicine, Professor of Rheumatology and Immunology, Chief, Division of Rheumatology and Immunology, Duke University School of Medicine, Durham, North Carolina

Thomas D. Sutton, Esq Leventhal Sutton & Gornstein, Trevose, Pennsylvania

Steven Taylor, Chief Executive Officer, Sjögren's Syndrome Foundation, Bethesda, Maryland

Elke Theander, MD, PhD Senior Consultant, Department of Rheumatology, Lund University, Malmö, Sweden

Elisa Rodriguez Trowbridge, MD Assistant Professor, Department of Obstetrics and Gynecology and Urology, Division of Female Pelvic Medicine and Reconstructive Surgery, University of Virginia, Charlottesville, Virginia

Frederick B. Vivino, MD, MS, FACR Chief, Division of Rheumatology, Penn Presbyterian Medical Center; Director, Penn Sjögren's Center; Associate Professor of Clinical Medicine, University of Pennsylvania School of Medicine, Philadelphia, Pennsylvania

Daniel J. Wallace, MD Clinical Professor of Medicine, Cedars-Sinai Medical Center, David Geffen School of Medicine at the University of California, Los Angeles, California

C. Keith Wilkinson, ND Naturopathic Doctor, Arthritis Health, Scottsdale, Arizona

Jeffrey Wilson, MD Rheumatology of Central Virginia Family Physicians, Lynchburg, Virginia

Ava J. Wu, DDS Clinical Professor, Sjögren's Syndrome Clinic, Department of Orofacial Sciences, University of California, San Francisco, California

PREFACE

In 1983, a small group of patients who were interested in gaining more knowledge about a little-known and medically under-recognized disorder met in a lecture room at Long Island Jewish Medical Center in New Hyde Park, New York. They were led by Elaine Harris, a patient who possessed the knowledge, determination, and vision to make a difference in the lives of a multitude of individuals who were touched in some way by Sjögren's syndrome. She was aided by three physician advisors—a dental medicine specialist, an ophthalmologist, and a rheumatologist—and donations of time and effort by staff and physicians at local area hospitals. This, nearly 30 years ago, began what would become the Sjögren's Syndrome Foundation (SSF), now recognized to be the premier international organization supporting education, patient services, and research in Sjögren's. *The Sjögren's Book* is the flagship publication of the organization and represents the broad clinical, scientific, and patient support scope of the modern SSF under the stewardship of CEO Steve Taylor and staff.

This edition of *The Sjögren's Book* updates and expands upon previous editions and in doing so offers 39 chapters that span the spectrum of Sjögren's issues that confront patients, family members, and healthcare providers alike. Like its predecessors, this edition of *The Sjögren's Book* is designed as a reference for patients, their caregivers, and clinicians of all stages of training and specialties and is intended not only to provide factual knowledge but also to encourage communication regarding Sjögren's.

The contributors to this edition represent a large cadre of national and international experts involved with research, diagnosis, and treatment, and living with Sjögren's. This edition of *The Sjögren's Book* will be a valuable resource to those involved with all aspects of Sjögren's and we hope will stimulate collaboration among those caring for individuals with Sjögren's as well as stimulate new ideas leading to research in the pathogenesis of and therapy for this prevalent disorder.

Steven E. Carsons, MD
Founding Member, Sjögren's Syndrome Foundation Medical
and Scientific Advisory Board, and Chief, Division of Rheumatology,
Allergy and Immunology, Winthrop-University Hospital
Professor of Medicine
SUNY, Stony Brook

INTRODUCTION: WHY WRITE A BOOK ON SJÖGREN'S?

Daniel J. Wallace

One American in 70 has a mysterious condition known as Sjögren's syndrome. While the disease was named 70 years ago after a Swedish ophthalmologist described its salient features, until recently Sjögren's resided in a nosologic purgatory, with its manifestations misunderstood, underappreciated, and ignored. An international consensus has finally been derived regarding what the term *Sjögren's* means. Now that organized science has finally come to terms (literally) with the syndrome, a number of insights elucidated by Sjögrenologists have been rapidly forthcoming. The collective wisdom of these investigators has recently resulted in the publication of prescient findings that serve to emphasize the importance of research into this area and will have implications far beyond the syndrome itself. It is our hope that researchers, clinicians, physicians, allied health professionals, and dentists as well as patients and their families will be able to use this resource.

Why should we write a book on Sjögren's? It is an autoimmune condition that affects the whole body, especially musculoskeletal and glandular tissues. It can exist as a primary condition or be a concomitant feature of rheumatoid arthritis, systemic lupus erythematosus, scleroderma, or other rheumatic disorders. According to the National Institutes of Health, 14.7 to 23.5 million people in the United States have an autoimmune condition, and 120 such conditions have been identified to date. Up to 4 million of these individuals have Sjögren's, according to the National Arthritis Data Workshop estimates, which would make the perception that it is uncommon incorrect. Its prevalence varies internationally from 0.1% to 4.8% of a general population. Sjögren's does not have a strong focus in medical education. Its symptoms are subtle and can be intermittent or nonspecific. It has been estimated that symptoms are present for a mean of 6 to 7 years before it is properly diagnosed. This is unfortunate because a delayed diagnosis drastically alters quality of life. For example:

1. Patients report greater fatigue, pain, depression, and cognitive function than their peers.
2. A survey showed that primary Sjögren's affects patients in the following way: 52% report effects on physical function, 46% on intimacy, 41% on career, 45% on daily life, 41% on social life,

and 39% on mental well-being, with similar numbers reported for those with secondary Sjögren's.

3. The majority of patients have serious dental complications (e.g., caries), and 38% report significant musculoskeletal impairments.

More importantly, 5% to 10% of those with primary Sjögren's develop a lymphoproliferative malignancy. Sjögren's is almost unique among autoimmune disorders in its ability to result in lymphoma in certain cases. This link could be exploited by researchers to help us understand many of the common immunological features shared by cancer and autoimmune disorders.

Although Sjögren's is the second most common autoimmune condition affecting the musculoskeletal system, it ranks eighth in terms of research funding. Studies aimed at finding the cause of and cure for this disease will ultimately save taxpayers billions of dollars in lost wages and productivity as well as improve the lives of many. We hope that our efforts will result in increased awareness and greater understanding of this underappreciated syndrome.

The editor gratefully acknowledges the help of Katherine Hammitt, Vice President of Research for the Sjögren's Syndrome Foundation, for rounding up difficult-to-access statistics on the impact of the syndrome in the United States. The sources supporting this data are available from the national office upon request.

Daniel J. Wallace, MD
Clinical Professor of Medicine
Cedars-Sinai Medical Center
David Geffen School of Medicine at the
University of California, Los Angeles
September 2010

PART ONE

INTRODUCTION AND DEFINITIONS

1

Sjögren's Syndrome Foundation

THE PATIENTS' AND PROFESSIONALS' KEY RESOURCE AND ADVOCATE

Steven Taylor, CEO, Sjögren's Syndrome Foundation

Being diagnosed with Sjögren's can be a relief for some and a little frightening for others. It can be a relief because the patient finally has a diagnosis that he or she has been searching for on average over 6 years. The diagnosis can be frightening for others because they received a diagnosis for a disease they know nothing about and have never heard of. That is where the Sjögren's Syndrome Foundation (SSF) can help.

For healthcare professionals, Sjögren's syndrome is sometimes a challenging disease to treat and manage. Often patients present differently, have different complications, and need different treatments depending on the severity and progression of their disease. The SSF can help with that, too.

Founded in 1983, the SSF has been helping patients, their families, and healthcare professionals maneuver through the maze we all know as Sjögren's. This maze is different for each person and often for each healthcare professional. That is why the SSF has developed a wealth of materials, resources, and services that can help.

Patient Resources

As a patient, you may need materials to help you understand, manage, or live with Sjögren's, or you may need them to help your loved ones understand what Sjögren's is. The SSF has both. The SSF continues to develop materials to help patients understand the various complications of Sjögren's. We have patient education fact sheets on numerous symptoms, brochures on dry eye, dry mouth, and Sjögren's and produce a monthly newsletter for patients. You can visit www.sjogrens.org to see our materials and learn more about the SSF and how to receive our monthly newsletter.

The SSF redesigned its website to better meet the needs of patients and healthcare professionals. By visiting our site, you will find all of our downloadable materials. You will also find comprehensive information about Sjögren's, tips for living with Sjögren's, as well as information about SSF activities and support groups.

In addition to our website and printed materials, the SSF hosts patient educational conferences in various cities around the United States to help patients get first-hand education from leading Sjögren's physicians around the United States. In addition to our conferences, the SSF manages 80-plus support groups around the United States. Each support group is managed by a local Sjögren's patient who volunteers to organize meetings and help support local patients. To learn more about conferences and support groups, visit our website or contact the SSF.

Professional Resources

In addition to our patient resources and materials, the SSF has also focused on expanding resources for healthcare professionals—from our various patient-ready materials to our support for Sjögren's research to the launching of our healthcare professional newsletter, the *Sjögren's Quarterly*.

With the introduction of our newly updated website, the SSF launched a professional resource page that has information about various resources available for professionals. From camera-ready patient materials to research information to our downloadable brochures, the SSF continues to support healthcare professionals.

Most impressively, the SSF has invested over $1 million in Sjögren's research since 2003. We have funded programs in genetics, gene expression, the immune system, potential regeneration of glands, cognitive symptoms, and the many other complications in Sjögren's, just to name a few. We have supported projects at institutions around the United States, including launching our innovative concept grant, which rewards the most innovative application with a $50,000 grant per year for 2 years. Support of such studies entices new researchers to Sjögren's, keeps current researchers devoted to Sjögren's, and sparks novel ideas that other researchers can build upon. And all of these programs provide hope toward finding potential treatments for Sjögren's and ultimately unlocking the mystery of Sjögren's to find a cure.

In 2010, the SSF launched a major initiative to develop clinical practice guidelines that will establish a baseline for physicians to follow when treating Sjögren's. These guidelines will provide a comprehensive document that will cover management and treatment of ocular, oral, and systemic manifestations of Sjögren's. These guidelines will be the first of their kind for Sjögren's and will change the course of Sjögren's treatment by healthcare professionals.

Finally, the SSF launched its healthcare professional newsletter, the *Sjögren's Quarterly*. This newsletter is printed four times a year and distributed free to healthcare professionals. Each issue reviews the latest in Sjögren's research and features a clinical corner sharing a healthcare professional's experience in treating various aspects of Sjögren's. In addition, the SSF reviews scientific conferences and updates professionals on clinical trials being conducted in Sjögren's.

Advocate for Patients

The SSF advocates for Sjögren's patients by representing their voice on numerous coalitions as well as working toward increasing awareness for Sjögren's throughout the United States. The SSF serves on many volunteer coalitions on such topics as autoimmune diseases, cost of prescription products, healthcare reform, and government funding for research. All coalitions must meet our standards, but most importantly they must ensure that our Sjögren's voice will be heard in the discussion. In addition to these volunteer coalitions, the SSF has also been fortunate to be invited to serve on prestigious committees and boards, including those managed by the National Institutes of Health, National Health Council, professional societies, and other government and private agencies. Through these coalitions, the SSF has been able to increase awareness for Sjögren's as well as ensure that our disease is represented in legislative bills, government guidelines, and research appropriations.

Most impressively, after a 5-year project, the SSF was successful at getting Sjögren's listed with our own guidelines for Social Security Disability. This change will ensure that patients who qualify for disability will be reviewed based on Sjögren's guidelines and not by a more general category. This language change was monumental for Sjögren's since not all autoimmune diseases have their own guidelines.

The SSF also organizes community events that help increase awareness for Sjögren's. These events include not only participating in local health fairs throughout the United States but also hosting over 20 additional special events to help raise funds for our research and education programs. Most importantly, they help to increase awareness by having local volunteers promote our events, solicit sponsors, and encourage friends and families to attend. In 2010, the SSF raised over $400,000 from our special events and attracted over 2,000 participants.

And finally, the SSF advocates on patients' behalf at healthcare professional conferences each year. From the American College of Rheumatology to ocular and dental conferences, the SSF continues to host presentations and panels to educate professionals on Sjögren's.

Our Hope

In 1983, when Elaine Harris founded the SSF, she believed in the basic premise that it would always help Sjögren's patients by supporting education, increasing awareness, and supporting research. And nearly 30 years later, the SSF operates under the same premise of helping patients. Before beginning any new project, initiative, or program, our staff and volunteers must always be able to answer the same question, "How will this help patients?"

We must also thank all of the volunteers, past and present, who have helped to get the SSF to where it is today. Each of them has selflessly given his or her time and talents to help advance the mission of the SSF. Thanks to them, we have seen new treatments, new research concepts being developed, and additional educational opportunities offered for patients. In the past few years alone, we have seen great advancements for Sjögren's patients. And with your help, we can continue to make the same rapid advancements we have seen in the past few years. I thank you in advance for supporting the SSF by volunteering your time and donating to our campaigns. With your support, we will make Sjögren's a household name!

2

What Is Sjögren's?

Arthur I. Grayzel, MD, MACR

In this chapter, Sjögren's syndrome will be described and classified by means of its signs, symptoms, autoimmune features, and autoantibodies. This material is intended to be an overview, with both the concepts and specific findings to be explained in more detail in the following chapters.

Definitions: Is Sjögren's Syndrome a Disease?

Why isn't Sjögren's syndrome a disease? It really is, when viewed from a current perspective. A syndrome, as defined in the *Random House Dictionary*, is "a group of symptoms that characterizes a disease," whereas a disease, according to *Stedman's Medical Dictionary*, is "a pathologic entity characterized by two of these criteria: a recognized etiologic agent, an identifiable group of signs and symptoms, or consistent anatomical alterations." Sjögren's has an identifiable group of signs and symptoms and consistent anatomical alterations.

Signs and Symptoms

What are the signs and symptoms of Sjögren's? The most distinctive ones, and those originally described by Henrik Sjögren, are dry eye and dry mouth due to a lack of tear production and a lack of saliva. The actual symptoms in the eye include a gritty sensation, the sense of a foreign body in the eye, or itching; redness; and an increased sensitivity to light that may make reading or watching television difficult. The symptoms of lack of saliva may include difficulty chewing, swallowing, and speaking, and severe, progressive dental caries. Patients find they are continually sipping water. These distinctive symptoms have also been called the sicca syndrome (from the Latin *siccus,* meaning "dry").

Other organs in the body that secrete moist material, usually as a form of mucus, can also participate in this sicca syndrome and produce troublesome symptoms in patients with Sjögren's. Among these organs are the lungs, the upper airways such as the nose and throat, the vagina, and the skin. These symptoms, however, are not used to define the disease.

Finally, since Sjögren's is, as we shall see, a chronic inflammatory disease, patients complain of symptoms common to all inflammatory diseases, such as chronic and profound fatigue, as well as symptoms common to all chronic diseases, such as depression. These symptoms, while real and often disabling, are too nonspecific to define the disease.

Primary and Secondary Sjögren's

Henrik Sjögren also reported that 13 of the original 19 patients he described had arthritis. Arthritis in patients with Sjögren's resembles rheumatoid arthritis, but there is usually less swelling. On the other hand, 15% to 30% of patients with unequivocal rheumatoid arthritis may develop Sjögren's. This situation can be the source of much confusion and has led to the concept of primary and secondary Sjögren's. Patients have secondary Sjögren's when they also have another autoimmune disease—most commonly rheumatoid arthritis (RA) or systemic lupus erythematosus (SLE), but a large number of other autoimmune diseases qualify as well (Table 2–1).

Inflammation of the Glands

Patients with Sjögren's may have enlarged or swollen lacrimal or salivary glands. When biopsy samples are taken from such glands and examined microscopically, the glands can be seen to be infiltrated by white blood cells. These cells include B cells or antibody-producing lymphocytes, activated T lymphocytes, and macrophages. Together these cells produce a localized inflammation that is ultimately capable of destroying the gland. This inflammatory process is similar, if not identical, to that involving the islets of the pancreas in type 1 diabetes mellitus, the synovial membrane lining the joints in rheumatoid arthritis, and the tissues specifically involved in the other

TABLE 2–1
Diseases Associated with Secondary Sjögren's

Rheumatoid arthritis
Systemic lupus erythematosus
Scleroderma
Vasculitis
Polymyositis/dermatomyositis
Primary biliary cirrhosis

autoimmune diseases. The inflammatory infiltration of white blood cells can also be seen in the very small salivary glands that line the lower lip. These minor salivary glands are very easy to biopsy and are very helpful in making the diagnosis of Sjögren's. It is useful to make the diagnosis early because glands that have been invaded but not yet destroyed have enough residual glandular tissue to respond to medication that stimulates salivary flow.

Autoimmunity

Autoimmune diseases are so named because in these diseases the B lymphocytes produce antibodies to, and the T lymphocytes are activated by, proteins or protein–nucleic acid complexes that are a normal component of the body's own cells. The underlying reason for this abnormal immune response is not completely known, nor in the case of Sjögren's has the specific protein in the glandular tissue been identified for certain, but enough is known to definitely classify Sjögren's as an autoimmune disease. A hallmark of autoimmune diseases is the production of antibodies circulating in the blood that are characteristic for the specific autoimmune disease in question. This is true in Sjögren's, in which antibodies to one or both of two protein–RNA complexes, called Ro (also called SSA) and La (SSB), are present in more than 60% and 40%, respectively, of the serum from patients with Sjögren's. These autoantibodies are also commonly found in the serum of patients with SLE, thereby strengthening the concept of Sjögren's as an autoimmune disease.

The International Classification Criteria for Sjögren's

As we can see, Sjögren's fulfills the definition of a disease. It has a definite and almost unique set of sicca symptoms, a definite anatomic-pathologic basis, and a well-defined pair of autoantibodies. Still, Sjögren's is not easy to diagnose and until very recently was not easy to define in a way that would enable patients with Sjögren's to be studied as a uniform group. An international committee of experts was assembled, under the auspices of the Sjögren's Syndrome Foundation, to formulate diagnostic criteria so that patients who could be universally considered to have Sjögren's could be entered into clinical trials and other forms of research (Table 2–2). These classification criteria now define how one decides that a patient has unequivocal Sjögren's. Early in the disease, patients who actually have Sjögren's may not meet all of the criteria, so the diagnosis and treatment of any individual patient is a matter of clinical judgment.

It is important to rule out diseases that might also produce typical Sjögren's findings. These conditions include:

- Previous radiation to the head and neck
- Lymphoma

TABLE 2–2
Revised European-American Criteria for the Classification of Sjögren's Syndrome

1. Ocular symptoms (1 of 3)
   - Dry eyes for >3 months
   - Sensation of a foreign body in the eye
   - Use of artificial tears >3 times a day
2. Oral symptoms (1 of 3)
   - Dry mouth for >3 months
   - Swollen salivary glands
   - Need liquids to swallow
3. Ocular tests (1 of 2)
   - Unanesthetized Schirmer's ≤5 mm/5 minutes
   - Vital dye staining
4. Positive lip biopsy (focus score ≥1/4 mm²)
5. Oral tests (1 of 3)
   - Unstimulated salivary flow rate ≤0.1 mL/minute
   - Abnormal parotid sialography
   - Abnormal salivary scintigraphy
6. Positive anti-SSA and/or SSB

Diagnosis of secondary Sjögren's syndrome requires established connective tissue disease and one sicca symptom plus 2 of 3 objective tests for dry mouth and dry eye (items 3–5).
Modified from *Ann Rheum Dis.* 2002;61:554–558.

- ¤ Sarcoidosis
- ¤ Hepatitis C infection
- ¤ HIV infection (AIDS)
- ¤ Graft-versus-host disease
- ¤ Medications that can cause dryness

Summing Up

Sjögren's is a relatively common and serious autoimmune disease that involves an inflammatory immune destruction of the lacrimal and salivary glands, producing a well-defined set of symptoms connected with dry mouth and dry eye. Constitutional symptoms such as fatigue, joint pain, and depression are also common.

FOR FURTHER READING

Bloch KJ, Buchanan WW, Wohl MJ, Bunim JJ. Sjögren's syndrome, a clinical, pathological and serological study of 62 cases. *Medicine.* 1965; 44: 187–231.

Vitali C, Bombardiere S, Jonsson R, et al. Classification criteria for Sjögren's syndrome: a revised version of the European Criteria proposed by the American European group. *Ann Rheum Dis.* 2002; 61: 554–58.

3

Who Develops Sjögren's?

Katy M. Setoodeh, MD, and Daniel J. Wallace, MD

Since Sjögren's is a syndrome and a disease, ascertaining how many people have it and elucidating its epidemiologic features have proven to be difficult undertakings. Although there are a variety of reasons for this, the most important is that an international consensus on how to define Sjögren's has only recently been agreed upon. This chapter will review how many people have Sjögren's and the principal identifying features of those individuals as well as issues relating to genetic predisposition.

How Many People Have Sjögren's?

Most professionals trained in estimating the numbers of people with a disorder do so in terms of prevalence or incidence. Prevalence is defined as the number of individuals per 1,000,000 people with a condition, while incidence is the number per 1,000,000 who are diagnosed in a given year. Some papers have published figures based upon self-reported dry eye or dry mouth with arthritis. Others have relied upon older definitions of Sjögren's, which could include dry eye, dry mouth, and arthritis; some of these cases could have occurred as a consequence of viral infections such as AIDS or hepatitis. If we restrict ourselves to autoimmune Sjögren's, the Sjögren's Syndrome Foundation estimates that more than 4 million people in the United States (out of 330 million) have it. This breaks down to one person in 70.

Where did these numbers come from? In the United States, approximately 0.5% of the population, or 1 person in 200, meets the criteria for primary Sjögren's. To these 1.4 million Americans, we next add the numbers of those who fulfill the criteria for other autoimmune conditions and who also have Sjögren's. Approximately 30% overall of individuals with rheumatoid arthritis (3 million), systemic lupus erythematosus (1 million), and scleroderma-related disorders fulfill definitions for Sjögren's, as do other musculoskeletal conditions that are autoimmune diseases (1 million). Thus, 1.5 million of these

5 million brings the total to 2.9 million. How does one account for the remaining 1.1 million? The answer is simply because Sjögren's is underreported. Many people (especially those with mild Sjögren's) never bother to complain to their doctor about their symptoms, or their healthcare professional may attribute their symptoms to other causes.

Age, Race, Geography, Sex, and the Environment

The mean age of onset of Sjögren's is the early 50s. Less than 5% of Sjögren's patients are under the age of 20, and nearly all of these have anti-Ro/SSA antibodies. Sjögren's is probably found in all races and ethnicities to a similar extent, although this has not been well studied. In the past decade, published studies estimating the prevalence of the disease in China, Spain, Slovenia, Finland, Greece, and the United States have demonstrated strikingly similar results. In all of these surveys, 90% to 95% of people with primary Sjögren's were female. The percentage is slightly lower in secondary disease. But for all practical purposes, signs and symptoms of Sjögren's in males and females are the same.

Studies indicate that there is a relationship between hormones and auto-immunity. Hormonal influences no doubt play a role in the female predominance of the syndrome, but this issue has not been adequately explored. While chemical or environmental exposures play a role in other rheumatic disorders associated with Sjögren's, with the exception of sun sensitivity (which is directly related to antibodies to anti-Ro/SSA), no specific chemical or occupational endeavor correlates with the presence of Sjögren's. One exception would be increased symptoms of Sjögren's among individuals residing in regions with a dry climate.

Primary and Secondary Sjögren's

Patients with primary Sjögren's by definition lack the obvious distinguishing features of rheumatoid arthritis, systemic lupus erythematosus, or sclero-derma. These include deforming arthritis, malar and discoid rashes, and tight skin. However, compared to individuals with secondary Sjögren's, there are certain features noted more commonly in primary Sjögren's. These consist of Raynaud's phenomenon (color changes in the hands with cold exposure), salivary gland enlargement, swollen lymph nodes, anti-Ro/SSA and anti-La/SSB positivity, central nervous system dysfunction, and the potential for developing lymphoma (44 times greater than in healthy individuals).

Sjögren's, Genetics, and Other Autoimmune Diseases

Sjögren's syndrome can run in families. One Sjögren's patient in eight will have a relative (usually female) with the condition. Only a handful of reports of identical twins with Sjögren's have been published; clearly the genetic factors regulating inheritance of the disease are complex and multifactorial. A first-degree relative (parent, sibling, or child) of someone with Sjögren's has a 1% to 3% risk of developing the syndrome. Actually, these relatives have a much higher risk for being diagnosed with autoimmune thyroid disease or lupus than Sjögren's. In some studies, up to 30% of Sjögren's patients have Hashimoto's thyroiditis or are hypothyroid. Other autoimmune conditions found in 1% to 30% of Sjögren's patients include lupus, rheumatoid arthritis, scleroderma, inflammatory myositis, type 1 diabetes, and multiple sclerosis. Occasionally, family members of Sjögren's patients have antinuclear antibodies, rheumatoid factor, and anti-Ro/SSA on blood testing without any symptoms or evidence of autoimmune disease. Certain members of a series of genetic markers present on the surface of cells known as human leukocyte antigen (HLA) haplotypes also predispose individuals to Sjögren's.

Summing Up

¤ One American in 70–85 has Sjögren's, evenly divided between primary and secondary disease.
¤ This population is overwhelmingly female and middle-aged.
¤ Sjögren's patients are at increased risk of having another autoimmune disorder, developing lymphoma, or having a family member with an autoimmune disease.
¤ No geographic, racial, environmental, or ethnic risk factors have been associated with primary Sjögren's syndrome.

FOR FURTHER READING

Garcia-Carrasco M, Ramos-Casals M, Rosas J, et al. Primary Sjögren's syndrome: clinical and immunologic disease patterns in a cohort of 400 patients. *Medicine (Baltimore).* 2002; 81: 270–80.

Helmick CG, Felson DT, Lawrence RC, et al. Estimates of the prevalence of arthritis and other rheumatic conditions in the United States. *Arthritis Rheum.* 2008; 58: 15–25.

Pillemer SR, Matteson EL, Jacobsson LT, et al. Incidence of physician-diagnosed primary Sjögren's syndrome in residents of Olmstead County, Minnesota. *Mayo Clin Proc.* 2001; 76: 593–99.

Ramos-Casals, M, Brito-Zeron P, Font J. The overlap of Sjögren's syndrome with other systemic autoimmune diseases. *Semin Arthritis Rheum.* 2007; 36: 246–55

Taiym S, Haghighat N, Al-Hashimi I. A comparison of the hormone levels in patients with Sjögren's syndrome and healthy control. *Oral Surg Oral Med Oral Pathol*. 2004; 97: 579–83.

Thomas E, Hay EM, Hajeer A, Silman AJ. Sjogren's syndrome: a community-based study of prevalence and impact. *Br J Rheumatol*. 1998; 37: 685–86.

PART TWO

THE PATHOPHYSIOLOGY
OF SJÖGREN'S

4

Pathogenesis of Sjögren's

Ian R. Mackay, MD, FRCP, FRACP, FRCPA, FAA

The classic form of Sjögren's disease (or syndrome, see below) is now attributable to autoimmunity—that is, an aberrant immune response to a bodily constituent of the affected individual (self). However, the causal immunopathological and other pathways that determine the occurrence of autoimmune diseases, and particularly Sjögren's, remain so unclear that specifying contributors to pathogenesis seemed at first rather a daunting task. Yet on rereading Henrik Sjögren's 1933 monograph, there was comfort in the realization of the great advances in knowledge of autoimmunity since his time. A previous edition of this handbook questioned whether the time had come for "Sjögren's disease" to replace "Sjögren's syndrome" as the preferred usage. This time *has* come, since Sjögren's syndrome has become a distinct entity defined as a lymphocyte-mediated lacrimal exocrinopathy with autoimmune expressions, and due to a cell-destructive lymphoproliferation that terminates either in lacrimal acinar obliteration, or B-cell lymphoma. Usage of "Sjögren's disease" is adopted here, and other types of conjunctival-oral dryness remain as "sicca" syndromes. The particular problem of "facsimiles" of Sjögren's disease presented by patients chronically infected with certain viruses (HIV, HCV) is mentioned later. This chapter, insofar as possible, will present overall consensus views and, as well, a few personal opinions.

A Glance at Sjögren's Contribution

The classic monograph by the Swedish ophthalmologist Henrik Sjögren *Zur Kenntnis der Keratoconjunctivitis Sicca* emanated from a doctoral thesis published in German in 1933 and translated in 1943 by Bruce Hamilton of Hobart, Australia. The content eventually came to world attention in the 1950s (Fig. 4–1). Dr. Sjögren's "point of entry" was recognition of pathology affecting the cornea of the eye, for which he used an earlier term *keratitis filiformis,* and which he correctly inferred was the result of a secretory failure of degenerated

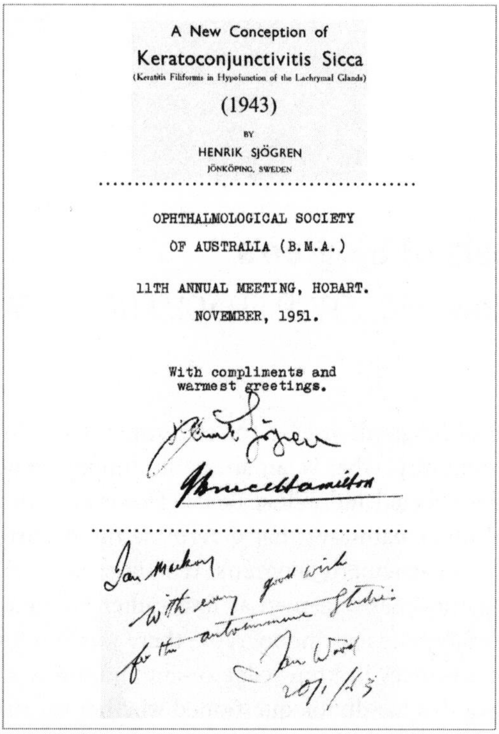

A New Conception of
Keratoconjunctivitis Sicca
(Keratitis Filiformis in Hypofunction of the Lachrymal Glands)
(1943)
BY
HENRIK SJÖGREN
JÖNKÖPING, SWEDEN

OPHTHALMOLOGICAL SOCIETY
OF AUSTRALIA (B.M.A.)

11TH ANNUAL MEETING, HOBART.
NOVEMBER, 1951.

With compliments and
warmest greetings.

FIGURE 4–1 **An Historical Memoir.**

Montage showing frontispiece of 1943 translation of Henrik Sjögren's 1933 monograph in German on his eponymous disease, his signature on a notice of a meeting in Hobart, Tasmania, in 1951 of the Ophthalmological Society of Australia (B.M.A.) indicating that he attended, together with Bruce Hamilton of Hobart who translated Sjögren's monograph in 1943. This copy was donated to Sir Ian Wood, first Head of the Clinical Research Unit of the Hall Institute in Melbourne, who later donated it to the present author in 1963.

lacrimal exocrine glands. He emphasized the distressing ocular dryness and discomfort, demonstrated objectively by the Schirmer procedure and by dye (Rose Bengal) staining of the cornea, and so he coined the term *keratoconjunctivitis sicca* for the disease.

His monograph includes case notes on 19 patients, all middle-aged to elderly women, most with longstanding symptoms suggesting a pathology evolving over many years. The symptom of oral dryness often accompanied dry eyes, and a peripheral arthritis coexisted in 13 of the 19 case descriptions. The monograph is profusely illustrated with 56 photomicrograph figures, of which the last 12 depict inflammatory cell infiltrates in lacrimal glands. The figures and accompanying text repeatedly refer to infiltration with numerous "round cells" but with no comment on their possible origin or significance.

Dr. Sjögren was unaware of, or neglected previous relevant observations, including the salivary-oral components of the syndrome and the swellings of and round cell infiltration into lacrimal and salivary glands described in 1892 by Johann von Mikulicz-Radecki from Prussia, as well as failing salivary secretion and conjunctival dryness described in 1926 by Henri Gougerot from France. The likelihood that the Sjögren and Mikulicz syndromes were expressions of the same disease was formally proposed by Morgan and Castleman in 1953. Understandably, given this was 1933, Dr. Sjögren did not address the possibility that the lacrimal-salivary affliction was due to autoimmunization, although such had been described as early as 1904 by Donath and Landsteiner in the context of the hemolytic disease, paroxysmal cold hemoglobinuria.

In fact, after 1904, autoimmunization as a disease process underwent a 40-year-long eclipse to the degree that any suggestive clinical or experimental pointer towards it during this time became discounted or neglected. However, from the late 1940s, there were many observations, some deliberate and others fortuitous, that led to its gradual acceptance as a pathogenetic reality, counterintuitive as it was. Autoimmunity as the cause of Sjögren's disease (among many others) was canvassed from 1958. Indeed, the ubiquity of autoimmune pathology thereafter was to become regarded as one of the major surprises of 20th-century medicine Further, the infiltrating "round cells" described by Mikulicz and Sjögren are now seen as crucial contributors to pathogenesis, as described later. Thus, in the span of just 77 years—within my own lifetime— these cells have been identified phenotypically as members of various well-defined functional subsets of lymphocytes and monocytes that normally provide for the immunological security and defense of the body, but abnormally are potently cytodestructive, as illustrated in autoimmune organ destruction and rejection of tissue transplants.

Functional Basis of Normal and Pathological Immune Responses

The occurrence of autoimmunization calls for comment on the *modus operandi* in health and disease of the immune system that functions as a complex, highly precise "recognition machine." It comprises three interdependent elements, *innate, adaptive,* and *regulatory,* that interact in defense against microbial or other attack while sparing self.

Innate immunity depends on cellular components (dendritic cells, monocytes, and macrophages) and humoral components (complement and lectins). It is inflexible, having evolved for an immediate response to regularly harmful pathogens and depends on recognition of "pathogen-associated molecular patterns" (PAMPS) by "pattern-recognition receptors" (Toll-like receptors [TLR]) present on the surface of phagocytic cells. Although innate immunity would not be expected have any capacity for anti-self reactivity, it does become anomalously activated by some endogenous components, including the orderly disposal of products of cell death, a process called apoptosis. Activation of TLRs with release of inflammatory mediators occurs in the initial stage of adaptive immune responses including autoimmune responses.

Adaptive immunity normally is functionally triggered after initial activation of the innate immune system by a foreign pathogen. It evolved, first, to meet the need for a more highly diverse immune system to combat the myriad extrinsic environmental challenges and, second, to provide for memory to enhance responses after a past exposure. It leads to production of various functionally different subsets of lymphocytes that are generated by a developmental diversification of their antigen receptors and an accompanying acquisition of other functionally active surface molecules. The ensuing component lymphocytes are all descendents of progenitor cells originally derived from the bone marrow. These cells mature in the primary lymphoid tissues wherein there is random re-assortment of genes that encode their antigen receptors. This bestows a recognition repertoire adequate for innumerable molecular (antigenic) configurations of harmful pathogens.

Adaptive immunity differs from innate immunity by reason of an exquisitely specific responsiveness and a capacity for clonal amplification of activated cells. The constituent lymphocytes are the progeny of either specifically reactive T lymphocytes (having matured in the thymus) that subserve cell-mediated immunity, or B lymphocytes (having matured in the bone marrow) that secrete humoral antibodies. Normally, adaptive immunity is robustly protective, but the constituent lymphocyte can become very harmful when these happen to acquire a capacity for anti-self reactivity and invasiveness of tissues, as in autoimmune diseases, or reactivity with normally harmless constituents of the environment, as in allergic diseases.

Regulatory immunity needed to evolve in order to facilitate termination of a no-longer-needed adaptive response, and also to limit responses to "self" (auto) antigen, that is, to confer immune tolerance which can be either "central" or "peripheral." Central tolerance develops within the primary lymphoid organs, for T cells in the thymus, and and for B cells in the bone marrow. In these sites, nascent autoreactive lymphocyte become clonally eliminated before their exit to the periphery, a process called "negative selection". Peripheral tolerance depends on the generation in the thymus of a particular subset of T lymphocytes called regulatory T cells (Tregs). These cells operate after their exit from thymus to the periphery by a capacity for recognition and deactivation of self-reactive cells that have escaped prior negative selection. There also exist subsets of B lymphocytes with a regulatory capability, of which the best-known secretes anti-antibodies (known as anti-idiotypic antibodies) capable of shutting off potentially harmful immune responses.

Normal Immune Responses: Prototypic for an Autoimmune Response?

Normally, three sequential steps occur after the lodgement of an immunogenic (antigenic) foreign particle or microorganism in a peripheral tissue: *recognition/initiation, induction/maintenance,* and *elimination/termination.* This is shown in Figure 4–2. If an autoimmune response to a self antigen were to occur, this same sequence would eventuate, although this is not fully established.

1. RECOGNITION/INITIATION

Any potentially injurious foreign particle (antigen) is identified by phagocytic cells of the innate immune system, dendritic cells and macrophages, that are constitutively present in most tissues. This antigenic particle undergoes endocytosis and degradation and is accompanied by a pro-inflammatory milieu that favors immune induction, and there is migration of antigen-laden dendritic cells to a regional lymph node. Self molecules can be likewise sampled by dendritic cells, but this is harmless under non-inflammatory conditions and even confers tolerogenic properties on such dendritic cells.

In regard to autoimmunity, and Sjögren's in particular, it is not known whether antigen recognition, immune induction, and initiation of a pathogenic

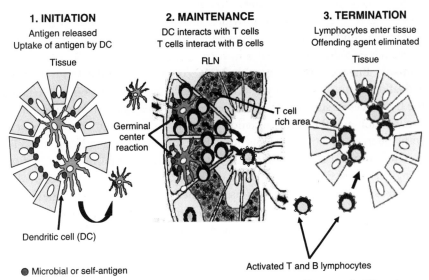

1. INITIATION
Antigen released
Uptake of antigen by DC

Tissue

2. MAINTENANCE
DC interacts with T cells
T cells interact with B cells

RLN

3. TERMINATION
Lymphocytes enter tissue
Offending agent eliminated

Tissue

Germinal
center
reaction

T cell
rich area

Dendritic cell (DC)

● Microbial or self-antigen

Activated T and B lymphocytes

FIGURE 4–2 **Events that may Determine Anti-Lacrimal Autoimmune Response in Sjögren's Disease.**
A simplified depiction of the presumed stages in the pathogenesis of the destructive autoimmune lacrimal adenitis in Sjögren's disease. Proof of the nature and site of initiation of these events awaits the identification of the critical provocative autoantigenic molecule(s) (see text).

response actually does proceed in the same way, but there is no reason to think otherwise.

The initial provocative event is likely to be a microbial or viral invasion that causes an infectious salivary-lacrimal adenitis: the Epstein-Barr herpes-type virus (EBV) has been long suspected although never actually convicted. Whatever the infection might be it could, given a genetically susceptible background, contribute by either causing release of autoimmunogenic cell degradation products, or by displaying constituents that sufficiently resemble or mimic a host product to generate an anti-self response (see below).

2. INDUCTION/MAINTENANCE

Dendritic cells bearing endocytosed and potentially antigenic fragments have as their destination a lymph node or spleen, known as the secondary lymphoid tissues. Dendritic cells are directed by "traffic signals", small molecules called cytokines, lymphokines and chemokines, and their particular receptors, to sites in the lymph node wherein immune induction can occur following an effective contact with a responsive T or B lymphocyte. Such lymphocytes are continually patrolling through the peripheral lymphoid tissues from the bloodstream.

In the T-cell-rich areas of the lymph node, dendritic cells bearing endocytosed antigen "present" this antigen to a responsive T lymphocyte with a cognate antigen receptor (TCR), provided that the antigen has been degraded within the dendritic cell to short peptides that associate within the cell with molecules encoded by the major histocompatibility complex (MHC, HLA in humans). Engagement by a peptide-MHC combination of the TCR results in activation of the T lymphocyte – this is called "MHC restriction." Thereafter, the influences of stimulatory cytokines result in the T cell undergoing clonal proliferation and then differentiation of descendent cells into various subsets with different functional properties. These subsets are identifiable by cell-specific surface markers, called CD, followed by a numeral. Among the first recognized were the CD4+ and CD8+ subsets of T cells. The CD4 subset, also known as T-helper (Th) cells by reason of their collaborative capabilities comprises several different families, Th1, Th2, Th17, Tfh, and Treg, each of which secretes functionally different cytokine messengers, called lymphokines. CD8+ T-cells also secrete lymphokines, but primarily are directly cytotoxic.

B lymphocytes after activation by antigen mature differently; this occurs within germinal centers in lymph nodes. The B-cell antigen receptor, which is identical with the binding site of the antibody that the B cell produces, makes contact with large conformational surfaces of the antigen. Such contact, together with activating lymphokines such as the B-cell stimulator BAFF (see below) and other helper lymphokines from CD4+ Th cells, provide stimuli for hypermutation among genes that encode the B-cell receptor (BCR), so resulting in successive "refinements" of the specificity of antigen recognition, known as affinity maturation of the antibody product. Self-reactive B cells inevitably arise during these events but, normally, there are processes in place to eliminate B cells with this undesirable reactivity.

In regard to autoimmunity, the proviso is needed that there must be a thymic tolerance defect (see below) that will allow self reactive T lymphocytes to enter and persist in the circulation. Given this, inductive events similar to those that occur with a foreign antigen can occur in the draining regional lymph node. Thus, for example, in autoimmune diabetes, in both NOD diabetes-prone mice and humans, an islet cell autoantigen (insulin or glutamate decarboxylase) is demonstrable in pancreatic lymph nodes, and likewise (as thyroglobulin) in regional (cervical) lymph nodes in human autoimmune thyroiditis in. For Sjögren's, there are of course no data yet, since the initiating antigen is unidentified, regional lymph nodes are seldom studied, and animal models are not sufficiently close.

3. TERMINATION/ELIMINATION

After maturation of the normal adaptive immune response in a lymph node, various subsets of effector T and B lymphocytes activated for specific reactivity with the provocative antigen exit to the periphery and "home" to wherever in the body this antigen is located. CD4+ Th cells release inflammatory lymphokines, CD8+ T cells exert direct cytotoxicity, and B cells secrete neutralizing antibodies, so acting in concert to eliminate the antigen and terminate the respons. However in regard to autoimmunity, there is a crucial difference: autoantigen is constitutively irremovable, and elimination/termination is not attainable. Instead, there are successive rounds of re-stimulation of lymphocytes by autoantigen, setting up an intrinsically self-perpetuating autoimmune process. Moreover, immune inductive processes can extend from the regional node to the affected tissue itself, appearing there as ectopic lymphoid tissue. Dr. Sjögren's book (Fig. LI) depicts this characteristic feature of autoimmune histopathology in the setting of lacrimal disease.

Immune Tolerance and Relation to Autoimmunity

Self and foreign antigens are necessarily "processed" differently by the immune system since there are "contrivances," in the words of Paul Ehrlich in 1901, to prevent this unphysiological occurrence—he called it *horror autotoxicus*. Yet, adept as immunologists may be in minting new linguistic coinage, they failed for 40 years to derive a satisfactory term for this immunological inertness to self, until MacFarlane Burnet in Melbourne referred to it as *immune tolerance* in 1949. The hard facts and shifting theories of immune tolerance are beyond our scope herein, but we can say that tolerance may operate at all three stages of the immunization process.

Inthe first stage, *endocytosis of antigen peripherally*, tolerogenic properties can be acquired by dendritic cells following the uptake under non-inflammatory conditions of a self rather than a foreign antigen. In the second stage, *induction/maintenance of the response in the regional lymph node*, an important tolerogenic influence is the antecedent elimination (called negative selection) from thymus or bone marrow of potentially self-reactive T or B lymphocytes, so removing such cells from the peripheral repertoire and ensuring that activation by exposure to autoantigen bearing dendritic cells does not occur. In the third stage, *elimination/termination in the periphery*, interaction of immune effector cells with autoantigen can be nullified by inhibitory effects of regulatory T cells. Insufficiencies (mostly of genetic origin) of these various mechanisms of tolerance explain the escape of self-reactive lymphocytes from the thymus, their circulation within the peripheral T-cell pool, and their unimpeded damaging contact with autoantigen in the periphery, lacrimal and salivary glands in the case of Sjogren's disease.

Immunophenotypic Features of Sjögren's Disease

Why exactly is Sjögren's readily classifiable as autoimmune? It does in fact quite closely fulfill conventional properties of an autoimmune disorder, according to these typical features.

1. *Female sex predominance* (9:1). All 19 of Sjögren's cases were women.
2. *Clustering with other autoimmune disorders.* This occurs in autoimmunity within a single affected individual, or among direct relatives, and is seen in humans and experimental animal models. Two broad disease clusters are recognized, thyroid-associated organ-specific, and lupus-associated multisystemic. Sjögren's may cluster with either but, notwithstanding its localization to exocrine glands, aligns preferentially with the multisystemic group and particularly with rheumatoid arthritis as noted by Dr. Sjögren, and also with systemic lupus erythematosus (SLE); it is attributed to a sharing of genetic background.

Sjögren's disease is called "primary" when it coexists as a stand-alone and "secondary" when occurring together with another autoimmune disease, but this is an artificial division that provides no useful clinical or causal insights, and is dispensable. Sjögren's has many and varied extra-glandular expressions (see other chapters), with some affecting epithelial tissues other than lacrimal and salivary glands, and thus has been called an "autoimmune epithelitis; the lack of evidence for an epithelium-specific autoantigen weighs against this idea.

3. *Polyclonal hypergammaglobulinemia.* Levels of immunoglobulin (Ig) G in serum exceed 20 grams/Liter, but neither the immunogenic stimulus nor the antigenic reactant(s) for this IgG increase have been discerned.

4. *Disease-characteristic autoantibodies in serum.* These are prominent features, albeit not including an exocrine epithelium-specific autoantigen. The two major autoantibodies, *anti-SS-A/Ro and anti-SS-B/La*, react with closely related autoantigens identified independently in the late 1950s, and hence they have different names: SS-A, also called Ro, and SS-B, also called La. (Ro and La follow a early convention of naming new autoantigens from the surname letters of the donor of the reactive serum.) Both antigens are cytoplasmic- and nuclear-located ribonucleoproteins (RNPs) that, in association with ribonucleic acids, participate in transcriptional activities required for protein synthesis within the cell. The many uncertainties about these autoantibodies to Ro and La include (a) the stimulus for their formation; b) their (relative) specificity for lacrimal and salivary autoimmunity despite their presence in all cells of the body noting that anti-SS-A/Ro is frequent too in SLE); (c) their contribution to the elevated IgG in serum; and (d) their functional effects if any, noting intriguing data on fetal cardiac damage after placental transfer of autoantibody (usually anti-SS-B/La, see below) from an autoantibody-positive mother.

Alpha-fodrin, another reactant with Sjögren's disease sera, is a cytoskeletal type of protein enriched in exocrine acinar epithelial cells, but the modest frequency of reactivity seems insufficiently high for it to be considered diagnostically or pathogenetically significant.

M3 muscurinic acetyl choline receptors (M3 AchRs are expressed by acinar cells of exocrine secretory glands. These are reactants for an interesting type of autoantibody, anti-M3 AChR, that has functional effects on parasympathetic neurotransmission, either inhibitory or initially agonistic with later exhaustion and secretory failure, and so would contribute to sicca features. Assays to demonstrate interference with M3 AChR transmission are rather tedious, tending to limit applicability to research laboratories.

Rheumatoid factor (RF) is an IgM class autoantibody traditionally associated with rheumatoid arthritis, but it is also frequently detected in Sjögren's disease as well, and in certain other inflammatory diseases too. RF is specifically reactive with an autoantigen on the Fc piece of the IgG molecule and is of interest by reason of the frequent clinical association of Sjögren's disease and rheumatoid arthritis, suggesting that there are shared genetic causes.

5. *Tissue deposits of immune complexes of antigen, antibody, and complement.* Such deposits characterize multisystem autoimmune

diseases, typically SLE, in which they are nephritogenic i.e. damaging to the kidneys. Immune complex deposits do not appear relevant to the glandular lesions of Sjögren's but may cause some of the extra-glandular features.

6. *Dense lymphoid infiltration into the affected tissue.* As recorded in Dr. Sjögren's book, lymphocytic (round cell) infiltration occurs to such a degree that exocrine glandular tissue is obliterated and replaced by residual cystic ductular elements and myoepithelial structures; the infiltrates resemble ectopic lymphoid tissue and indicate a B-lymphocyte drive that can evolve to B-cell lymphoma. The infiltrating lymphocytes comprise B cells, activated CD4+ T cells, including Th1 and Th17cells, and cytolytic CD8+ T cells; however, a better definition of the proportions of these cell types in affected glands is needed. The autoantigenic reactants (targets) of antibodies secreted by infiltrating B cells include anti-Ro and anti-La but are otherwise undefined, so the immune mechanisms of acinar cell destruction remain unclear

7. Genetic *association with HLA alleles.* This is a characteristic of many autoimmune diseases, with Sjögren's no exception. The main association (among Caucasians) is with the HLA class II allele DR3; the relative risk for Sjogren's conferred by DR3 is about seven-fold. As mentioned, antigenic activation of T cells requires that the inducing peptide antigen be "presented" in association with an MHC/HLA molecule by a specialized dendritic cell; this association also necessary if that peptide antigen becomes a T-cell target on the acinar cell surface in the destructive phase of the autoimmune response. But from here, in Sjogren's, the trail peters out, since data are insufficient on how association between a particular HLA risk allele and an autoantigenic peptide can facilitate disease development. Suppositions are that the binding affinity of autoantigenic peptides with the hypervariable region of the beta chain of an HLA molecule, whether over-efficient or under-efficient, influences the selection of the peripheral T cell antigen repertoire that is biased towards autoimmunity.

8. *Increased levels in serum and tissues of cytokines (including BAFF).* A lymphokine-mediated inflammatory response is a feature of autoimmune tissue damage in general and is characteristically seen in Sjögren's. The pro-inflammatory lymphokines include interleukin (IL)-1-beta, IL-6, tumor necrosis factor (TNF)-alpha, and interferon (IFN)-gamma. Much interest centers on BAFF (B-cell activating factor of the TNF family), also called B Lymphocyte Stimulator (BLyS), a powerful driver of B-cell development and survival, and an activator of T cells as well. The contribution of BAFF to Sjögren's, and to its

companion diseases rheumatoid arthritis and SLE is reflected by highly raised levels of BAFF in blood. Also, mice that are transgenic recipients of the BAFF gene have overproduction of BAFF and so provide a close disease model of Sjogren's. However, the exact causal al relationships between excessive BAFF production and Sjögren's disease expressions need more investigation.

9. *Responsiveness to immunomodulatory therapies.* A response to prednisolone is a cardinal feature of autoimmune disease, but is not well met in Sjogren's. However a biological (monoclonal antibody) therapy that depletes B lymphocytes (rituximab) appears promising.

10. *Experimental models in animals replicate the human counterpart.* In general there are highly illustrative models of autoimmunity in animals, usually mice, that either occur spontaneously or are experimentally inducible by immunization with a disease-relevant antigen, or by a molecular genetic manipulation. A model of Sjögren's, unlike certain other experimental diseases, is not inducible by immunization with lacrimal gland extracts, consistent with the idea that a salivary/lacrimal specific autoantigen might not exist. Thus a search elsewhere is needed for the immunogenic provocation of the natural disease. Models of Sjogren's that are available include (a) that developing spontaneously in autoimmune-prone diabetic (NOD) mice but independent of the usual diabetes/insulitis in that strain, and (b) that generated in BAFF transgenic mice, informing that BAFF "overdrive" with proliferation and enhanced survival of B cells is sufficient to induce disease. Disappointingly, these disease "replicas" lack the autoantibody profile (anti-Ro and anti-La) of the human counterpart.

When All is Said and Done: What Actually Causes Sjögren's Disease?

The major factors are diathesis (i.e., genetic loading) and a triggering event referred to as "environmental" and an unquantifiable element of random chance (bad luck).

First, the genetically based autoimmune predisposition *per se* can be nominated as an etiology. This accrues from female gender, HLA risk alleles and an inheritance, from both parents of a suite of relatively low- risk "tolerance-autoimmunity" genes of which each individually exerts little effect but cumulatively contribute to a high-risk for disease. Notably the normal complex function of the mammalian immune system requires an estimated several hundred genetic elements of which each could be susceptible to mutations carried in the germline and therefore heritable. Such mutations are being increasingly revealed in vatious autoimmune diseases by genome-wide association scans (GWAS) in collaborative studies on large disease populations.

Of the risk alleles for autoimmunity defined so far, some are shared among many autoimmune diseases and so confer an overall risk, whereas others act in various ways to direct the autoimmune process to particular sites and are therefore relatively disease-specific. So, as well as the better known susceptibility genes associated with female gender (regulation of estrogen production, those on the X chromosome) and genes encoding the highly polymorphic MHC (HLA) molecules there are lower-risk polymorphisms of genes that encode molecules involved with innate immune functions, cellular traffic, inter- and intra-cellular signaling, immune regulation/tolerance, immune effector activities and the orderly disposal of products of tissue degradation i.e. apoptosis. Future applications of GWAS to large populations of patients with Sjogren's should prove very informative.

Second, the initiating (triggering) process is usually related to "environment," meaning some infectious or toxic insult. There are two possibilities here: a) An infectious agent carries and exposes a molecular sequence(s) that sufficiently resembles "self" that the immune response to this sequence spreads to a self reactivity This "molecular mimicry" theory has had an enduring appeal to immunologists, perhaps beyond the quality of the assembled evidence. b) Any type of tissue destruction that causes spillage of cellular contents, particularly under conditions of defective apoptosis, could expose self antigens to a genetically "sensitive" immune system. Notably, there are various inherited disorders of apoptosis that predispose to autoimmunity in experimental mice and in humans. A telling example relevant to Sjögren's is the congenital heart rhythm block in babies born of mothers carrying the Sjögren's autoantibodies, anti-Ro/La. Fetal heart muscle cells (cardiocytes) undergo natural apoptosis in the course of developmental cardiac remodeling during which intracellular Ro and La become translocated to the cardiocyte surface. Thus Ro/La can become reactants for anti-Ro/La transmitted via the placenta in maternal blood, with cardiotoxic consequences. Perhaps some anomaly of apoptosis of acinar cells is present in adult carriers of anti-Ro/La who, after some type of lacrimal injury, develop the exocrinopathy of Sjögren's. This is supported by the presence in affected lacrimal glands of numerous BAFF-driven B lymphocytes with specificity for the Ro/La antigens. Similarly, in the autoimmune liver disease primary biliary cirrhosis, there is a biochemical impairment of apoptosis that affects cholangiocytes lining small biliary ductules such that the culprit autoantigen (pyruvate dehydrogenase complex E2 subunit) resists apoptosis and becomes promiscuously exposed in apoptotic blebs on the surface of such cells.

Third, an element of random chance enters consideration, since all of the multiple genetic and environmental provocations may appear equally operative in relatives A and B, yet relative A develops Sjögren's disease and relative B does not, or does so later in life, or develops another form of autoimmunity. There are complex issues here, such as epigenetics, somatic mutations, cellular interactions in the generation of immune responses, and others.

The nature of normal immune responsiveness and the aberrations characteristic of autoimmune Sjögren's disease are summarized in table 4-1.

Chronic Lacrimal-Salivary Adenitis Simulating Sjögren's Disease

There is an exocrinopathy particularly affecting lacrimal and salivary glands that simulates Sjögren's disease in a few patients chronically infected with either human immunodeficiency virus (HIV) or hepatitis C virus (HCV). Admittedly a nosological dilemma, it seems injudicious to link such cases with autoimmune Sjögren's disease as described herein: alternative designations could be "HIV- or HCV- related exocrinopathy." This takes cognizance of wide

TABLE 4–1
How Sjögren's Disease Influences and is Influenced by the Immune System

1. The normal immune response consists of three components

   A. **Innate immunity:** microbial products (or products of cell death, apoptosis) cause release of cytokines and pro-inflammatory agents via Toll-like receptors (TLR)

   B. **Adaptive immunity:** normally a protective response triggered by activation of innate immunity and providing memory of prior exposures leading to enhanced secondary specific responses carried out by T and B lymphocytes (white blood cells)

   C. **Regulatory immunity:** required for natural immune tolerance and dampening or ending a no-longer-needed adaptive response

2. Under certain circumstances, this entire system becomes dysfunctional, leading to autoimmunity as demonstrated herein

   A. A potentially injurious foreign particle (likely a microbe, also known as an antigen) alerts a pattern recognition receptor (e.g., a TLR of the innate immune system).

   B. Fragments (autoantigens) derived from the degradation of normal cells (self) activate T cells and stimulate B cells to produce antibodies to self (i.e., autoantibodies).

   C. Tolerance is not achieved and thus chronic inflammation ensues.

   D. Activated T lymphocytes and autoantibodies react damagingly with lacrimal antigens—T lymphocytes produce inflammatory factors and antibodies form immune complexes, all resulting in lymphocyte infiltration and further inflammation.

3. Additional immune associations specific to Sjögren's disease

   A. Increased prevalence in patients with other autoimmune disorders such as lupus, rheumatoid arthritis, and thyroiditis

   B. Female prominence and specific genetic associations

   C. Increased incidence of Sjögren's disease-specific autoantibodies (e.g., anti-Ro, -La) and nonspecific autoantibodies (e.g., ANA, rheumatoid factor) too

   D. Response to anti-inflammatory regimens

   E. Replication of the above inflammation/autoimmune scenario in animal models

   F. Presumed but not proven sequence of events shown in Figure 4–2 as follows:

      i) To be initiated in exocrine (lacrimal) gland itself

      ii) To develop in lymph nodes wherein T and B lymphocytes become activated

      iii) To be executed in lacrimal glands by activated T and B lymphocytes that infiltrate into glands, react with (unknown) autoantigen, and destroy the glands

differences in pathogenesis, and requirement for modern biotherapies, in Sjögren's disease and these virus-related exocrinopathies.

A Last Word on Sjögren's "Round Cells"

We know, or think we do, that the infiltrating "round cells" described by Sjogren are autoimmune-reactive lymphocytes that do all the damage, relentlessly, until the acinar tissue is entirely destroyed leaving only ductular remnants. These lymphocytes comprise variable proportions of activated Th1 and Th17 CD4 T cells secreting inflammatory cytokines, CD8 cytolytic cells, and autoantibody-producing B cells (see above), all likely generated autonomously *in situ* by the ectopic lymph node-like structures that develop within affected exocrine glands.

Yes, indeed, much knowledge has accrued since 1933 when Henrik Sjögren published *Zur Kenntnis____*. But much more is needed!

FOR FURTHER READING

Bolstad AI, Jonsson R. Genetic aspects of Sjögren's syndrome. *Arthritis Res.* 2002; 4(6): 353–59.

Chen W, Konkel JE. TGF-beta and "adaptive" Foxp3(+) regulatory T cells. *J Mol Cell Biol.* 2010; 2(1): 30–6.

Chiorini JA, Cihakova D, Ouellette CE, Caturegli P. Sjögren syndrome: advances in the pathogenesis from animal models. *J Autoimmun.* 2009; 33(3–4): 190–6.

Clancy RM, Neufing PJ, Zheng P, et al. Impaired clearance of apoptotic cardiocytes is linked to anti-SSA/Ro and -SSB/La antibodies in the pathogenesis of congenital heart block. *J Clin Invest.* 2006; 116(9): 2413–22.

Jones DT, Monroy D, Ji Z, et al. Sjögren's syndrome: cytokine and Epstein-Barr viral gene expression within the conjunctival epithelium. *Invest Ophthalmol Vis Sci.* 1994; 35(9): 3493–504.

Mackay IR. The etiopathogenesis of autoimmunity. *Semin Liver Dis.* 2005; 25(3): 239–50.

Manoussakis MN, Moutsopoulos HM. Sjögrens syndrome. In: Rose NR, Mackay IR, eds. *The Autoimmune Diseases.* Elsevier Academic Press, 2006: 401–15.

Mavragani CP, Moutsopoulos HM. The geoepidemiology of Sjögren's syndrome. *Autoimmun Rev.* 2010; 9(5): A305–10.

Nagata S, Hanayama R, Kawane K. Autoimmunity and the clearance of dead cells. *Cell.* 2010; 140(5): 619–30.

Plenge R. GWASs and the age of human as the model organism for autoimmune genetic research. *Genome Biol.* 2010; 11(5): 212–9.

Tengner P, Halse AK, Haga HJ, et al. Detection of anti-Ro/SSA and anti-La/SSB autoantibody-producing cells in salivary glands from patients with Sjögren's syndrome. *Arthritis Rheum.* 1998; 41(12): 2238–48.

Youinou P. Tenth International Symposium on Sjögren's syndrome. *Autoimmunity Rev.* 2010; 9(9): 589–634.

5

Genetics and Sjögren's Syndrome

John A. Ice, MD, Christopher J. Lessard, PhD,
and Kathy L. Moser, PhD

Genetics broadly refers to the study of genes, which control the physical traits that are passed from parents to their offspring. Genes determine observable features such as hair and eye color. They also determine how our bodies will metabolize medications, what hormones we produce, and, perhaps most importantly, our innate predisposition to develop certain diseases. Indeed, all of the genetic information required to govern functions of the human body is contained in approximately 22,000 genes. Furthermore, the expression of all diseases is influenced to some degree by the genetic makeup of each individual.

Genes determine physical traits by essentially serving as an instruction manual that guides how cells function. Other cellular components (primarily proteins) are produced that carry out the work of a cell based on the information provided by genes. Differences in traits such as hair or eye color result from changes or variants in the information contained within the relevant gene. Some variants are like typos in the instruction manual, where mistakes can cause significant problems. Other variants have very little, if any, consequence. Humans naturally carry millions of variants across all 22,000 genes, and these variants are not only what make each human unique (except in the case of identical twins), but they also hold the key to understanding why some individuals are more vulnerable to developing autoimmune diseases, such as Sjögren's syndrome. Thus, the goals of genetics research are to identify which specific genes cause a disease and to understand how the variation in those genes leads to clinical manifestations.

Simple Versus Complex Genetic Diseases

Family studies can be helpful in genetics research. Many diseases that are obviously "genetic," such as cystic fibrosis, Huntington's disease, sickle cell anemia, and hundreds more that are typically rare in human populations, follow predictable inheritance patterns in families, and reflect very basic principles of genetic inheritance. In these cases, the cause can be traced to a single gene with alterations in the genetic code that lead to disease. Here, the disease is considered genetically "simple." In contrast, for at least a third of Sjögren's patients, a look at family history provides some evidence to support a role for inherited factors as a root cause, but the patterns are not so obvious. Clues from families of Sjögren's patients may include the presence of other members with Sjögren's syndrome, or more commonly, other members with either another autoimmune disease or immunological problems that suggest an underlying genetic link. The patterns of how Sjögren's-related disease manifestations are inherited usually vary from one family to the next and often appear to be random.

The differences in patterns of inheritance between Sjögren's and genetically simple diseases, such as cystic fibrosis can be largely explained by how complex the underlying genetic causes are that contribute to the risk of developing disease. We know with certainty that multiple genes are important in Sjögren's. How they work together to cause disease is undeniably complex. However, there are many details we do not yet understand. How many of the approximately 22,000 genes in humans play a role in Sjögren's? Do certain combinations of risk genes result in more severe disease or a specific feature of disease such as lymphoma? How do other factors, such as diet, exposure to UV light, infections, age, race, and gender, interact with susceptible genetic backgrounds to influence the disease risk? Are there genes that increase the risk of developing more than one autoimmune disease? Furthermore, we expect that the set of genes that increase the risk of developing Sjögren's will not always be the same for every individual.

Recent progress in understanding basic human genetics, coupled with powerful laboratory tools to tackle these questions for complex diseases, has been nothing short of revolutionary. Many common diseases, such as diabetes, many cancers, and most autoimmune diseases, are genetically complex. For many of these diseases, dozens of disease genes have now been identified, and extensive effort is under way to understand more precisely how the variations in those genes lead to disease.

The importance of genetics and understanding how genes work also can be seen in many other aspects of our society. We have modified the genes of livestock and crops to make them heartier and more resistant to diseases, spliced genes into bacteria to produce life-saving medicines, revolutionized the science of criminal forensics, and developed new methods of diagnosing and treating complicated illnesses. Current research in Sjögren's uses cutting-edge technology to investigate the genetic and environmental triggers that lead to the development of Sjögren's. While research into this disease has lagged behind when compared with other autoimmune diseases, we are on the precipice of many significant and novel findings that will lead us to reinterpret our understanding of Sjögren's. An accurate and detailed understanding of what causes Sjögren's will certainly lead to the development of better tools for diagnosis and treatment for patients afflicted with this disease.

Early Genetic Discoveries

In the 1850s, Gregor Mendel, an Augustinian priest and scientist, undertook experiments to study the heritability of the physical characteristics of pea plants and unknowingly laid the foundation for modern human genetics. As he painstakingly documented the physical traits, or phenotypes, of successive generations of pea plants, he established that some unknown element conveying physical characteristics was passed from the parent plants to their offspring in mathematically predictable ratios. His observations led to the establishment of Mendel's Laws of Inheritance, rules that accurately predicted how physical traits would manifest in subsequent generations and paved the way for the discovery of that unknown heritable element: the gene. Mendel's work remained largely unknown for more than three decades until it was rediscovered at the turn of the 20th century by the botanists Hugo de Vries and Carl Correns, who were studying plant hybridization. By this time scientists had identified a variety of cellular components and hypothesized that structures called chromosomes were the key to understanding the patterns of trait heritability that Mendel described. It was not until 1915, however, that scientist Thomas Hunt Morgan proved that chromosomes carried genetic information from parents to their offspring.

We now know there are 23 human chromosomes. Each individual inherits one set of 23 chromosomes from the father and another set from the mother such that the offspring essentially receives two copies of the full set of genetic information. This is important in cases where a carrier of a detrimental gene located on one chromosome may be "rescued" by the second normal copy inherited from the other parent. Expression of some traits may be obviously derived from one parent, while other traits may show influences from both parents. In 1944, Oswald Avery, Colin MacLeod, and Maclyn McCarty determined that deoxyribonucleic acid (DNA) is the molecule responsible for inheritance. Landmark studies in 1953 by scientists James Watson, Francis Crick, and Rosalind Franklin defined the molecular structure of DNA, at last giving scientists the ability to explain precisely how DNA carries genetic information.

From Genetics to Cellular Functions

DNA is normally present inside a cell as a double-stranded, helical-shaped molecule (Fig. 5–1). DNA strands contain four chemical building blocks called nucleotides. The four building blocks are adenosine (A), cytosine (C),

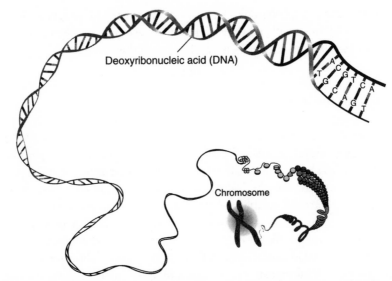

FIGURE 5–1 DNA Exists in a Condensed State within the Chromosome when not Undergoing Replication or Gene Expression. Note the pairing of A-T and C-G nucleotides on the double-stranded DNA molecule.

guanine (G), and thymine (T). Like a winding staircase, pairs of the four nucleotides form the "steps" and are linked in tandem along two phosphate/sugar backbones. The order of these nucleotides along a stretch of DNA is critical and acts much like letters in an alphabet to form the basis of how information is conveyed. The full genetic code, or DNA sequence, along all 23 chromosomes in humans consists of about 3 billion A, T, C, or G nucleotides. Abnormalities or changes in the order of any of the 3 billion nucleotides can range from having no effect on cellular function to having devastating effects on health or even life.

A gene is defined as a specific segment of a DNA strand that carries the instructions for producing a certain protein. Examples include genes that code for insulin, hemoglobin, collagen, antibodies, blood clotting factors, interferons, hormone receptors, and thousands more proteins used by the body to carry out needed functions. A gene may range in size from about 500 nucleotides to about 2.5 million nucleotides.

There are large segments of DNA that are in between genes and do not directly contain the genetic code for proteins. These regions were once called "junk" DNA, but scientists are now learning that many of the secrets of how genes work, such as when to produce a protein or how much of a protein should be produced, lie in the sequences found in these intergenic regions.

If a protein is needed, the corresponding gene becomes active and the DNA will be used as a template for cellular machinery that copies the gene sequence into a sister molecule called RNA (ribonucleic acid). Hundreds to thousands of copies of the active gene may be produced in a given cell. The RNA strands then serve as messengers that carry the code, or sequence copied off the DNA, from the nucleus of the cell, where the chromosomes are housed, to the location of the cell where proteins are then made.

Understanding regulation of gene activity is a major component of genetics research. How much RNA is made from a gene, how long the RNA molecule survives inside a cell before degradation occurs, how fast a protein is produced from the messenger RNA, and other complex processes occur that serve to regulate when and how much of a protein is made. Furthermore, certain genes are active only in certain cell types, at certain times in development, or in response to certain environmental conditions. The regulation of RNA function is determined to a great extent by the specific sequences of DNA between genes. These regions are called "non-coding" and are extremely important to normal cellular functions. Overall, the DNA sequences between genes contain the majority of all genetic variation present in humans. Interestingly, one theme that is emerging from genetic research in many complex diseases is that the majority of genetic associations with diseases are due to sequence variants in these regulatory regions and not directly in the gene coding segments.

Following production of RNA molecules when a gene becomes active, proteins are produced in a process called translation. Scientists have deciphered the code that is used in translation between the molecular language of genes and amino acids. This has led to many important discoveries about protein structure and function. Proteins are also linear molecules made of chains built from 20 possible amino acids. The order of amino acids in a protein chain is derived directly from the coding sequence of nucleotides in the DNA for the relevant gene via the messenger RNA molecules. Short sequences of three nucleotides, referred to as codons, correspond to any of 20 specific amino acids, somewhat analogous to translating a set of instructions from one language to another (Figs. 5–2 and 5–3). During translation, chains of amino acids are linked together into a protein molecule based on the order of the codons. For example, insulin and hemoglobin are both composed of amino acid chains, but the order in which the amino acids are linked together is different. Once a protein is made, the amino acid composition determines how the protein may fold or take on a non-linear shape, where the protein goes inside the cell, if the protein should be secreted, and many other functional capabilities such as binding to DNA or other proteins.

Genetic Effects on Disease

Important genetic variants have now been identified for over 2,200 human disorders. There are numerous ways in which the structure and function of

RNA codon table

1st position		2nd position				3rd position
		U	C	A	G	
U		Phe	Ser	Tyr	Cys	U
		Phe	Ser	Tyr	Cys	C
		Leu	Ser	stop	stop	A
		Leu	Ser	stop	Trp	G
C		Leu	Pro	His	Arg	U
		Leu	Pro	His	Arg	C
		Leu	Pro	Gln	Arg	A
		Leu	Pro	Gln	Arg	G
A		Ile	Thr	Asn	Ser	U
		Ile	Thr	Asn	Ser	C
		Ile	Thr	Lys	Arg	A
		Met	Thr	Lys	Arg	G
G		Val	Ala	Asp	Gly	U
		Val	Ala	Asp	Gly	C
		Val	Ala	Glu	Gly	A
		Val	Ala	Glu	Gly	G
		Amino acids				

Ala: Alanine
Arg: Arginine
Asn: Asparagine
Asp: Aspartic acid
Cys: Cysteine
Gln: Glutamine
Glu: Glutamic acid
Gly: Glycine
His: Histidine
Ile: Isoleucine
Leu: Leucine
Lys: Lysine
Met: Methionine
Phe: Phenylalanine
Pro: Proline
Ser: Serine
Thr: Threonine
Trp: Tryptophane
Tyr: Tyrosisne
Val: Valine

FIGURE 5–2 The Molecular Language of Genes is based on Sequences of Three Nucleotides, known as a Codon, Corresponding to an Amino Acid. When DNA is copied into RNA, T nucleotides are substituted for a uracil, or U. In this table, the codon UUU corresponds to the amino acid phenylalanine, while the codon CCG corresponds to the amino acid proline. The codon UAA does not code for an amino acid, but rather generates a stop signal that ends further addition of amino acids to the growing protein molecule.

DNA can contribute to disease. Most changes to DNA sequence occur as DNA is being replicated when cells grow and divide or as a result of exposure to damaging elements, such as UV radiation, oxidative stress, or carcinogenic chemicals. In either case, complex cellular mechanisms exist to help prevent or repair detrimental changes. However, the proteins involved in DNA repair or replication may mistakenly add or insert an extra nucleotide, or inappropriately delete a nucleotide (Fig. 5–4). By far the most common type of DNA

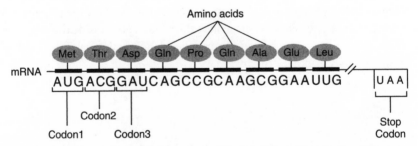

FIGURE 5–3 Example of a Nucleotide Sequence and the Translation of Each Codon of the Molecular Language into a String of Amino Acids that will make the Final Protein.

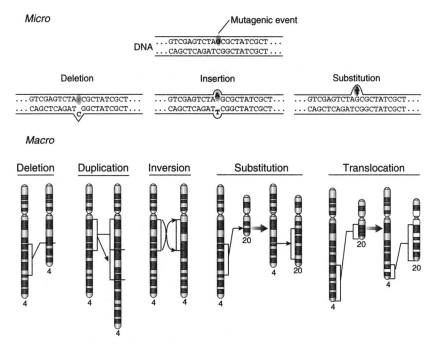

FIGURE 5–4 Examples of the Types of Variants that can occur in DNA Sequences.

sequence variation is a single nucleotide substitution, commonly called a single-nucleotide polymorphism (SNP, pronounced "snip"). Millions of SNPs have been identified. These types of variants are the ones most often associated with complex diseases.

Sometimes DNA sequence variations occur on a larger scale, where portions of chromosomes might be deleted, duplicated, inverted (flip-flopped), or translocated (swapped), possibly leading to losses, gains, or disruptions of genetic information that have widely varying effects (Fig. 5–4). Sometimes during cellular division, entire chromosomes are either added or lost, leading to odd numbers of chromosomes. These chromosomal deletions or additions typically result in massive losses or gains of genetic information, and most are incompatible with life. One addition that is compatible with life is trisomy 21, where three copies of chromosome 21 lead to the condition known as Down's syndrome.

Changes, or variants, in the DNA sequence can sometimes have profound effects on the order of amino acids and may lead to significant problems. Such changes can cause a protein strand to be truncated if an abnormal "stop" codon is introduced by mutated DNA sequence, a faulty protein may no longer be able to bind to other proteins or receptors properly, or other normal protein modifications may be interrupted, such as the attachment of other molecules necessary for normal function. Many variants simply change the amount of protein that is produced.

A classic example of a DNA variant that changes the structure and hence function of a protein in a dramatic way is in sickle cell anemia. In this case, a single nucleotide in the DNA sequence is switched from an A to a T. This leads to an amino acid substitution during production of the hemoglobin protein. The resulting protein structure is altered, which causes red blood cells to manifest a "sickle" shape that is stiff, does not move easily through blood vessels, and leads to a shorter life span of the cells, causing anemia. This single gene disorder is present in individuals who have inherited two copies of the abnormal hemoglobin gene. Individuals who inherit one normal copy and one abnormal copy carry the sickle cell "trait" but do not exhibit full-blown disease.

Sometimes changes in the DNA sequence are beneficial. For example, individuals who carry the sickle cell trait are more resistant to malaria infections. This happens because the parasite that causes malaria cannot infect those cells that carry the abnormal hemoglobin protein. This balance between the advantages or disadvantages to the health of human populations derived from DNA sequence variations has developed over thousands of years. For many of the autoimmune diseases, one theory for why they develop is in part based on the idea that "selection" for immune response genes that were once strongly protective for infections and other environmental assaults has persisted in humans and may now be detrimental under circumstances where such robust responses are not required.

In addition to the basic nucleotide sequence, DNA and the proteins it interacts with can undergo permanent chemical and structural modifications that have an effect on when and under what circumstances a gene is expressed or silenced. This adds an additional layer of complexity for understanding how genes contribute to disease. Epigenetics is an emerging field that studies how these heritable modifications that do not involve changes in the nucleotide sequence lead to altered gene expression. This area of research is relatively new, but studies are revealing that epigenetic processes are important in many disorders, including autoimmune diseases.

The Tools of Genetics Research

With over 30 million SNPs and over 12,000 other sites along the human DNA sequence that are known to vary in humans, identifying those that are relevant to disease is a significant challenge in complex diseases such as Sjögren's. For SNPs, the essence of identifying the variants that are most likely to contribute to disease often involves comparing the frequency of a specific nucleotide at a specific site between patients (cases) and healthy individuals (controls). For example, one individual may have a base pair of C-G at a particular location on a particular chromosome, whereas another individual may have a base pair

Individual 1

Chr 2 ...CGATATTCCTATCGAATGTC...
copy1 ...GCTATAAGGATAGCTTACAG...

Chr 2 ...CGATATTCCCATCGAATGTC...
copy2 ...GCTATAAGGGTAGCTTACAG...

Individual 2

Chr 2 ...CGATATTCCCATCGAATGTC...
copy1 ...GCTATAAGGGTAGCTTACAG...

Chr 2 ...CGATATTCCCATCGAATGTC...
copy2 ...GCTATAAGGGTAGCTTACAG...

Individual 3

Chr 2 ...CGATATTCCTATCGAATGTC...
copy1 ...GCTATAAGGATAGCTTACAG...

Chr 2 ...CGATATTCCTATCGAATGTC...
copy2 ...GCTATAAGGATAGCTTACAG...

Individual 4

Chr 2 ...CGATATTCCTATCGAATGTC...
copy1 ...GCTATAAGGATAGCTTACAG...

Chr 2 ...CGATATTCCCATCGAATGTC...
copy2 ...GCTATAAGGGTAGCTTACAG...

Individual 5

Chr 2 ...CGATATTCCCATCGAATGTC...
copy1 ...GCTATAAGGGTAGCTTACAG...

Chr 2 ...CGATATTCCTATCGAATGTC...
copy2 ...GCTATAAGGATAGCTTACAG...

Individual 6

Chr 2 ...CGATATTCCCATCGAATGTC...
copy1 ...GCTATAAGGGTAGCTTACAG...

Chr 2 ...CGATATTCCTATCGAATGTC...
copy2 ...GCTATAAGGATAGCTTACAG...

FIGURE 5–5 Example of Single Nucleotide Polymorphisms (SNPs). Note the variations at the same location on the two copies of the same chromosome (chr) among various individuals.

of T-A at the exact same chromosomal location (Fig. 5–5). If the C nucleotide is present at that site 58% of the time in cases compared to 42% of the time in controls, the C variant in the DNA sequence may be associated with disease. Further, studies can then test if the associated variant that is more common in patients causes altered expression or structure of the relevant protein, which then could lead to important changes in the biological function of the cell. Likewise, differences in the frequency of other types of variants (insertions, deletions, etc.) between cases and controls may also indicate an association with disease.

To date, a small number of studies in Sjögren's have focused on testing approximately 20 or so of the estimated 22,000 genes for genetic associations. Moreover, the genes tested thus far have typically been evaluated for association with only a very small number of SNPs and have thus not been comprehensively assessed. Thus, the number of variants potentially contributing to Sjögren's is substantial and the genetic architecture is virtually unexplored. We have much work to do.

Fortunately, extraordinarily powerful tools to perform far more comprehensive studies are now available and being applied to numerous diseases, including Sjögren's. These new tools have been developed at a rapid pace over the past two decades and allow us to quickly collect and analyze genetic data. For example, genotyping refers to the genetic typing that must be done in individuals in order to determine which nucleotide is present at a given site in the DNA. The current technology for genotyping allows data for over 1 million known SNPs to be determined in a single experiment. These studies are generally focused on identifying variants that are common in most human populations.

Over just the past few years, this technology has allowed scientists to perform much more informative genetic studies. More than 30 large-scale genetic studies have been completed for autoimmune diseases, including systemic lupus erythematosus (SLE), rheumatoid arthritis (RA), type 1 diabetes, Crohn's disease, psoriasis, and celiac disease. Dozens of new genetic associations have been established, opening up exciting new avenues for further research and providing fundamental new insights into the causes of these diseases. Interestingly, genes that are indisputably associated with multiple autoimmune diseases are common and may eventually help explain why various autoimmune traits or different autoimmune diseases can be found within families.

For sites in the DNA sequence that vary but with low frequency and are considered rare (i.e., occur in less than 1% of individuals), determining the entire genetic code for a gene or gene region is often necessary. This is done through a process known as sequencing. Advances in this technology are also under rapid development. Within the next decade, we will be able to fully sequence an individual's entire DNA sequence for costs that are considered feasible. Thus, the rate at which we can accumulate and study genetic information is changing dramatically.

Another important tool that has helped advance genetic research is gene expression microarrays. Using RNA extracted from blood or other cell types, scientists are able to identify which genes are active and measure the levels of RNA being produced for each gene. The key to these experiments is that essentially every gene is tested at the same time. This serves scientists in many ways, but one important type of study is to compare gene expression between patients and healthy controls. Surprising results are common in these types of studies because new genes or biological pathways are often implicated that had not been previously considered relevant to disease. Hundreds to thousands of genes can be differentially expressed, providing important clues for potential genetic associations, possible new diagnostic markers, or new therapeutic targets that should be developed. The importance of innate immune responses that involve interferons and other proteins that provide antiviral protection in Sjögren's patients has been a common finding in several studies using these tools.

Genetics of Sjögren's Syndrome

Although very few genetic studies have been completed in Sjögren's, there are a few genes that are convincingly associated. Since the 1970s, scientists have noted a clear association between Sjögren's and genes involved in the human leukocyte antigen (HLA) system. HLA genes, which are located on chromosome 6, code for proteins that reside on the surface of cells and are essential to proper immune function. They play a major role in recognition of "self" proteins in humans. The strongest associations between HLA and Sjögren's have been found in the HLA class II molecules, *HLA-DQ* and *HLA-DR*. These particular molecules are highly variable in humans, which reflects the wide variety of nucleotide sequences that are present in these genes. In Sjögren's patients, certain variants in *HLA-DR* are more frequent that may alter functions such as how these molecules bind to foreign antigens presented to T cells.

Other genetic investigations in Sjögren's to date have focused efforts on genes that have been previously linked to RA and SLE. Two genes, *STAT4* and *IRF5*, have been found that are associated with Sjögren's as well as RA and SLE. Both genes code for proteins that play an important role in innate immune responses. Researchers are now studying how the variants in these two genes may dysregulate biological pathways that involve interferons, as shown in gene expression studies mentioned previously. Once the details are understood, researchers may then be able to use this information to develop therapeutics that correct the problem.

The Future of Sjögren's Research

We expect that Sjögren's will be similar to many of the related autoimmune diseases such as SLE or RA, and more than 100 genes will be important in contributing to disease manifestations. Single variants (SNPs) will probably account for most of the genetic effects, but insertions, deletions, and other types of variants could possibly be involved. Once the catalogue of genetic variants associated with Sjögren's is developed, researchers will focus on how those genetic changes lead to altered biological functions.

Genes that play a role in development and control of autoimmune responses, such as cytokines, interferons, antibodies, and receptors on T cells or B cells, are all good candidates. Other genes, such as those involved in the production and secretion of saliva or other exocrine gland functions, are also possible candidate genes. Genes with variants that cause lymphomas to develop, neurological dysfunction, or many of the other possible disease manifestations described throughout this book may also be discovered.

To successfully apply the powerful genetic tools that have been developed over the past few years, researchers will need thousands of samples and comprehensive clinical information from Sjögren's patients for comparison with healthy controls. Over 15 research sites around the world have joined together as the Sjögren's Genetics Network (SGENE) and are now conducting the first large-scale genetic studies in Sjögren's syndrome. As seen in so many other complex diseases, we have the tools and are on the path towards many new discoveries that will provide insight into the genetic causes of Sjögren's in the very near future.

TABLE 5–1

The Genetics of Sjögren's

1. The human body contains approximately 22,000 genes.

2. Whereas some diseases (e.g., cystic fibrosis) are simple conditions associated with a single gene, Sjögren's syndrome is a complex disorder associated with multiple genes. Dozens are expected to be identified in the near future.

3. The development of Sjögren's is influenced by DNA sequence variants that include single nucleotide substitutions (or polymorphisms, termed SNPs) and epigenetics, where chemical modifications or environmental factors alter gene expression without changing the nucleotide sequence.

4. Some of the genetic associations in Sjögren's patients include human leukocyte antigens (HLA), STAT4, and *IRF5*. The former involves the adaptive immune system and latter two influence the innate immune system.

5. Genetic associations lead to various problems with the production or function of proteins, which ultimately are responsible for expression of the clinical manifestations of Sjögren's.

6. A consortium of researchers has recently been formed to accelerate our ability to identify genetic associations and understand how they lead to development of Sjögren's.

Summing Up

In the past few years there has been a concerted, coordinated effort to ascertain which genetic markers are important in Sjögren's syndrome. We now know that there are dozens of Sjögren's susceptibility genes that influence the innate and adaptive immune systems. Additionally, environmental and infectious factors play a role in altering genetic expression. Table 5–1 explains how our current knowledge base is being expanded. We hope that someday these insights will lead to the prevention, amelioration, or treatment of the syndrome.

FOR FURTHER READING

Altshuler D, Daly MJ, Lander ES. Genetic mapping in human disease. *Science.* 2008; 322(5903): 881–8.

Baranzini SE. The genetics of autoimmune diseases: a networked perspective. *Curr Opin Immunol.* 2009; 21(6): 596–605.

Cobb BL, Lessard CJ, Harley JB, Moser KL. Genes and Sjögren's syndrome. *Rheum Dis Clin North Am.* 2008; 34(4): 847–68.

Feero WG, Guttmacher AE, Collins FS. Genomic medicine—an updated primer. *N Engl J Med.* 2010; 362(21): 2001–11.

Moser KL, Kelly JA, Lessard CJ, Harley JB. Recent insights into the genetic basis of systemic lupus erythematosus. *Genes Immun.* 2009; 10(5): 373–9.

6

Sjögren's Syndrome

AN IMMUNOLOGICAL PERSPECTIVE

Robert I. Fox, MD, PhD

Sjögren's syndrome is an autoimmune disorder that develops when one's genetic predisposition combines with environmental or infectious factors. Further, there are *neural* and *hormonal* influences that influence the onset and severity of the disease.

The immune process may involve only the salivary and lacrimal glands (leading to dryness) or may involve additional organs, including nerve, muscle, joints, lung, kidney, gastrointestinal organs, and/or skin. There is a high frequency of associated fibromyalgia, a poorly understood condition that has symptoms of fatigue and vague cognitive changes. Although the pathogenesis of Sjögren's remains unclear, it involves the immune system in a manner that leads to an imbalance of inflammatory transmitters in the glands, tissues, and nerve fibers. Chapter 5 by Moser et al. outlines recent advances on specific genes associated with Sjögren's.

This chapter reviews the two basic portions of the immune system:

1. The *acquired* (or HLA-DR-dependent) immune system associated with autoantibody production
2. The *innate* (HLA-DR-independent) system responsible for many of the symptoms occurring in Sjögren's

We will also review how genetic factors interact with environmental factors to alter the hormonal and neural system and thus produce Sjögren's symptoms.

There are several important "take-home" points regarding the immune system and Sjögren's that will help us understand symptoms, current therapies, and approaches to develop new therapies:

    ◻ Biopsies of the salivary or lacrimal gland typically show that only about 50% of the ducts and acini are destroyed in Sjögren's patients, so one of the key questions is: *Why are the residual glands not functioning at optimal level?*

¤ Salivary and lacrimal functions, namely the production of tears and saliva, are part of a "functional" circuit that includes the central nervous system (midbrain and cortex of the brain), which in turn controls the blood vessels and glandular function;

¤ Saliva and tears are more than just water, as they contain a complex mixture of proteins, carbohydrates, and mucins to provide the lubrication required for movement of the mucosal membranes (including eyelids and tongue in the mouth).

¤ At the level of the salivary or lacrimal gland, as well as in the extra-glandular tissues, there is a complex interaction of immune cells that release a series of inflammatory factors that interfere with normal glandular function; type I interferon is an important part of this process.

¤ Sjögren's patients have more aggressive lymphocytes than in patients with other autoimmune disorders, which is reflected in an elevated frequency of lymphomas or infiltration into other organs such as nerves, lung, or kidney.

The Interaction of Genetic and Environmental Factors

Inherited genes are important, but not enough to explain why patients develop Sjögren's. In this chapter, we will often group certain results of studies of Sjögren's and systemic lupus erythematosus (SLE), since the genetic and nongenetic factors appear to have a great deal in common, and the data available for SLE are more extensive than those for Sjögren's at present. Indeed, the symptoms and pattern of autoantibodies are often overlapping, and the medications are frequently similar. However, the differences between Sjögren's and SLE will also be discussed below.

Physicians and patients have long recognized that simply having suscepti-bility genes is not enough to guarantee the emergence of clinical disease. The simplest example is the lack of concurrence of Sjögren's or SLE in identical twins:

¤ Each identical twin shares the same genome but has different exposure to environmental agents and slightly different ways in which their genes are activated (or rearranged) as they respond to infections and hormonal changes.

¤ If only genetic factors were required, then we would expect that if one twin develops Sjögren's, then the other twin would always develop Sjögren's as well.

¤ Although the second identical twin does have an increased risk for development of Sjögren's (the concordance rate), the observed frequency of Sjögren's (or SLE) in the other twin is only about 20% to 25%.

¤ So, roughly speaking, only about 20% of the disease can be considered strictly genetic (i.e., encoded by a person's genome), and the other 80% is due to some other factors such as environmental influence, including exposure to infections or hormonal changes.

Even though there is a great deal of enthusiasm surrounding genomic sequencing, we must remember that the best we will do in terms of prediction is what nature has provided us in the form of identical twins. We do not want to minimize the important role of new advances in genetics, however, and Chapter 5 outlines advances in identifying important genes and the interaction of genes (a field called proteomics).

To summarize, the study of genetics of Sjögren's has allowed the identification of different genes that vary from very important to those that play a weaker role, as assessed by a genetic measure called the *relative risk association*. Each individual will have some combination of these genes, and in the presence of the environmental trigger, an "immune mistake" will occur in which the body attacks some portion of glands or other tissues in a pattern characteristic for each Sjögren's patient.

Long before we ever started genetic studies, it was clear that one of the most important genes was gender, as 90% of Sjögren's patients are female. However, the specific genes on the X chromosome have been difficult to identify. One of the important genes identified in animal models was called the "Toll receptor," and this molecule helps link immune response to different environmental antigens as discussed below. However, sex hormones also play an important role in modulating the effect of many other genes involved in inflammation. In those males who have Sjögren's, there is an increased frequency of an extra X chromosome (a condition called Klinefelter's syndrome). However, only a few males with Sjögren's have the extra chromosome, so that cannot be the whole story. Current research is trying to identify the specific mechanisms of hormonally responsive genes (particularly because of their role in progression of certain cancers), but this task has remained difficult to translate into useful therapies for Sjögren's or other autoimmune diseases.

The second strongest gene (or cluster of genes) is located on the sixth chromosome in a region that was first identified during the early days of organ transplantation. These genes are called human lymphocyte antigen (HLA) genes. When a person is typed for donation of an organ (such as liver or kidney), both the donor and recipient are tested for their HLA genes since a match will greatly decrease the chance of organ rejection. Subsequent studies have identified a series of additional genes on chromosome 6 that also contribute by encoding additional proteins, including one that was named "complement" (since it complemented the activity of antibodies) and other inflammatory mediators or receptors for those mediators. Thus, the take-home lesson here is that:

> Each SS patient has a series of genes, and when that genetically predisposed individual encounters certain environmental and hormonal stimulation, a "mistake" may be made that leads to the initiation and perpetuation of clinical symptoms of Sjögren's or SLE.

A schematic that shows the timeline is shown in Figure 6–1. The patient starts with the genetic tendency (i.e., female and perhaps HLA-DR3, discussed below). This predisposes the patient to make a particular set of autoantibodies, which we measure in blood tests such as the *anti-nuclear antibody* (ANA) and the antibody to *Sjögren's-associated antigen A* (SS-A), which we now recognize as two different proteins with molecular weight 60,000 and 52,000 respectively. Some patients make antibodies against only the 60,000 molecule, others against only the 52,000 molecule, but most patients make antibodies against both.

In some patients, a second Sjögren's-associated antigen called SS-B, with molecular weight 45,000, is also found. These antigens are detected in clinical blood tests. The ability of patients to make particular antibodies is closely correlated with the particular HLA-DR (and associated genes) that they have inherited. These antibodies may be present for many years prior to the onset of any clinical disease; indeed, many patients with these antibodies may never develop clinically significant disease. This is shown schematically in Figure 6–1.

The SS-A and SS-B are proteins that are derived from dying cells (a process called apoptosis). It has been hypothesized that some viruses damage particular

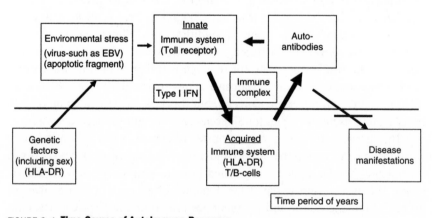

FIGURE 6–1 **Time Course of Autoimmune Response.**
1. Environmental stress is interpreted in context of genetic factors.
2. Antibodies precede disease.
3. Presence of antibody does not mean disease.

cells in the salivary gland, leading to the release of the SS-A and SS-B proteins, and that immune response against "self antigens" becomes a self-perpetuating autoimmune response in genetically predisposed individuals. Later in this chapter we will discuss some of the environmental agents and "apoptotic" fragments that contribute to the immune process.

The (HLA-DR-Dependent) Acquired Immune System

The genome encodes two type of immune response. The part that involves "immune memory" and is associated with the antibodies characteristic of Sjögren's is called the *acquired* immune system. This is the part of the immune system first identified as being important in tissue transplantation. These histocompatibility genes are made of DNA and encode a series of proteins called HLA genes (Fig. 6–2). The HLA antigens were named in the order of their discovery—thus the first ones were called HLA-A, and then HLA-B, HLA-C, and finally HLA-D.

The most important of these transplantation genes for the development of Sjögren's or SLE was found to be HLA-D. The genes encoded by the HLA-A and B have a slightly different structure than the structure of HLA-D (Fig. 6–2). In recognition of the importance of the HLA-D region and its control of autoantibody production, the acquired (transplantation-like) portion of the immune system is also called the HLA-DR-dependent part of the immune system.

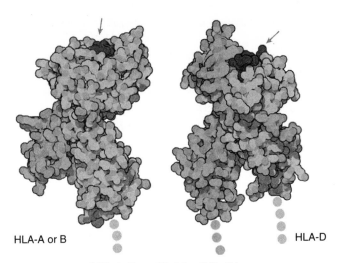

HLA-A or B   HLA-D

FIGURE 6–2 **The Histocompatibility Antigens Bind Small Peptides.**
HLA-A or B
HLA-D

The function of these histocompatibility genes is similar to a plate that holds food in an orientation that can be recognized by certain immune lymphocytes that "come to the table." In Figure 6–2, you can see that the histocompatibility molecule holds the small string of about 12 amino acids (called peptides) in a particular formation (shown by the red molecule held in a groove). The stabilization of the peptide allows efficient recognition of the molecule by other immune cells. If the peptide correctly fits with the immune receptor (generally on the surface of the T cell or B cell, as discussed below), then the lymphocyte will be stimulated and will make an immune response. This ability to present (or not present) a peptide to the other immune cells is one of the key regulatory steps of the immune system.

Each individual inherits one copy of chromosome 6 from each parent and each contains one copy of HLA-DR. So the patient has two chances to be a responder (i.e., a binder of peptide), or a non-responder if neither of the histocompatibility antigens efficiently binds with the peptide. These histocompatibility genes are different in different individuals (like brown eyes or blue eyes) but have many more choices (as if we could have a hundred different types of eye color). Further, the distribution of these HLA-D antigens is quite different in distinct ethnic populations, and this may help explain the different frequency and clinical manifestation in different countries.

One of the surprising findings of the study of immunology is that a key role for the immune system is the "disposal" of fragments of dead cells that may die as a result of "natural causes" or after a viral infection. We create about a billion new cells per day and an equal number die a "normal death." The debris from these dead cells must be removed and "digested" so the protein and nucleic acid building blocks can be reused to form the new cells. Indeed, one of the immune system's most important functions is to dispose of cell debris.

One of the leading theories of autoimmune disease is that a mistake in processing of the fragments from dead cells is a key stimulus to autoimmune disease. Rather than simply disposing of the dead cell material, a mistake is made and the dead cell's material is identified as foreign and the immune system is activated (as if it were a foreign graft or invading virus). For example, in Sjögren's patients the characteristic Sjögren's antibody is anti-SS-A antibody, and immune responses against SS-A protein may have a role in perpetuating the damage to the glands and other tissues.

SS-A is a normal nuclear protein found in all cells, and its job is to "chaperone" another protein into the cell's cytoplasm. However, this protein (and its associated RNA molecule) is particularly difficult for the immune system to break down, and thus SS-A may accumulate after a cell dies. This buildup may result in a stimulus to the immune system. Part of that reaction is the formation of antibodies to SS-A, which is a characteristic laboratory finding in many Sjögren's patients.

To summarize, the contribution of the "acquired immune system," auto-immunity is caused when self antigens cannot be properly removed by the immune system, and the residual protein is inappropriately bound to the HLA-D molecule (Fig. 6–3). This in turn stimulates a cascade of other immune factors that constitute the "acquired" immune system. This includes production of autoantibodies and the release of inflammatory factors that are measured when we try to assess the activity of the disease, such as the level of anemia, sedimentation rate, or attack of the immune system on organs other than the salivary and lacrimal glands. Many of the medicines now used in autoimmune disease were initially developed to prevent organ rejection in the "transplant" model. These include prednisone, hydroxychloroquine, methotrexate, and many others.

The (HLA-DR-Independent) Acquired Immune System or the "Innate" Immune System

We noted above that the acquired (HLA-DR) system was important but that it could not explain the entire story. In parallel with the search for an understanding of organ transplantation, other scientists were trying to understand the immune system's response to infectious organisms. Why do we get fevers, muscle and joint pains, and fatigue that we associate with feeling "flu-ish"? This led to recognition of a different part of the immune system that did not involve the HLA-DR system. It was called the "innate" (inborn) or the HLA-DR-independent immune response.

In autoimmune disorders such as Sjögren's or SLE, there is a close mutual stimulation of the innate and the acquired immune system. To assess disease activity and understand symptoms of Sjögren's, it is necessary to understand both arms of the immune system.

The acquired immune system is important, but it takes about 2 to 3 weeks after a foreign infection for this system to recognize the invader and make the appropriate T-cell, B-cell, and antibody responses. With most infections, we would have succumbed long before—assuming it was not an infection we recognized from a prior encounter and had an "acquired" immune memory.

Thus, studies of our response to infections such as pneumococcal infection led to recognition of a separate branch of the immune system called the innate (HLA-D-independent) system. The acquired system (defined by HLA-D) and the innate system work closely together to defend us from external infections—but when they function together in excess, the result may be autoimmunity, such as Sjögren's or SLE.

The innate immune system provides our first line of defense to bacteria and viruses. It consists of a different set of cells, such as *macrophages* and *dendritic cells,* that are not dependent on HLA-D proteins for their response.

Instead, it has evolved a series of receptors that can immediately recognize particular proteins, sugars, or nucleic acids that are common to many pathogens in the environment. Indeed, many of the symptoms such as fever or muscle aches that we feel in response to viruses or bacteria derive from the immediate release of inflammatory hormones from the cells of the innate immune system. A further consequence of stimulating the innate immune system is the stimulation of the acquired immune system described above. It is the perpetual mutual stimulation of the innate (HLA-D-independent) and the acquired (HLA-D-dependent) systems that characterizes autoimmune disorders such as Sjögren's and SLE.

The Relationship between Sjögren's and SLE

The immunological features and clinical features of Sjögren's and SLE show a great deal of overlap. However, there are distinct differences that are important. Perhaps the easiest way to simplify this overlap is to consider SLE a disease where the "organ" damage is done by autoantibodies.

- This refers to the binding of an autoantibody to a self antigen, which is mistaken for a foreign protein.
- The autoantibody may be directed against an antigen (i.e., protein) located on the surface of a red blood cell (leading to hemolytic anemia), a platelet (leading to a condition called thrombocytopenia), or the skin (leading to certain types of rashes).

Also, autoantibodies may bind to circulating proteins or DNA to form "immune complexes," which can then lodge in the kidney (leading to glomerulonephritis) or in blood vessels (leading to vasculitis). The immune complex

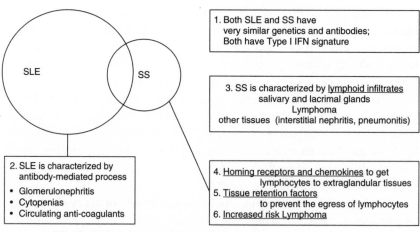

FIGURE 6–3 **What Is the Relationship Between SLE and SS?**

Box 6–1

Sjögren's Syndrome at a Glance

- An autoimmune disorder characterized by severely dry eyes and dry mouth due to lymphocytic infiltrates
- Prevalence for primary Sjögren's: 0.1% to 0.3% of adult females
- Female-to-male ratio is 9:1.
- Two peak ages of onset—in the 30s and in the 50s
- Many older patients diagnosed with "SLE" actually have Sjögren's.
- Pediatric Sjögren's may be part of spectrum of juvenile rheumatoid arthritis.

Box 6–2

Sjögren's Syndrome at a Glance

- Patients have a characteristic HLA-DR (extended haplotype): in Caucasians, it is extended DR3
- The genetic background is different in distinct ethnic groups (Chinese, Japanese, Greeks), but these groups have similar antibody profiles.
- The autoantibody profile is similar to subset of SLE.

Box 6–3

- Increased mortality risk, particularly due to lymphoproliferative complications
- Quality of life—equated with moderate angina
- "Disability" predominantly due to fatigue and cognitive "limitations"
  - Dry eyes limit work, especially at computer.
  - Dry mouth limits sleep and social interaction.

can bind an additional protein called "complement" and trigger an additional inflammatory cascade that is part of the innate immune system.

The pattern of antibodies found in SLE has a great deal of overlap with those found in Sjögren's. It is important to think of SLE as a series of different clinical syndromes that each has its characteristic autoantibodies (each associated with a distinct HLA-DR), and that one of the SLE subsets (characterized by HLA-DR3) has the closest overlap with Sjögren's. The HLA-DR3 subset of SLE has the antibody to SS-A, and these patients have Sjögren's-like symptoms, often termed "Sjögren's secondary to SLE."

In addition to immune complex features that characterize SLE in some Sjögren's patients, Sjögren's is also characterized by dryness of the eyes and mouth. This is due to the infiltration of the glands by lymphocytes (Fig. 6–4). Since the glands of most individuals do not have any lymphocytic infiltrates, we must consider Sjögren's a disease of "aggressive" lymphocytes where they get into tissues where they do not belong. This aggressive tendency can become very pronounced, where the salivary glands have become massively infiltrated and the patient may have developed a lymphoma (Fig. 6–5).

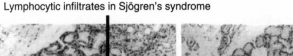

Lymphocytic infiltrates in Sjögren's syndrome

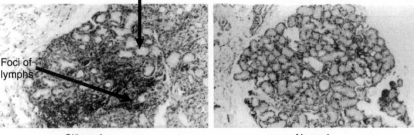

Foci of
lymphs

Sjögren's   Normal

FIGURE 6–4 **Lymphocytic Infiltrates in Sjögren's Syndrome**
Sjögren's Normal

Sjögren's syndrome – with parotid enlargement

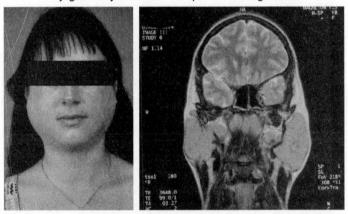

FIGURE 6–5 **MRI not used much for Diagnosis of Sjögren's Itself but is of value in Investigating Causes of Persistent Salivary Gland Swelling.**
However, with the increasing availability of scanners, and emerging evidence from Berlin and Japan, we may see this noninvasive technique being used more frequently for diagnostic purposes.

The Immunology of Clinical Symptoms in Sjögren's

More commonly, we see only the results of glandular infiltration of the lacrimal and tear glands that results in dry eyes (Fig. 6–6) and dry mouth with associated dental problems (Fig. 6–7). The surprising feature of this severe dryness is that the glands are not totally destroyed by the lymphocytic infiltrates.

Although we previously pointed out the lymphocytes that did form clusters in the gland, we now emphasize that about 50% of the glands remain visible. So one of the key questions in Sjögren's is: *Why are the residual glands not functioning at a high level?*

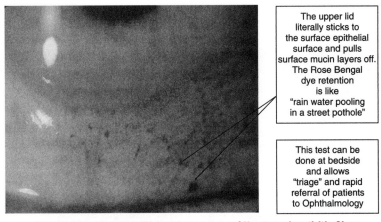

The upper lid literally sticks to the surface epithelial surface and pulls surface mucin layers off. The Rose Bengal dye retention is like "rain water pooling in a street pothole"

This test can be done at bedside and allows "triage" and rapid referral of patients to Ophthalmology

FIGURE 6–6 **Dryness Results in the Clinical Appearance of Keratoconjunctivitis Sicca Characteristic of Sjögren's Syndrome.**
The upper lid literally sticks to the surface epithelial surface and pulls surface mucin layers off. The Rose Bengal dye retention is like rainwater pooling in a street pothole. This test can be done at bedside and allows "triage" and rapid referral of patients to Ophthalmology.

In other diseases, a kidney, liver, or lung may continue to function until the organ is over 90% damaged. Thus, we must conclude that in Sjögren's patients, the local release of inflammatory mediators within the gland causes the residual cells to be "paralyzed."

Studies in animal models indicate that the inflammatory mediators (such as type I interferon, tumor necrosis factor [TNF], and interferon gamma) greatly decrease the gland's ability to respond to neural stimulation. An example of a salivary gland biopsy with cells producing type 1 interferon is shown in Figure 6–8. Also in this figure, the right-hand panel shows the "gene expression signature" from the lip biopsy from different individuals.

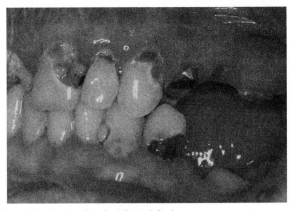

FIGURE 6–7 **Sjögren's Syndrome: Cervical Dental Caries.**

Normal lip biopsies lack type I interferon
gene signature

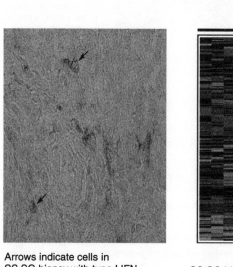

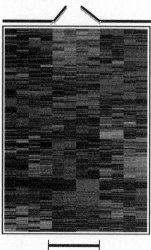

Arrows indicate cells in
SS SG biopsy with type I IFN

SS SG biopsy with type I IFN gene
profile

FIGURE 6–8 **Interferon (IFN) Type I in Salivary Gland Suggests a role in Sjögren's Syndrome.**
Arrows indicate cells in Sjögren's salivary gland biopsy with type I IFN.
Normal lip biopsies lack type I IFN gene signature.
Sjögren's salivary gland biopsy with type I IFN gene profile.

¤ The three columns on the left are from normals, the next three columns are from Sjögren's patients, and the three columns on the right side are from patients with dryness not due to Sjögren's.
¤ The pattern of colored bands indicates the strength of gene expression.
¤ In the middle columns (from the Sjögren's patients), the dark-green bands at the top of each column indicate a very high level of expression and show the characteristic pattern that is associated with response to type 1 interferon.

Thus, we see that different lip biopsies from Sjögren's patients all share a pattern of genes that are "upregulated" by type I interferon.

To re-emphasize this important point: One of the pivotal inflammatory molecules in both Sjögren's and SLE is type I interferon. This molecule is normally produced by the innate immune system in response to infection. It leads to low-grade fevers, fatigue, joint and muscle pain, and all of the symptoms we associate with having the flu. The presence of type I interferon leads to elevations of the erythrocyte sedimentation rate (ESR) and C-reactive protein (CRP) blood tests that we routinely measure in Sjögren's patients to assess activity. When the lymphocytes infiltrate the salivary or lacrimal gland, they paralyze the gland's response to normal stimuli. Thus, the gland may be

Box 6–4
Genetic Predisposition in Sjögren's to Type I Interferon

In genome-wide screens, association of IRF5 alleles and Stat 4 is associated with predisposition to development of Sjögren's.

only 50% destroyed, but the residual glandular tissue is unable to secrete adequately due to the presence of inflammatory mediators such as type 1 interferon.

However, most of us get over flu symptoms in a day or two, so the key question is: What leads to the persistence of production of the type I interferon signal in the glands and other tissues? This appears to be the link between the *acquired* (HLA-DR) and *innate* (non-HLA-DR) systems.

Perhaps an additional factor in causing Sjögren's is the finding that certain genes appear to increase the sensitivity of type 1 interferon production and response. Sjögren's patients have increased frequency of two of these genes, called interferon response factor 5 (IRF5) and a molecule that is closely bound to the type 1 interferon receptor (Stat 4) (Box 6–4).

Extraglandular Manifestations of Sjögren's

Although Sjögren's is characterized by dry eyes and dry mouth, some patients have rash, muscle pains (myalgia), joint pains (arthralgia), nerve pain (neuropathy), and fatigue. The lymphocytes leave their site of origin (the bone marrow) and travel through the bloodstream to various organs that may be involved.

In addition to the glands, we mentioned that other tissues, such as lung, kidney, skin, and nerves, might have lymphocytic infiltration. For this to occur, the lymphocytes must travel through the bloodstream until they reach the target organ. The lymphocytes know when to take the "exit ramp" off the "highway" of the bloodstream due to particular molecules on both the lymphocyte (called addressins, since they encode the address of the target organ) and molecules on the local blood vessels (called vascular adhesion molecules). The additional genes that lead to susceptibility to Sjögren's (and its extraglandular manifestations) play a key role in regulating this process of lymphocytes homing to the target organs.

Role of Antibodies Against SS-A and SS-B Antigens

The HLA-DR system encodes a tendency to make antibodies against the SS-A antigen, so a person born with the HLA-DR3 gene has a higher tendency to make the autoantibody. In salivary or lacrimal gland tissue that is damaged by virus or some other process, the SS-A antigen stimulates the immune lymphocytes that produce the antibody, which in turn binds to a normal cell chaperone called hYRNA. Although this molecular biology is esoteric, it is fun to see the probable "smoking gun" that perpetuates the process of Sjögren's.

This immune complex is able to stimulate the production of type I interferon, which in turn stimulates the production of more antibody to SS-A. A vicious cycle leads to the clinical picture that we know as Sjögren's or SLE. Of course, a myriad of other genes and hormones play a role in modulating this process. How to interrupt this cycle without crippling the important infection-fighting capacity of the body is a goal of current research.

Hormonal Influences

Estrogen activity may be involved in developing dry mouth and dry eye symptoms because of the following two factors:

1. Sjögren's affects women much more frequently than men.
2. The symptoms of dry mouth and dry eye are more prevalent in patients who are receiving hormone replacement therapy than those who are not.

Viruses, the Immune System, and Sjögren's

It is thought that some viral infections could have a role in the pathogenesis of Sjögren's by the following mechanism. After a virus or bacterium enters the body, an immune reaction is almost always activated. (Parasitic infections are less of a threat to us than they were to our forebears.) Thankfully, the infection is almost always defeated, and the person returns to normal health. Sometimes this initial response against the virus or bacterium becomes chronic because the body cannot clear the infection, and sometimes the immune response heads off in the direction of autoimmunity.

Examples of infections that can cause chronic problems include:

- Streptococci (a bacterium that can cause rheumatic fever)
- Human immunodeficiency virus (HIV)
- Hepatitis C virus (chronic hepatitis)

Indeed, hepatitis C virus can cause dry eye, dry mouth, and arthritis, all symptoms found in Sjögren's.

Epstein-Barr virus has been suggested as a possible activator or co-factor in the development of Sjögren's. Once we are infected with this virus, we remain infected for the rest of our lives, and nearly everyone is infected. The evidence for this virus being important in Sjögren's has not yet convinced most scientists, and it remains an idea that is not generally accepted.

Chronic **hepatitis C** can cause symptoms that are similar to Sjögren's (dry mouth, dry eye, and arthritis occurring in association with an enlarged parotid gland with lymphocytic infiltration). Anti-Ro and anti-La, which are present in the blood of Sjögren's patients, are typically absent in the blood of patients with chronic hepatitis C infection. Most experts in Sjögren's lean toward including hepatitis C as one of the differential diagnoses of dry eye–dry mouth syndrome, as other features distinguish it. Anti-Ro and anti-La are usually absent in hepatitis C patients, as are the usual pathologic findings of autoimmune Sjögren's.

Two **retroviruses**, HIV and human T-cell leukemia virus (HTLV-1), are known to be causes of a syndrome that presents with a clinical picture similar to that seen in Sjögren's. Those viruses affect males more than females, and the autoantibodies that define Sjögren's have not been found in the patients who carry those viruses. HLTV-1 may cause muscle deterioration and causes a condition with the unattractive name of tropical spastic paraparesis. This virus is endemic in some parts of the world.

The medical literature now has many, many reports describing the dry eye and mouth associated with HIV infection. Both Sjögren's and HIV infection have diffuse lymphocyte infiltration in the affected tissues. However, the kind of lymphocyte that dominates in HIV-infected patients tends to be different than those that dominate in Sjögren's. The characteristic autoantibodies, anti-Ro and anti-La, are typically not found in HIV-infected patients. There are other gene-related differences as well. Consequently, HIV-infected patients are not usually considered to have Sjögren's, but there is some disagreement among doctors on this point.

The Functional Circuit That Links Ocular/Oral Symptoms and Secretory Function

To understand the spectrum of disorders that contribute to dry eye and mouth, it is important to recognize that these symptoms result from an imbalance in a functional circuit that controls lacrimal and salivary function. The functional circuit can be considered to start at the mucosal membrane (either the ocular surface or buccal mucosal surface) where the patient has decreased aqueous secretions (Figs. 6–9) and 6–10). These highly innervated surfaces send unmyelinated nerves to specific regions of the midbrain, termed the lacrimatory and salvatory nuclei. This midbrain region sends signals to the cortex, where dryness is sensed, and receives input from cortical centers that reflect input such as depression or stress reactions associated with dryness. The clearest evidence

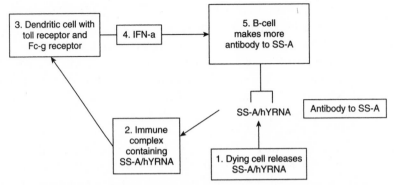

FIGURE 6–9 **The Vicious Cycle of Innate and Acquired Leads to IFN Type I (Links Genetic and Autoantibody Response).**

of these cortical inputs is the classical Pavlovian response of salivation in response to other cortical stimuli.

After the midbrain receives input from the mucosa and higher cortical centers, efferent (outgoing) nerves that innervate the glands using cholinergic neurotransmitters (especially acetylcholine and vasoactive intestinal peptide) and blood vessels using adrenergic (adrenalin-containing) neurotransmitters are activated. The presence of inflammatory infiltrates in the glands contributes to inadequate secretory response not only by destruction of glandular elements, but also by interfering with effective release of neurotransmitters by the nerves in the end organ and the response of the glandular cells at the level of post-receptor signaling. As a result, there is decreased activation of the receptors that subsequently produce the energy source for water transport.

Thus, a key point in the pathogenesis of Sjögren's is the observation that the salivary and lacrimal glands are not totally destroyed and local

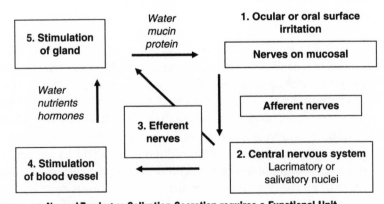

FIGURE 6–10 **Normal Tearing or Salivation Secretion requires a Functional Unit.**

immune-generated release of cytokines, autoantibodies, and other chemicals leads to dysfunction of the residual glands.

Although rheumatologists are talking about autoantibodies and acute phase reactants, the patient has complaints about dry, painful eyes and mouth.

In the initial stages of the disorder, patients are describing increased friction as the upper eyelid traverses the globe or the tongue moves over the buccal mucosa. For example, the upper eyelid normally traverses the globe on a carpet of lubricating tear film, composed of a mixture of aqueous and mucous secretions. When the aqueous tear or saliva component is deficient, the patient senses increased friction. The friction between the upper lids can be great enough so the surface components of the conjunctiva adhere to the upper lid and are torn off by upper-lid motion. Defects of the surface mucin layer are detected by the retention of Rose Bengal (a characteristic test for keratoconjunctivitis sicca [dry eye]). The ocular surface becomes a site of chronic inflammation, similar to a wound. From these regions arise unmyelinated afferent (incoming) nerves, which eventually end in specific regions of the midbrain, including the lacrimatory/salvatory nuclei. Neural signals are subsequently sent to the cortex, where pain is sensed.

Fibromyalgia or "Central Sensitization"

In addition to dry eyes and dry mouth, some of the most disabling symptoms for Sjögren's patients are fatigue and vague cognitive dysfunction. These symptoms do not correlate closely with our normal laboratory tests such as ESR or CRP (which are products of the innate immune system). Indeed, the symptoms of fibromyalgia are reminiscent of the "flu" or "jet lag," but the patient does not quickly bounce back. Studies in animal models and using new-generation magnetic resonance techniques have suggested that subtle interplay of inflammatory products in particular portions of the brain influences the function of nerves responsible for alertness and muscle pain. Since these symptoms are also found in many patients with depression, it is not surprising that many medications useful in depression are also useful in fibromyalgia.

A further finding is that there is a poor correlation between the findings of patient's pain in the nerves and muscles (i.e., muscle tender points) and the results of biopsies of nerve and muscle. This is currently being attributed to the fact that the nerve fibers from the "periphery" must travel up to the spinal cord, where they are joined through structures called ganglia. The nerve signal then ascends the spinal cord to particular portions of the brain that sense pain. Equally important, the brain sends signals down the spinal cord that "dampen" pain receptors, and this is also an important target for certain medications. Medications used in fibromyalgia are also used in peripheral neuropathy associated with diabetic neuropathy, since they help stabilize the neurotransmission along this critical pathway that the patient ultimately senses as pain.

Thus, the concept of fibromyalgia has now been upgraded to "central pain sensitization" to reflect the importance of how pain signals are transmitted.

However, we cannot emphasize strongly enough that fibromyalgia is the "elephant in the room." Many therapeutic trials have failed to understand that patients' quality of life may depend more on how their brain senses the dryness than the millimeters of tears that are generated, or that overall functional status depends strongly on the muscle pain, nerve pain, and "energy" level, which are not reflected in other measurements of glandular or inflammatory activity.

Summing Up

Sjögren's syndrome results from the interaction of genetic and environmental factors. It is likely that multiple genes interact to predispose an individual to Sjögren's. However, even when all of the genes are present (as in identical twins), it is clear that other (presumed) environmental factors play a role, since less than 20% of identical twins are concordant for the disorder.

No single environmental agent has been identified, despite an intensive 50-year search. It is more likely that many different agents can stimulate the

TABLE 6–1

Important Components of the Immune System in Sjögren's

1. **White blood cells**
   a. Granulocytes—promote acute inflammation
   b. Lymphocytes—promote chronic inflammation
      i. T cells (memory cells)
      ii. B cells (promote production of autoantibodies)
2. **Proteins**
   a. Albumin—carrier proteins, decreased in chronic disease
   b. Globulin—levels increased in inflammation
      i. Alpha globulins
      ii. Beta globulins
      iii. Gamma globulins—IgG, IgM, IgD, IgA, and IgE
3. **Important autoantibodies in Sjögren's**
   a. Anti-SSA, also known as anti-Ro
   b. Anti-SSB, also known as anti-La
   c. Rheumatoid factor
   d. Antinuclear antibody
   e. Anti-muscarinic receptor antibody

innate immune system, which is a primitive immune system, and thus prime the more sophisticated acquired immune system to perpetuate the autoimmune process. The molecules that define the innate system and the acquired immune system and that link the two systems are the subjects of intensive research. It is hoped that an understanding of these molecular events will lead to a new generation of therapies for patients.

FOR FURTHER READING

Cobb BL, Lessard CJ, Harley JB, Moser KL. Genes and Sjogren's syndrome. *Rheumatic Disease Clin North Am.* 2008; 34: 847–68.

Daniels TE. Sjogren's syndrome: clinical spectrum and current diagnostic controversies. *Adv Dent Res.* 1996; 10: 3–8.

Delaleau N, Jonsson MV, Appel S, Jonsson R. New concepts in the pathogenesis of Sjogren's syndrome. *Rheumatic Disease Clin North Am.* 2008; 34: 833–46.

James JA, Harley JB, Scofield RH. Role of viruses in systemic lupus erythematosus and Sjogren's syndrome. *Curr Opin Rheumatol.* 2000; 13: 370–6.

Manoussakis MN, Moutsopoulos HM. Sjogren's syndrome: current concepts. *Adv Intern Med.* 2001; 47: 191–217.

Vitali C, Bombardieri S, Jonsson R. Classification criteria for Sjogren's syndrome: a revised version of the European criteria proposed by the American-European Consensus Group. *Ann Rheum Dis.* 2002; 61: 554–8.

7

What Causes Exocrine Dysfunction in Sjögren's?

Janine Austin Clayton, MD, Serena Morrison, MD,
and Philip C. Fox, DDS

Sjögren's syndrome affects the exocrine glands, the moisture-producing glands of the body. The cardinal symptoms of Sjögren's are dry eye (called keratoconjunctivitis sicca [KCS]) and dry mouth (termed xerostomia), affecting greater than 90% of patients. These symptoms are due to altered function of the lacrimal and salivary glands, which produce the tears and saliva. Other moisture-producing glands are affected as well, and this leads to other sicca symptoms such as dry skin, nose, and throat and vaginal dryness. What causes this exocrine dysfunction? In this chapter, the normal functions and disease-related dysfunction of the lacrimal and salivary glands affected in Sjögren's will be discussed and current theories about the causes of the dryness will be considered.

The Lacrimal Gland

Since the source of human tears is the lacrimal gland, it is important to know its normal anatomy and structure. The lacrimal gland is located underneath the upper eyelid on the outer side near the temple. There are two lobes of the lacrimal gland, the palpebral and the orbital. Some smaller, accessory lacrimal glands are located in the conjunctiva (the transparent membrane that covers the white part of the eye and that gets red when irritated) (Table 7–1).

The lacrimal glands should constantly be producing tears while we are performing our normal activities. Their purpose is to lubricate and protect the surface of the eye. We are usually unaware of these tears, called basal tears. Reflex or emergency tears are produced to flush and lubricate the eye quickly if a particle or chemical gets into the eye. Some people with dry eye have painful episodes due to decreased amounts of basal tears, but because their lacrimal gland is not completely damaged, they can still produce a normal amount

TABLE 7–1
Exocrine Glands

1. Lacrimal glands (produce tears)
   a. Consist of palpebral lobe, orbital lobe, and accessory glands
   b. Tear film layers: mucous, aqueous, lipid
2. Salivary glands (produce saliva)
   a. Consist of parotid, submandibular, sublingual, and minor glands
   b. Secretions (mucous and serous)

of reflex tears. They may even think they have excess tearing when in fact they have dry eye. This is because as their eyes dry out from a lack of basal tears, their eyes start to hurt, and this triggers production of emergency tears.

In Sjögren's, the lacrimal gland does not produce a sufficient volume of tear fluid. In addition, the tears produced are abnormal in their consistency and composition and do not lubricate or protect the surface of the eye well. For example, the tears are unstable and often evaporate faster than normal, leaving dry spots on the surface of the eye. In addition, when reading or concentrating (such as when working on a computer), one blinks less, which allows the tear film to evaporate more readily. Dry eye can result in a decreased ability to read for extended periods of time.

TEAR FILM LAYERS

Tears have three major components: mucous, aqueous (or liquid), and lipid (or oil). These contents are arranged in layers, and the components of each layer must be healthy and in balance for the tears to function properly.

The *mucous layer* is the tear layer that is closest to the eye surface. Special cells that are found in the conjunctiva, called goblet cells, create mucin, which makes up this layer. This layer makes the tears slippery and anchors them loosely to the surface of the cornea for protection. It also helps prevent infection by keeping bacteria from sticking to the surface of the eye.

The *aqueous layer* is the liquid component of the tears and hydrates the mucous layer to form a sort of tear gel. The aqueous layer is produced by the lacrimal gland and also lubricates and enhances the spreadability of the tear film. The aqueous layer contains proteins such as lysozyme and lactoferrin, which act as antimicrobials and protect the eye from bacteria.

Tiny sebaceous (oil-producing) glands, called meibomian glands, are located along the margin of the eyelids, adjacent to the lashes. They produce the outermost *lipid layer* of the tear film, which enhances tear stability and retards evaporation of the tears. If the lipid layer is completely removed, the rate of evaporation is increased fourfold.

Salivary Glands

Sjögren's also affects the salivary glands. The principal glands of salivation are the parotid, submandibular, and sublingual glands, which are located in front of the ears, under the jaw, and under the tongue, respectively. When these glands are functioning well, they can produce 800 to 1,500 milliliters of saliva each day. In addition, there are hundreds of minor salivary glands located throughout the oral cavity just below the mucosa that provide a small but constant flow of saliva to moisten and lubricate the surface. These minor glands are particularly important for comfort during the majority of the day when the major glands are not stimulated by oral stimulatory activities (such as eating).

The salivary glands produce two major types of secretions. The first is the serous secretion, which is watery. The second type is the mucous secretion, which is thicker and more viscous and contains mucin for lubricating and protection.

Saliva is critical for protection of the oral cavity. The mouth is laden with bacteria, fungi, and viruses that can cause infection, destroy tissue, and promote cavities (dental caries). Saliva contains numerous components that are antimicrobial and help to control or destroy these organisms. Also, the flow of saliva helps wash away the bacteria and food particles that the bacteria require to survive. Saliva is also important to nourish the mucosa, maintain the teeth, and support other oral functions such as chewing, swallowing, and taste.

Both the eye and the mouth encounter microbial and environmental irritants on an ongoing basis. Both the eyes and mouth need lubrication as well, since they are constantly in motion. Saliva and tears contain all the necessary elements to protect and lubricate the surfaces of the eyes and mouth.

Theories of How Dryness in Sjögren's Develops

The production of tears and saliva is a complex process that is still being defined at a molecular level. There are many steps involved in the production of these fluids, and disruption of this process at any stage can reduce the amount of the secretions and alter their composition. Nerve fibers going into the glands, the acinar gland cells (the cells that transport fluid from the blood), the ductal cells (which transport exocrine fluids to the body surface), the stromal cells (which support the acinar cells), and even sex hormones all play a major role in the production of saliva and tears. All aspects of these systems need to be functioning and in concert with each other for normal tear and saliva production. At this time, the causes of Sjögren's are not known. Increasing knowledge is available about the mechanisms of lacrimal and salivary dysfunction, but the underlying triggers and initiating events remain elusive. However, many theories exist and are being investigated actively.

DECREASE IN GLANDULAR CELL OUTPUT

The lacrimal and salivary glands are exocrine glands. This type of gland has special cells, acinar cells, that transport fluid to the ducts, which, in turn, produce some components and modify these secretions. For the acinar cells to transport fluid, their relationship with the supporting stromal cells needs to be exact. If this relationship is disrupted, secretion will decline.

Damage to these special gland cells can occur with an autoimmune event. For unknown reasons, in Sjögren's patients lymphocytes (the body's immune defense cells) are attracted to and retained in the salivary and lacrimal glands. Once the lymphocytes gather in the exocrine glands, they multiply, become activated, and form the focus of inflammation. This inflammation is an attack by the body directed on itself. For example, the lymphocytes release compounds called cytokines that can injure the acinar cells and can even cause the stromal cells to dysfunction and fail to support the acinar cells. As a result, the gland cells become damaged and may undergo apoptosis or other forms of cell death. When an acinar cell dies, it releases its contents, and this can lead to even more inflammation. Damaged gland cells do not produce normal amounts or quality of fluid secretions. In the salivary glands, the lymphocytic inflammation is most dense surrounding duct and nerve cells and there is selective loss of the acinar cells. However, it has been shown that even normal-appearing acinar cells do not function optimally in involved glands.

NERVE FUNCTION DISRUPTION

Normally, signals sent through the nerve fibers to an exocrine gland cause it to secrete. Damage to or dysfunction of the nerves can lead to surface dryness by disturbing the fluid production and release. The salivary and lacrimal glands have a direct link to the brain through these nerve fibers.

There are a number of ways in which the nerves may be involved in Sjögren's. In one scenario, there is confusion in signaling, in that even though the sensory input is intact and signals that tears or saliva need to be produced, the appropriate signal is not transmitted and the tears and saliva are not made. Drugs can also cause this confusion at the brain level; that is why many medicines often have the side effect of dry mouth and dry eye.

The second situation is that the correct message *is* transmitted through the nerves, but the response is aberrant. One possibility is that cytokines produced by the lymphocytes at the site cause paralysis in these nerves. The result is that the glands that are supposed to be stimulated fail to receive the message to make tears and saliva, although they are capable of doing so.

A third possibility (in the eye) involves the cornea and its connection to the neural centers. If for some reason the cornea's nerves are not working well, as occurs with dryness, then no message will be sent to the brain that tears are needed. Without the message that a problem exists, the brain does not know to send a message to the lacrimal gland to increase secretions. Any interruption of this feedback loop, which some researchers call a servomechanism, can decrease the amount of secretions.

SEX HORMONES

Another factor to be considered is the role of sex hormones. It is known that autoimmunity is more prevalent in women than men. In Sjögren's, the female-to-male ratio is about 9:1. Could this be because of sex hormones? Women normally have higher levels of estrogen and lower levels of androgens than men, and eye tissue has components that specifically bind sex hormones. It has been found that with a decrease in local androgens, the inflammation mentioned above goes unchecked. A certain amount of androgens are required to maintain a non-inflamed state in exocrine glands. For example, androgens decrease the production of autoantibodies, and estrogens tend to promote inflammation. Some studies have even found that menopausal hormone replacement therapy (with estrogen and progestin) is associated with dry eye in postmenopausal women. While there is strong evidence for a role for sex hormones in lacrimal dysfunction in animal models of Sjögren's syndrome, the situation is not clear in the salivary glands.

AUTOIMMUNE THEORIES

In the previous section, we talked about how damage to the lacrimal and salivary glands, a problem with the nervous system, or a disturbance in the level or balance of sex hormones could result in dryness. One prevalent theme for the cause of the damage is autoimmunity. But what triggers the autoimmunity? Scientists are investigating many theories: that the cause of Sjögren's autoimmunity may be an infectious trigger, a genetic factor, environmental, or a combination of factors.

Extension of the Inflammatory Theory: Apoptosis

Apoptosis is the process by which a cell is programmed to self-destruct. If cells do not die when they are supposed to, problems result. Cells that keep growing and dividing can become tumors and may be malignant. What does this have to do with Sjögren's? In Sjögren's, when the lymphocytes arrive at the fluid-producing lacrimal or salivary gland, instead of just passing through, they are activated and signal the immune system to initiate an attack. That is a problem in itself. The second problem is that the lymphocytes are supposed to die at some point but sometimes do not undergo natural death or apoptosis. The lymphocytes accumulate in the glands and keep stimulating the immune system to attack the glands. An accumulation of lymphocytes, called a focus, is characteristic in the exocrine glands of people with Sjögren's. This focus is a significant diagnostic finding when a lip biopsy of a minor salivary gland is performed while evaluating a subject for Sjögren's. An increased risk for Sjögren's may exist in people whose cells are resistant to apoptosis. Further, B-cell lymphomas are more common in primary Sjögren's than in non-patients, and this too may be related to the chronic B-cell hyperreactivity and limited apoptosis of these cells.

Conversely, increased apoptosis has been considered a cause of the exocrine damage in Sjögren's. The theory is that the ongoing autoimmune inflammation in the glands causes accelerated apoptosis, leading to the loss of essential acinar cells. While there is some evidence of increased apoptosis (particularly in some animal models) in Sjögren's, a consistent alteration compared to healthy glands has not been shown. It is unlikely that apoptosis is a significant cause of exocrine dysfunction in Sjögren's.

Infections

Infection with viruses such as hepatitis C, human lymphotrophic leukemia virus (HTLV-1), and human immunodeficiency virus (HIV) has been known to cause dry eye and mouth. Therefore, viral infection in general (not necessarily with the above viruses) has been suspected as a potential pathogenic mechanism for Sjögren's.

When viruses enter a cell, they can change the surface so that the normal cells now look like foreign invaders (such as bacteria). As a result of these changes, the cells are no longer recognized as "self," and the body's defenses attack them.

Another mechanism involves invading microbes, which sneak past the body's defenses by disguising themselves as native cells. If the normal microbial defenses recognize this, they will attack the invaders. Unfortunately, the true native cells are so similar to the masqueraded microbes that the defense cells cannot differentiate and therefore attack the native cells as well as the bacteria.

Epstein-Barr virus (EBV) has been investigated as a contributor to Sjögren's syndrome. The picture is not clear and the only evidence is indirect. EBV is found in almost all salivary glands, healthy or otherwise. Other viruses and bacteria have also been studied, but at present none has been identified as clearly involved in the pathogenesis of the syndrome.

Genetics

As mentioned above, the environment (such as viruses and bacteria) is a consideration for the cause of Sjögren's, but another major factor is a person's genetic background. Does something about the genetic makeup of someone with Sjögren's make him or her more susceptible to autoimmune disease? For unknown reasons, some patterns of genes make people more susceptible to autoimmune diseases than others. When certain interactions, as yet undefined, occur between the genes and the environment, then autoimmune diseases can be triggered.

Numerous studies have shown that certain gene frequencies lend a predisposition for Sjögren's. Association studies are ongoing, examining the genome and proteome of Sjögren's patients to look for a "signature," a pattern of alterations in gene and protein expression characteristic of the disorder. To date, many candidates have been identified, but a specific gene or genes has not been found definitively. One complicating factor is that many autoimmune conditions appear to share gene patterns. It has been shown, for example, that Sjögren's has a similar gene signature to systemic lupus erythematosus. However, it is likely that in the next few years a clear genetic pattern will be identified, which will be helpful in diagnosis of Sjögren's.

Summing Up

As Sjögren's is a complex disorder, it is unlikely that a single "cause" will be found. It is probable that a combination of factors leads to alterations in the immune system that in turn lead to the constellation of signs and symptoms that characterize Sjögren's. One can imagine that an infection or viral reactivation, even with a common virus such as EBV, in a host with a susceptible genetic makeup, combined with some environmental trigger or other illness, could lead to chronic immune stimulation and resulting B-cell hyperreactivity. This could result in lymphocyte accumulation in the exocrine glands and the subsequent series of events leading to exocrine dysfunction and dryness.

An intricate pathway exists to create the right amount, components, and consistency of tears and saliva. If this process is disrupted in any way, the production and components of the secretions can be altered. We know an autoimmune process is involved, but many possibilities exist as to why Sjögren's starts and how it damages the body. The cause of the body's attack on itself remains unclear, and a combination of infection and genetics is being investigated as a potential disease-inducing factor.

FOR FURTHER READING

Chiorini JA, Cihakova D, Ouellette CE, Caturegli P. Sjögren syndrome: advances in the pathogenesis from animal models. *Curr Opin Rheumatol.* 2009; 21(5): 465–70.

Cobb BL, Lessard CJ, Harley JB, Moser KL. Genes and Sjögren's syndrome. *Rheumatology (Oxford).* 2006; 45(7): 792–8.

Dawson LJ, Fox PC, Smith PM. Sjögren's syndrome—the non-apoptotic model of glandular hypofunction. *Cornea.* 2000; 19(5): 644–49.

Lee BH, Tudares MA, Nguyen CQ. Sjögren's syndrome: an old tale with a new twist. *Immunol Rev.* 2010; 237(1): 264–83.

Manoussakis MN, Kapsogeorgou EK. The role of intrinsic epithelial activation in the pathogenesis of Sjögren's syndrome. *J Autoimmun.* 2010; 35(3): 219–24.

Mariette X, Gottenberg JE. Pathogenesis of Sjögren's syndrome and therapeutic consequences. *Curr Opin Rheumatol.* 2010; 22(5): 471–7.

Nikolov NP, Illei GG. Pathogenesis of Sjögren's syndrome. *Arch Immunol Ther Exp (Warsz).* 2009; 57(1): 57–66.

Pflugfelder SC, Solomon A, Stern ME. The diagnosis and management of dry eye: a twenty-five-year review. *Cornea.* 2000; 19(5): 644–9.

Townsend MJ, Monroe JG, Chan AC. B-cell targeted therapies in human autoimmune diseases: an updated perspective. *Rheum Dis Clin North Am.* 2008; 34(4): 847–68.

PART THREE

WHERE AND HOW CAN THE BODY BE AFFECTED BY SJÖGREN'S?

8

Generalized Symptoms and Signs of Sjögren's

Steven E. Carsons, MD,
and Nehad R. Solomon, MD, FACR

Although Sjögren's syndrome is a disorder primarily recognized as causing dry eyes and dry mouth, it is a complex disease that may be accompanied by a myriad of extra-glandular (outside of the glands) symptoms. These may include constitutional symptoms such as fatigue, achiness, fever, adenopathy (swollen glands), myalgias (muscle pain), and weight loss. Although dryness in Sjögren's is predominantly of the eyes and mouth, it too may affect areas external to the tear and salivary glands such as the skin, respiratory tract, and vaginal lining. Patients with Sjögren's also may suffer from shortness of breath, cough, joint pain and swelling, rashes, gastroesophageal reflux, muscle weakness, urinary dysfunction, peripheral or central nervous disease, and autoimmune thyroid disease. This chapter will focus on the many extra-glandular signs and symptoms that may be associated with Sjögren's (Table 8–1), whereas the next chapter will focus on the specific organ manifestations.

TABLE 8–1
General Extra-glandular Symptoms and Signs of Sjögren's Syndrome

Symptoms	Signs
Fatigue	Adenopathy
Myalgias	Rash
Fever	Mouth sores
Cough	Raynaud's
Shortness of breath	Weight loss
Dysphagia	Synovitis
Reflux	Diminished reflexes
Vaginal dryness	Cracked skin
Dysuria	Hives
Achiness	Vasculitis

(Continued)

TABLE 8–1

General Extra-glandular Symptoms and Signs of Sjögren's Syndrome (Cont'd)

Symptoms	Signs
Joint pain	Pneumonitis
Muscle weakness	Hypokalemia
Numbness	
Tingling	
Depression	
Itchy skin	
Epigastric pain	
Nocturia	
Renal colic	
Painful intercourse	

Constitutional Symptoms

Constitutional symptoms (generalized aching, fatigue, alterations in temperature) are common in Sjögren's and may be due in part to the overactive immune response and persistent inflammation. High levels of autoantibodies circulating in the body mediate this inflammatory immune response. Fatigue may be caused by several factors, including poor sleep due to discomfort associated with nocturnal dryness or thyroid dysfunction as well as inflammation.

Skin Manifestations

The skin is a common site where signs of Sjögren's occur. Some symptoms and signs involving the skin include dry skin as well as a whole host of rashes and discoloration. When the glands in the skin are affected by Sjögren's, the result is dryness, which may occur in about 50% of patients. This dryness can often lead to flaking, cracking, and fissuring. Cracks in dry skin can lead to infection, with areas of the skin becoming reddened and tender.

When blood vessels in the skin become inflamed due to white blood cells infiltrating and destroying their walls, the result is called vasculitis. A vasculitis rash resembles red spots located over the lower extremities. Skin vasculitis usually occurs over the course of several years following the diagnosis of Sjögren's. Occasionally the rash may be raised, may display a deep reddish-purple hue, and may be painful. This is referred to as palpable purpura. Hypergammaglobulinemic purpura is another type of skin rash, which is an orange-brown color. This results from high levels of immunoglobulin (antibody) circulating in the blood. These immunoglobulins are proteins commonly found in the blood of Sjögren's patients and in high quantity cause the blood to be thicker than normal and cause the red blood cells to leak through the superficial blood vessels of the skin.

Urticaria or hives may also occur in some patients with Sjögren's. These may differ from typical hives in that they may not always itch, may be tender, and may be persistent. A unique set of rashes, originally described in patients with lupus, may occur in Sjögren's and are common in patients with anti-SSA (Ro) and anti-SSB (La) antibodies. These rashes are called subacute cutaneous lupus (SCLE). One is called annular and looks like a series of red rings. The other is called papulous-squamous and is scaly, looking somewhat like psoriasis. Their presence does not necessarily imply that the patient has systemic lupus.

Another common sign seen in Sjögren's is Raynaud's phenomenon, which is a three-part response that classically occurs when extremities are exposed to the cold. Generally, the fingers will initially turn white as blood vessels constrict. They will then turn blue as a result of pooling of blood in the veins, and finally red when fresh blood re-enters the region. Raynaud's phenomenon is seen not only in Sjögren's but also in a variety of other connective tissue disorders.

Respiratory Symptoms

The upper airway, which includes the mouth, nose, and throat, and the lower airway, including the windpipe and lungs, are commonly involved in Sjögren's. The internal linings of the upper and lower airways, which contain mucus-secreting glands, become flooded with lymphocytes (white blood cells) and fail to function properly, leading to dryness. Mucous gland dysfunction may result in laryngotracheobronchitis, which is a chronic inflammatory condition involving the voice box, windpipe, and bronchial tubes. As a result of this inflammation, patients often experience a dry cough. An inability to clear the mucus may result in an infection such as bronchitis or pneumonia. Pneumonia manifests itself with fever, chills, and cough being the predominant symptoms.

In addition to pneumonia, patients with Sjögren's may experience shortness of breath due to a condition known as interstitial pneumonitis. This is an inflammation of the supporting tissue around the alveoli (air sacs) of the lungs caused by the autoimmune process. This is a slow process that occurs over years and is not due to infection. This type of lung involvement is usually found by x-ray, CT scanning, and pulmonary function testing.

Musculoskeletal Pain

Approximately 50% of patients with Sjögren's will experience episodes of joint pain during the course of their disease. These episodes may present as symptoms of arthralgias (joint pain), morning stiffness, or intermittent swelling of the joints referred to as synovitis. X-rays generally tend not to show destructive changes. Many patients will already have a diagnosis of rheumatoid arthritis (RA) (or lupus or scleroderma) before the onset of classic Sjögren's symptoms; this subset of patients is referred to as having secondary Sjögren's syndrome. In fact, when Dr. Sjögren first described the symptoms of dryness, it was in a group of patients who had an established diagnosis of RA. Having said this, it is important not to mistake symptoms of joint pain, which is a common manifestation of Sjögren's that may precede the symptoms of dryness, as being always due to RA.

Gastrointestinal Symptoms

Sjögren's also may involve the gastrointestinal tract, leading to symptoms of esophageal reflux and dysphagia. Reflux, which is the regurgitation of acid into the esophagus, is thought to result from the inappropriate relaxation of the lower esophageal sphincter (valve). This may be due in part to a dysfunction in the autonomic nervous system, which controls the valve. Lymphocytes infiltrating the nerves may be the cause of this dysfunction. The classic symptom of reflux is burning or discomfort in the epigastric area (mid-chest). Excessive acid in the mouth, in addition to the existing dryness, can also commonly result in mouth sores and contribute to tooth decay.

Dysphagia (difficulty swallowing) is thought to occur by one of two mechanisms. The first is due to dryness of the pharynx and esophagus leading to functional inability to swallow. The second mechanism may be due to an actual dysfunction in the movements of the esophagus controlled by the autonomic nervous system. The resultant clinical symptoms include nausea and epigastric pain.

Inflammation of the pancreas may be seen in association with Sjögren's but is rare. Symptoms include nausea, fever, and burning abdominal pain with a radiation to the back.

Liver disease also has been reported in some patients with Sjögren's. Such diseases include autoimmune hepatitis and primary biliary cirrhosis. Patients with these diseases are frequently asymptomatic and are diagnosed by routine laboratory testing. With progression of liver disease, some signs and symptoms include pruritus (itching), predominantly of the palms and soles, jaundice (yellowing of skin), and malabsorption of fat, leading to loose or greasy stools.

Signs of Kidney Involvement

Patients who have kidney involvement may present with symptoms of muscle weakness as a result of an electrolyte imbalance known as hypokalemia (low potassium). This electrolyte imbalance may also lead to the development of kidney stones, which often present with symptoms of renal colic. Renal colic is recurrent, sharp back pain in the area of the kidney. Interstitial cystitis, which is a nonbacterial (sterile) inflammation of the bladder, can also been seen in Sjögren's and presents with symptoms such as night-time urination, suprapubic pain, and dysuria (pain on urination). Inflammation of the kidney tubules may lead to an inability of the kidney to concentrate the urine properly. This may cause frequent urination of urine that is too dilute.

Symptoms and Signs of Nervous System Involvement

The nervous system may be involved in as many as 25% to 50% of patients with Sjögren's. Symptoms of peripheral neuropathy include numbness, tingling, and burning of the extremities. This may also on rare occasion lead to difficulty with balance. Peripheral neuropathy also can result in symptoms of extremity weakness or abnormal gait. On physical exam, reflexes may be absent.

A cranial neuropathy may also be seen in primary Sjögren's syndrome. The cranial nerves arise from the brain. One of the most common nerves to be affected is the trigeminal nerve, which supplies sensation to the face and the surfaces of the eyes as well as to the organs of taste and smell. When this nerve is affected, the result may be facial pain or a loss of sensation, taste, or smell. On rare occasion the central nervous system may also be involved, resulting in symptoms resembling those of multiple sclerosis, such as difficulty with speech, balance, blurry vision, movement, and coordination, as well as fine motor skills.

Depression has not been formally studied in Sjögren's but is frequently reported. In a survey devised by the Sjögren's Syndrome Foundation, depression was reported in about 29% of patients who responded. This depression is thought to be independent of thyroid disease or fibromyalgia.

Lymphoma

Lymphoma is another rare but serious complication of Sjögren's. It may present as persistent fever, weight loss, and swelling of the salivary glands as well as the glands of the neck, armpits, or groin. Because salivary gland swelling is common in Sjögren's, the physician should be aware of any unusual increase in gland swelling or any new or unusual swelling or mass in the head, neck, armpit, or groin.

Association with Thyroid Abnormalities

Thyroid disease is not uncommon in Sjögren's. The common symptoms of a hypofunctional thyroid include weight gain, cold intolerance, deepening of the voice, coarse hair, excessive fatigue, and depression. Hyperfunctional thyroid disease, known as Graves disease, may present with symptoms of sweating, palpitations, thinning of the hair, and weight loss. Autoimmune thyroid disease most often occurs independently of Sjögren's and is more frequent in relatives of patients with autoimmune disease.

Genital Complaints

As mentioned previously, dryness is the hallmark of this disease. This dryness also may occur on the vaginal surface, thereby decreasing the amount of natural lubrication and resulting in painful intercourse and vaginal burning. Excessive vaginal dryness also can result in various infections, including yeast (candida, monilia) infections.

Summing Up

The symptoms of Sjögren's syndrome are more than just dry eyes and dry mouth and include a whole array of symptoms encompassing the entire body. These symptoms may significantly impair a patient's quality of life; however, with prompt recognition and proper treatment, many of these symptoms may be largely ameliorated.

FOR FURTHER READING

Alexander EL, Arnett FC, Provost TT, et al: Sjögren's syndrome: association of anti-Ro(SS-A) antibodies with vasculitis, hematologic abnormalities, and serologic hyperreactivity. *Ann Intern Med.* 1983; 98: 155.

Alexander EL, Beall SS, Gordon B, et al. Magnetic resonance imaging of cerebral lesions in patients with Sjögren's syndrome. *Ann Intern Med.* 1988; 108: 815.

Gemignani F, Marbini A, Pavesi G, et al. Peripheral neuropathy associated with primary Sjögren's syndrome. *J Neurol Neurosurg Psychiatry.* 1994; 57: 983.

Goules A, Masouridi S, Tzioufas AG, et al. Clinically significant and biopsy-documented renal involvement in primary Sjögren's syndrome. *Medicine.* 2000; 79: 241.

Kassan SS, Thomas TL, Moutsopoulos HM, et al. Increased risk of lymphoma in sicca syndrome. *Ann Intern Med.* 1978; 89(6): 888–92.

Mialon P, Barthelemy L, Sebert P, et al: A longitudinal study of lung impairment in patients with primary Sjögren's syndrome. *Clin Exp Rheumatol.* 1997; 15: 349.

Ramos-Casals M, Brito-Zeron P, Font J. The overlap of Sjögren's syndrome with other systemic autoimmune diseases. *Semin Arthritis Rheum.* 2007; 36(4): 246–55.

Ramos-Casals M, Garcia-Carrasco M, Cervera R, et al: Hepatitis C virus infection mimicking primary Sjögren's syndrome: A clinical and immunologic description of 35 cases. *Medicine.* 2001; 80: 1–8.

Skopouli FN, Barbatis C, Moutsopoulos HM. Liver involvement in primary Sjögren's syndrome. *Br J Rheumatol.* 1994; 33: 745.

Theander E, Henriksson G, Ljungberg O, et al. Lymphoma and other malignancies in primary Sjögren's syndrome: a cohort study on cancer incidence and lymphoma predictors. *Ann Rheum Dis.* 2006; 65(6): 796–803.

Vrethem M, Lindvall B, Holmgren H, et al. Neuropathy and myopathy in primary Sjogren's syndrome: Neurophysiological, immunological and muscle biopsy results. *Acta Neurol Scand.* 1990; 82: 126.

9

The Internal Organs in Sjögren's

Fotini C. Soliotis, MD, MRCP,

Stuart S. Kassan, MD, FACP, FACR, and

Haralampos M. Moutsopoulos, MD, FACP, FRCP

In Sjögren's syndrome, the immune system primarily targets the salivary and lacrimal glands. However, the same immune process can also affect the major organs of the body, such as the lungs, heart, gut, liver, kidney, and nervous system. Major organ disease is only seen in one third of primary Sjögren's patients and can be divided into two categories depending on whether it manifests itself early (that is, together with the symptoms of dry eye and dry mouth) or later on, sometimes years after the Sjögren's diagnosis has been made.

Manifestations of lung and liver disease as well as one type of kidney disease (interstitial nephritis) occur early, around the time of diagnosis of Sjögren's, and are unlikely to occur later on. These diseases are characterized by a common immune process: an infiltration of the affected organ by a group of white cells called lymphocytes.

On the other hand, the less common type of kidney disease, glomerulonephritis, and the involvement of the peripheral nerves often occur later in the disease process and are not usually present at the time of diagnosis of Sjögren's. These two diseases also are characterized by a common immune process: inflammation of blood vessels, known as vasculitis, caused by the deposition of immune complexes (structures made up of antibodies) on the vessel walls.

Although disease of the major body organs is rarely severe or life-threatening in Sjögren's, it should nevertheless be diagnosed promptly so that effective treatment is given. This is one of the reasons why Sjögren's patients should be monitored by their physician on a regular basis.

Respiratory Tract

The entire respiratory tract can be affected in Sjögren's. Starting with the nose, thinning of the mucous membrane of the nose, or atrophic rhinitis, can occur, giving rise to nasal dryness. Moving down the airway, the voice box (larynx), windpipe (trachea), and bronchial tubes can become inflamed; this is known as laryngotracheobronchitis. The main symptoms of this condition are hoarseness, dry cough, wheezing, and shortness of breath.

Because there is less mucus produced in the airway, Sjögren's patients have difficulty clearing foreign material that has been inhaled into the respiratory tract. This can also contribute to the chronic inflammation of the bronchi and can predispose the patient to bacterial infections. Also, mucus can become stuck in the small bronchi, blocking the ventilation of a small segment of the lung. This can lead to the collapse of that lung segment (known as atelectasis).

Inflammation of the trachea and bronchi (tracheobronchitis) can be diagnosed by performing breathing tests known as pulmonary function tests. The patient blows into a tube connected to a machine that measures the flow of air in the bronchi. In this way the reduced flow of air in the bronchial tubes can be detected. In tracheobronchitis, a standard chest x-ray can be normal.

The use of room humidifiers can help relieve symptoms of mild tracheobronchitis. Also, prescribed nebulizers, which can deliver tiny water droplets into the small airways, can help. If the patient is wheezing or if the pulmonary function tests confirm blockage of airflow in the bronchi, then inhalers containing medications that dilate the bronchi can be prescribed. However, these are only partially effective, as they cannot clear the mucus blocking the bronchi. In this respect, drugs that break down mucus (mucolytics) may be of some benefit.

The lung itself can also become inflamed in Sjögren's (interstitial lung disease [ILD]). As the bronchi branch out, they end up in small air sacs known as the alveoli, where carbon dioxide is exchanged for oxygen. Around the alveoli there is supporting tissue known as the interstitium. This contains small blood vessels that take up the oxygen from the alveoli. If there is inflammation and scarring within the interstitium, then less oxygen can enter the blood within the lungs.

The symptoms of interstitial lung disease vary depending on the severity of the disease. In the early stages patients may have no symptoms or may complain of a dry cough and mild shortness of breath on exertion. In the late stages of severe ILD, which is rare, patients may have disabling breathlessness on exertion.

The chest x-ray may show a lacy or honeycomb type of shadowing within the lungs. Pulmonary function tests show impairment of gas transfer from the alveoli into the blood vessels and a reduced volume of air in the lungs. High-resolution computed tomography scans (HRCT) of the lungs are very useful in confirming the diagnosis. When looking at HRCT films, areas of inflammation appear as patches of white "ground glass" within the dark lungs. However, other lung conditions can mimic interstitial lung disease associated with Sjögren's, and therefore further investigations are sometimes necessary to confirm the diagnosis. In a procedure known as bronchoscopy, a tube can be inserted from the nose inside the lungs with the patient awake. Then a sample of bronchial secretions can be obtained and examined under the microscope. In ILD associated with Sjögren's, fluid from bronchial secretions typically contains numerous lymphocytes, which are cells involved in inflammation. Sometimes a lung biopsy, done either during bronchoscopy or through a chest incision under local anesthetic (open-lung biopsy), is needed to make the diagnosis.

The standard treatment for ILD is corticosteroids given either by mouth or intravenously. Depending on the response and on the severity of the disease, it may also be necessary to add other immunosuppressive drugs, such as azathioprine (Imuran, Azasan), cyclophosphamide (Cytoxan), or rituximab (Rituxan). If treated early, ILD does not cause any long-term disability.

Inflammation of the lining around the lung (pleurisy) can occur in Sjögren's. This condition is usually seen in patients with secondary Sjögren's and particularly in those suffering from systemic lupus erythematosus (SLE) or rheumatoid arthritis (RA). Pleurisy usually causes chest pain on breathing. Fluid can sometimes accumulate in the pleural space (pleural effusion), causing shortness of breath. Pleurisy is treated with nonsteroidal anti-inflammatory drugs or corticosteroids. Also, drainage of the pleural effusion may sometimes be necessary.

Very rarely, Sjögren's patients develop an abnormally high pressure in the pulmonary arteries, the vessels that carry blood from the heart to the lungs. This is known as pulmonary hypertension. The main symptom of pulmonary hypertension is shortness of breath on exertion. In Sjögren's, pulmonary hypertension can develop in isolation or as a result of ILD and lung scarring (fibrosis). Pulmonary hypertension can be diagnosed on a routine cardiac echocardiogram. To obtain an accurate measurement of the pulmonary artery pressure, the patient undergoes cardiac catheterization. Under local anesthesia, a thin wire is guided from the artery in the leg into the main aorta and then into the right side of the heart so that measurements of pressure can be taken. If left untreated, severe pulmonary hypertension can cause heart failure. Treatment of any underlying interstitial lung disease can help improve the degree of pulmonary hypertension. Current treatment of moderate to severe pulmonary hypertension in Sjögren's includes the use of anticoagulants, such as warfarin (Coumadin); endothelin receptor antagonists, such as bosentan (Tracleer); and phosphodiesterase-5 inhibitors, such as sildenafil (Revatio). In severe cases, a continuous infusion of intravenous epoprostenol (Flolan, Veletri) may be used.

Kidneys

The kidneys remove waste products from the blood and form urine. The most common kidney problem in patients with Sjögren's is inflammation of the tissue around the kidney filters, known as interstitial nephritis. Interstitial nephritis is found early in the disease and has a benign course. It generally causes mild deterioration in kidney function, manifested as a mild elevation in the plasma creatinine concentration. This usually requires no treatment. Progression to end-stage renal disease is a rare event.

When there is progressive deterioration of kidney function in a patient with Sjögren's, a kidney biopsy is often done. This involves taking a small piece of kidney tissue with a needle while the patient is awake but under local anesthesia. The tissue is examined under the microscope, and if the diagnosis of interstitial nephritis is made, a course of corticosteroids is given as treatment. Kidney function usually improves within a few weeks unless irreversible scarring in the kidneys has already occurred.

Interstitial nephritis can cause abnormalities in the kidney tubules, which are part of the kidney filtering mechanism. One such abnormality is renal tubular acidosis (RTA). In RTA the kidney tubules are unable to excrete acid in the urine. This can occur in up to 25% of patients with Sjögren's. As a result, the urine becomes more alkaline (high urine pH) and the blood becomes more acidic (low blood pH). This can lead to low levels of potassium in the blood and can give rise to kidney stones. Patients with RTA usually have no symptoms. Rarely, when the blood potassium level is very low, muscle weakness or even paralysis can occur. Also, recurrent pain in the loin area from kidney stones can sometimes be the presenting symptom. The treatment of RTA depends on its severity. If the potassium level is very low, then the patient is given potassium supplements. Alkaline agents (sodium bicarbonate) are given to correct the acidity of the blood to prevent the formation of renal stones.

Another rare abnormality of the renal tubules in Sjögren's is nephrogenic diabetes insipidus. In this condition the renal tubules become insensitive to the effects of antidiuretic hormone and as a result cannot concentrate the urine. Patients with nephrogenic diabetes insipidus complain of thirst and of passing large amounts of urine frequently. The diagnosis is suspected if the urine remains dilute when the patient is deprived of water (when a normal person becomes dehydrated, the kidneys try to save water by concentrating the urine). Nephrogenic diabetes insipidus can be treated by a number of means, including diuretics, nonsteroidal anti-inflammatory drugs, and a low-salt, low-protein diet.

The glomeruli, which also form part of the kidney filtering mechanism, are rarely affected in Sjögren's. Antibodies produced by the immune system become deposited on the glomeruli and cause inflammation (glomerulonephritis). As a result, the function of the kidneys deteriorates. This can be picked up on routine testing of a urine sample and by looking at the blood tests and observing a deterioration of kidney function. Symptoms include high blood pressure and leg swelling due to water retention (edema). Glomerulonephritis is rare in patients with Sjögren's and occurs mainly in patients who also have other overlapping conditions such as SLE, cryoglobulinemia (a condition whereby protein complexes circulating in the blood become deposited during cold weather), and vasculitis (inflammation of blood vessels). If left untreated, glomerulonephritis may lead to severe kidney failure. Therefore, in a patient with suspected glomerulonephritis, a kidney biopsy should be performed to confirm the diagnosis and assess the severity of the kidney disease. Treatment is then given in the form of corticosteroids as well as other immunosuppressive drugs such as cyclophosphamide (Cytoxan) or rituximab (Rituxan).

Inflammation of the bladder, known as interstitial cystitis, can occur in patients with Sjögren's. The symptoms are frequent urination and pain in the lower abdomen over the bladder area.

Gastrointestinal Tract

In Sjögren's, the exocrine glands of the gastrointestinal tract can also be affected. The cells lining the esophagus produce less mucus, and the esophagus becomes dry like the mouth. This can lead to difficulty in swallowing. Difficulty in swallowing can also be caused by abnormal contractions of the esophagus or by a lack of the normal contractions that move the food down the esophagus to the stomach. This condition, which can affect up to one third of patients with Sjögren's, is known as esophageal dysmotility.

The diagnosis of dysmotility is made by measuring the pressure inside the wall of the esophagus during swallowing (manometry). When the wall of the esophagus contracts abnormally, treatment is aimed at relaxing the smooth muscle of the esophagus. Nitroglycerine and calcium channel blockers may be helpful.

On the other hand, when the muscle tone in the wall of the esophagus is reduced, gastric juice moves up the esophagus, producing a burning sensation behind the breastbone (heartburn) and chest pain. This is known as gastroesophageal reflux. Prolonged reflux of acid results in chronic irritation of the esophagus (esophagitis). Mild reflux can be treated by the use of antacids. Antacids form a "raft" that floats on the surface of the stomach contents to reduce reflux and protect the lining of the esophagus. Severe gastroesophageal reflux and esophagitis are best treated by the use of drugs that reduce acid production by the stomach. These include H_2-receptor antagonists (ranitidine [Zantac]) and proton pump inhibitors (omeprazole [Prilosec]).

A proportion of patients with Sjögren's have reduced acid secretion by the stomach. This is a result of longstanding inflammation that destroys the cells that produce acid (chronic atrophic gastritis), an immune process similar to the one that destroys the salivary glands. Atrophic gastritis can cause indigestion (dyspepsia) and pain over the upper part of the abdomen. Diagnosis is made by endoscopy. This is performed by a gastroenterologist with the patient awake but slightly sedated. The stomach is visualized by inserting an elastic tube with a camera at its end (fiberoptic endoscope) inside the stomach. A biopsy often is taken to confirm the diagnosis. Unfortunately, once the acid-producing cells of the stomach are damaged, it is often too late to give any treatment.

However, other conditions associated with atrophic gastritis can be prevented. Destruction of the cells that produce acid in the stomach can prevent absorption of vitamin B_{12}, important in the production of red blood cells. Its deficiency can result in a form of anemia known as pernicious anemia. Pernicious anemia can be diagnosed by a simple blood test and can be successfully treated by monthly B_{12} injections.

In Sjögren's, involvement of other exocrine glands such as the pancreas can sometimes occur. Most of the time, this does not cause any symptoms. However, in some cases, the pancreas cannot secrete its digestive enzymes, and then diarrhea and steatorrhea (floating, fatty stools) occur. Pancreatic enzyme insufficiency can be treated by the regular administration of oral pancreatic enzymes.

Acute inflammation of the pancreas, known as pancreatitis, rarely has been described in Sjögren's patients. It presents with abdominal pain, nausea, and vomiting. Laboratory tests show elevation of amylase, an enzyme measured in the serum. Amylase is produced by the salivary glands as well as by the pancreas. A quarter of patients with Sjögren's may have a raised serum amylase level due to salivary gland inflammation rather than due to acute pancreatitis.

Liver

In studies of Sjögren's patients, approximately 6% have been found to have autoimmune liver disease. The main two conditions associated with Sjögren's are chronic active hepatitis and primary biliary cirrhosis.

Primary biliary cirrhosis (PBC) is a chronic disease that affects mainly middle-aged women. It is caused by inflammation around the channels that transport bile from the liver into the intestine, the bile ducts. As a result these ducts become blocked and bile builds up in the liver and spills into the blood. In the late stages of the disease, the liver becomes scarred. This is known as cirrhosis. In the early stages, the main symptoms of PBC are due to the accumulation of bile acids and salts in the blood. Patients complain of generalized itching and tiredness. Later on in the disease they develop jaundice (yellow tinge of the skin and the eyes), pale stools, and dark urine. In the late stages, cirrhosis can cause accumulation of fluid in the abdomen (ascites) and internal bleeding from buildup of pressure in the veins of the esophagus (esophageal varices).

The diagnosis is suspected when a patient with Sjögren's has the above symptoms and abnormal liver function tests. There is also a very specific blood test for the diagnosis of PBC, the presence of anti-mitochondrial antibodies.

However, a liver biopsy is usually necessary to confirm the diagnosis and to evaluate if the disease is in its early or late stages. This involves taking a small piece of liver, using a needle, under a local anesthetic.

The lack of bile salts in the intestine results in reduced absorption of fat and the fat-soluble vitamins A, D, E, and K. Vitamin D deficiency can result in weakening of the bones (osteoporosis) and fractures. Vitamin K deficiency can result in problems with blood clotting. Therefore, patients with PBC benefit from taking calcium plus vitamin D supplements to strengthen their bones, as well as vitamins A, E, and K.

Because the cause of PBC is not known, there is no curative treatment for the disease; the only definite treatment is liver transplantation. However, the prognosis of PBC varies greatly from one patient to another. Many patients lead active lives with few symptoms for 10 to 20 years. In some patients, however, the condition progresses more rapidly, and liver failure may occur in just a few years.

Ursodeoxycholic acid has been shown to improve liver function tests as well as reduce progression of the disease in patients with PBC. Treatment of pruritus is often a challenge in PBC. The mainstay is cholestyramine (Questran), a resin that forms a complex with bile acids in the intestine, promoting their excretion in the stools.

In chronic active hepatitis (CAH), the immune system continuously attacks the liver cells, and as a result scarring of the liver (cirrhosis) can occur. In general, CAH can be caused by hepatitis viruses, by drugs, or by an unknown mechanism that dysregulates the immune system. The last of these is the case in Sjögren's patients. CAH is suspected in a patient with Sjögren's when liver function tests become abnormal without the patient taking any new drugs. Evidence pointing toward an autoimmune active hepatitis is the finding of antibodies in the blood against smooth muscle or liver/kidney microsomes. Typical symptoms are fatigue, malaise, fever, and loss of appetite. The diagnosis is confirmed by liver biopsy. CAH can be treated by the use of steroids and other immunosuppressive drugs such as azathioprine (Imuran, Azasan).

Heart

Involvement of the heart is rare in primary Sjögren's. Some Sjögren's patients have been found to have a small amount of fluid around the heart, known as pericardial effusion. This is caused by inflammation of the lining around the heart (pericarditis). It is usually picked up by chance on routine ultrasound scanning of the heart, as most patients are asymptomatic. Patients with secondary Sjögren's who have lupus are more likely to develop pericarditis that gives rise to symptoms. This usually occurs during a lupus flare. The symptoms are typically of left-sided chest pain that changes with posture. When the patient is examined using a stethoscope, a characteristic sound, known as a "rub," can be heard at the left edge of the sternum. An electrocardiogram may show typical changes of pericarditis, and visualization of the heart using echocardiography reveals fluid around the heart. Lupus patients mostly develop small to medium-sized collections of fluid around the heart that have no bearing on the heart function. However, very rarely, if there is a large amount of fluid around the heart, it can impede the pumping action of the heart, and the patient can develop heart failure. Patients with RA and secondary Sjögren's can also develop pericardial effusions during a flare of the RA. However, it has been estimated that during the course of their disease, fewer than 10% of RA patients have a clinical episode of pericarditis.

Steroids are given to treat small to medium-sized pericardial effusions, whereas in the case of large effusions, draining of the fluid using a needle may be necessary.

Congenital Heart Block

When the fetus is inside the womb, its heart beats regularly as a result of its natural pacemaker. However, a condition known as congenital heart block can occur in which this pacemaker fails and the heart rate drops dangerously low. There are two types of congenital heart block: incomplete and complete. In complete heart block, insertion of an artificial pacemaker is necessary after delivery.

All babies born with congenital heart block have mothers who carry anti-Ro (SSA) antibodies, whereas 75% have mothers with anti-La (SSB) antibodies. Most of these mothers have these antibodies without having any symptoms of an autoimmune disease. These antibodies are thought to cross the placenta and bind onto the fetal heart, preventing the normal development of the pacemaker.

Up to 75% of Sjögren's patients have anti-Ro (SSA) antibodies and up to 40% have anti-La (SSB) antibodies. However, if a woman who has Sjögren's and anti-Ro antibodies becomes pregnant, the risk of having a fetus with congenital heart block is only 1% to 2%. If that woman also has anti-La (SSB) antibodies in addition to anti-Ro (SSA) antibodies, the risk of having a fetus with congenital heart block is 3%. The risk is much higher if she has previously given birth to another baby with congenital heart block. For this reason, the fetuses of anti-Ro- and anti-La-positive mothers need to be closely monitored after the 16th week of gestation for signs of heart block. If heart block is detected and is of the reversible form, treatment can be given with steroids that cross the placenta (dexamethasone).

There is a way of determining which mothers with anti-La (SSB) antibodies are protected from having a child with congenital heart block. This test involves taking a sample of blood from these mothers during pregnancy and measuring the activity of another group of antibodies, called anti-idiotypic antibodies, that bind to the anti-La (SSB) antibodies. Mothers who will give birth to a healthy child have high levels of anti-idiotypic antibodies. However, only certain research laboratories have the facilities to measure these anti-idiotypic antibodies as this test is new and not commercially available yet.

Nervous System

Patients with Sjögren's can have disease of the nervous system. The peripheral nerves that control sensation can be damaged by the immune system. This is known as sensory neuropathy. Patients with sensory neuropathy initially complain of numbness or tingling at the tips of their toes. Also, they may notice alterations in the appreciation of pain and temperature and a burning sensation. The problem is usually symmetrical. It can progress very slowly to involve the fingers of both hands. In most patients, the symptoms are mild and non-disabling. Approximately 40% of patients improve spontaneously.

The diagnosis is usually made by examination of the peripheral nerves. Patients may have reduced sensation in the hands and feet in a "glove and stocking" pattern. The reflexes may also be absent. However, the physical examination can be normal. The diagnosis is confirmed by electrical stimulation tests called nerve conduction studies. As most patients have mild symptoms, no specific treatment is usually given for peripheral sensory neuropathy in Sjögren's. For patients with severe symptoms, treatment may prove difficult. There are some therapies that can be tried, such as intravenous immunoglobulin or plasmapheresis.

Sometimes an individual nerve that controls the movement of one muscle can be affected, and this can result in weakness of the muscle. One such example is if a patient suddenly develops foot drop on one side. This is known as mononeuritis. The cause of this problem is inflammation in the blood vessel supplying the individual nerve or vasculitis. Vasculitis can be treated by the use of steroids or other drugs that suppress the immune system. If the treatment is given early, the nerve can recover from the damage and the muscle weakness can resolve.

The cranial nerves—that is, the nerves supplying the face—can also be affected in Sjögren's. Most commonly the sensory branch of the trigeminal nerve is affected. This supplies the sensation around the eyes, nose, cheeks, and mouth. In Sjögren's, the symptoms of trigeminal neuropathy are numbness or tingling around the mouth and the cheeks. The area around the eye is less commonly involved. Pain may be present but usually is not severe.

In carpal tunnel syndrome, a common complication in Sjögren's, inflamed tissue in the forearm presses against the median nerve, causing pain, numbness, tingling, and sometimes muscle weakness in the thumb and index and middle fingers. The symptoms are often worse at night. The diagnosis is confirmed by nerve conduction studies. Night splints can help alleviate the symptoms. Also, steroid injections into the carpal tunnel can give temporary relief for up to few months. Steroid injections can be repeated once or twice, but if the symptoms persist, surgery may be necessary. The surgical procedure, known as carpal tunnel decompression, involves making a small cut on the inside of the wrist to free the tissues that press the median nerve. This can be done under local anesthesia on an outpatient basis. It is usually very successful.

Sjögren's has been reported to affect the brain. However, this point will remain controversial until further studies are done. In studies of Sjögren's patients all over the world, a variety of neurological symptoms originating from the brain have been recorded. For example, some patients have been noted to have symptoms of epilepsy, stroke, multiple sclerosis, or Parkinson's disease. However, no consensus has been reached as to the proportion of Sjögren's patients affected by diseases of the brain. Although these neurological diseases are noted to occur in Sjögren's patients, they may not necessarily be caused by Sjögren's.

Some Sjögren's patients have been noted to have memory or concentration problems or symptoms of anxiety and depression. Again the percentages quoted in studies vary (7% to 80%). Part of the problem is that the symptoms can be quite subtle and not easily recognized. Memory or concentration problems can also sometimes be a manifestation of anxiety or depression, so patients have to be carefully evaluated by a psychologist or psychiatrist. If anxiety or depression is confirmed, therapy in the form of psychological counseling or drugs (antidepressants) may be of benefit. Also, patients with isolated memory or concentration problems may improve with the help of mental exercises prescribed by specially trained psychologists.

Summing Up

Major body organs can be affected in one third of primary Sjögren's patients. Involvement of the lungs usually produces mild symptoms not requiring more than symptomatic treatment. Interstitial lung disease occurs rarely and requires treatment with steroids and immunosuppressive drugs. Involvement of the kidneys can manifest as interstitial nephritis, which is usually benign and requires no treatment. Very rarely it may cause kidney damage, which can be reversed if treated early with steroids. More severe disease such as glomerulonephritis sometimes can occur, requiring treatment with steroids and immunosuppressive drugs. Esophageal dysmotility can cause difficulty in swallowing as well as acid reflux. The latter can be treated with drugs that reduce acid production by the stomach. More rarely, indigestion can be due to

TABLE 9–1

Organ Involvement in Patients with Primary Sjögren's

Organ	Complication	Percentage of Patients with Primary Sjögren's also Affected by this Complication
Lung	Interstitial lung disease	6%
Lung	Small-airway disease	23%
Lung	Pleurisy	2%
Kidney	Interstitial nephritis	9%
Esophagus	Esophageal dysmotility	36%
Heart	Pericarditis	2%
Liver	Primary biliary cirrhosis	4%
Nerves	Carpal tunnel syndrome	12%
Nerves	Peripheral neuropathy	2%

TABLE 9–2

Tools for Diagnosis of Internal Organ Involvement

Organs involved in Sjögren's	How to Diagnose if an Organ is Involved
Lung	Lung function test
	CT scan
Kidney	Urinalysis
	Blood tests
	Kidney biopsy
Esophagus	Manometry
Stomach	Gastroscopy
Pancreas	Blood tests
Liver	Blood tests
	Liver biopsy
Heart	Electrocardiogram (ECG)
	Blood tests
	Echocardiogram
Nerves	Nerve conduction studies
Brain	MRI scan

atrophic gastritis. This can result in pernicious anemia that can be treated with regular vitamin B$_{12}$ injections.

Primary biliary cirrhosis rarely occurs in association with Sjögren's and has a variable prognosis. Ursodeoxycholic acid can delay the progression of the disease. Chronic active hepatitis also rarely occurs, and it can be treated with steroids and immunosuppressive drugs. Pericarditis usually occurs in patients with secondary Sjögren's and SLE and can be successfully treated with steroids.

The most common disease of the peripheral nerves in Sjögren's is carpal tunnel syndrome. It can be treated with steroid injections or surgery. Peripheral sensory neuropathy can occur in Sjögren's, and it is usually mild and non-disabling. Very rarely vasculitis can result in mononeuritis, and this can be reversed after treatment with steroids and immunosuppressive drugs. Involvement of the brain is controversial. A variety of symptoms, such as memory problems, anxiety, and depression, are more common in Sjögren's patients. Other more severe symptoms of epilepsy, stroke, and multiple sclerosis have been reported and may possibly be caused by Sjögren's (Tables 9–1 and 9–2).

FOR FURTHER READING

Constantopoulos SH, Tsianos EV, Moutsopoulos HM. Pulmonary and gastrointestinal manifestations of Sjögren's syndrome. *Rheum Dis Clin North Am.* 1992; 18(3): 617–35.

Goules A, et al. Clinically significant and biopsy-documented renal involvement in primary Sjögren syndrome. *Medicine (Baltimore).* 2000; 79(4): 241–9.

Hatzis GS, Fragoulis GE, Karatzaferis A, et al. Prevalence and long-term course of primary biliary cirrhosis in primary Sjögren's syndrome. *J Rheumatol.* 2008; 35(10): 2012–6.

Kassan SS, Moutsopoulos HM. Clinical manifestations and early diagnosis of Sjögren syndrome. *Arch Intern Med.* 2004; 164(12): 1275–84.

Kaufman I, Schwartz D, Caspi D, Paran D. Sjögren's syndrome—not just sicca: renal involvement in Sjögren's syndrome. *Scand J Rheumatol.* 2008; 37(3): 213–8.

Mavragani CP, Moutsopoulos NM, Moutsopoulos HM. The management of Sjögren's syndrome. *Nat Clin Pract Rheumatol.* 2006; 2(5): 252–61.

Papiris SA, Tsonis IA, Moutsopoulos HM. Sjögren's syndrome. *Semin Respir Crit Care Med.* 2007; 28(4): 459–71.

Parke AL. Pulmonary manifestations of primary Sjögren's syndrome. *Rheum Dis Clin North Am.* 2008; 34(4): 907–20.

Skopouli FN, Barbatis C, Moutsopoulos HM. Liver involvement in primary Sjögren's syndrome. *Br J Rheumatol.* 1994; 33(8): 745–8.

Soliotis FC, Mavragani CP, Moutsopoulos HM. Central nervous system involvement in Sjögren's syndrome. *Ann Rheum Dis.* 2004; 63(6): 616–20.

Tzioufas AG, Moutsopoulos HM. Predicting autoimmune congenital heart block: is it feasible and how? *Rheumatology (Oxford).* 2007; 46(8): 1221–2.

Vassiliou VA, Moyssakis I, Boki KA, Moutsopoulos HM. Is the heart affected in primary Sjögren's syndrome? An echocardiographic study. *Clin Exp Rheumatol.* 2008; 26(1): 109–12.

10

The Central Nervous System and Sjögren's

VASCULITIS AND VASCULOPATHY

Elaine Alexander, MD, PhD

Introduction and Background

Neurologic disease in Sjögren's syndrome can affect any part of the central nervous system (CNS) and the peripheral nervous system, which includes the autonomic nervous system, resulting in a wide range of neurological damage and dysfunction. Although peripheral nervous system disease, as a potential neurological manifestation of Sjögren's, has been recognized since the initial monologue by Dr. Henrik Sjögren, CNS disease was not identified and appreciated as a neurological complication of Sjögren's until relatively recently. Subsequently, during the 1980s and 1990s, a multidisciplinary team of investigators and clinicians at a highly specialized referral center, Johns Hopkins Medical Institution in Baltimore, Maryland, sequentially described the clinical spectrum, neurodiagnostic assessment, and immunopathogenesis of neurological disease in Sjögren's and began to explore optimal management and treatment regimens. These observations will be briefly summarized in this chapter and placed in the context of confirmatory observations by other U.S. and international investigators. An impressive body of evidence has developed that indicates that neurological disease in Sjögren's is yet another manifestation of an underlying immunologically mediated disorder.

Initially, the description of neurological disease in Sjögren's was met with healthy skepticism by both clinicians and patients, since it could not be understood how such a broad spectrum of neurological disease occurring in a disorder as common as Sjögren's could have been largely overlooked and under-recognized for so many years. The potential reason could well be that the serial observations and description of neurological complications of Sjögren's were made at a major medical referral center with extensive and unique interactive collaboration between investigators in multiple disciplines, particularly rheumatology/immunology and neurology. The diagnosis of many Sjögren's patients with neurological complications who presented to neurologists, and other physicians unfamiliar with the manifestations of Sjögren's was commonly overlooked.

Prevalence of Neurological Disease in Sjögren's

The actual prevalence of neurological disease in the general Sjögren's population is unknown. Large, prospective, longitudinal, appropriately controlled, epidemiologic studies have not been performed. Frequency estimates vary depending on several circumstances, including the Sjögren's population studied, the clinical setting (i.e., highly specialized referral centers, less specialized academic centers, or clinical practice settings), the interest and expertise of the evaluating investigators or clinicians, and the extent and sophistication of the neurological evaluation.

Clinical Spectrum

Clinical manifestations of CNS disease in Sjögren's are multiple and diverse and can span the entire CNS neuroaxis, which includes the brain, spinal cord, and optic nerves. Any region of the brain may be involved: cerebral cortex (frontal/prefrontal, parietal, temporal, occipital regions), periventricular/subcortical regions, basal ganglia, thalamus, midbrain, cerebellum/pons, and medulla/brain stem. Likewise, any region of the spinal cord may be involved (cervical, thoracic, and lumbar). Finally, the optic nerves, which are part of the CNS, can be affected. More than one area may be involved in an individual patient. The clinical signs and symptoms that develop in Sjögren's depend on the location, size, and number of the involved regions of the brain, spinal cord, or optic nerves.

CNS disease involving the brain in Sjögren's can be categorized as **focal** (i.e., discrete neurological deficits) and/or **nonfocal** (i.e., diffuse with psychiatric and/or cognitive dysfunction). Individual patients may have both focal and nonfocal CNS disease. The neurological abnormalities may be subtle, usually of insidious onset, or, less often, changeable and of acute or subacute presentation. Early in the course of neurological disease, neurological symptoms or deficits are characteristically mild and transient and often resolve, with return to baseline function. With time, however, CNS disease manifestations may become multifocal, recurrent, and, in some cases, chronic and progressive. There can be long disease-free intervals between successive neurological events.

FOCAL CNS DISEASE

The spectrum of focal neurological involvement is well described in multiple Hopkins publications from the 1980s and 1990s and subsequently confirmed in small case series and case reports by other U.S. and international investigators. Focal neurological deficits involving the brain include motor (i.e., monoparesis, hemiparesis, paraparesis, and quadriparesis) and/or sensory loss (i.e., hemisensory, monosensory, or truncal sensory deficits), aphasia/dysarthria, gaze disturbances, and cortical blindness. Seizure disorders are most commonly petit mal (absence) or temporal lobe (psychomotor) in type. Grand mal seizures, focal motor seizures, status epilepticus, and epilepsy partialis continua have been less uncommonly observed. Movement disorders include tremors (involuntary and intentional), dystonias, pseudoathetosis, choreoathetosis, dyskinesias/akinesias, gait disturbances, ataxia (truncal and appendicular), and syndromes resembling or indistinguishable from classical Parkinson's disease and Huntington's disease. Cerebellar deficits occur in association with other focal neurological deficits but also may occur alone, resulting in isolated spinocerebellar degeneration syndrome. Uncommonly, brain stem syndromes have been described.

The spinal cord also may be involved in CNS disease in Sjögren's patients. Acute transverse myelopathy, often recurrent, and chronic progressive myelopathy can occur. Optic nerve involvement (optic neuritis or ischemic optic neuropathy) can occur alone or accompany spinal cord involvement. In fact, a subset of CNS-SS patients can have neurological presentations and disease manifestations clinically and neurodiagnostically indistinguishable from multiple sclerosis (MS). Neurogenic bladder may accompany these clinical presentations or occur alone. Less commonly, Brown-Séquard syndrome and lower motor disease, resembling amyotrophic lateral sclerosis (ALS), have been observed. Major stroke syndromes of acute onset are distinctly unusual but do occur in Sjögren's.

NONFOCAL CNS DISEASE

Nonfocal (diffuse) manifestations of brain involvement include aseptic meningoencephalitis, which can recur. Acute or subacute encephalopathy is an alarming complication of CNS-SS and, if recognized, usually responds to treatment. A spectrum of cognitive impairment can occur in Sjögren's ranging from mild (brain fog, mild cognitive impairment) to severe (frank dementia of the subcortical type and rarely resembling Alzheimer's disease).

What Does the Spectrum of CNS Manifestations Tell Us About Etiopathogenesis?

Describing the many potential CNS manifestations of Sjögren's also serves as the springboard for the consideration of the pathogenesis of the disorder and a discussion of the neurodiagnostic approach to evaluation of the

CNS-SS patient. The large body of clinical investigation that has been conducted on CNS-SS has been done in academic research settings. While the data from these investigations have formed the fundamental basis for understanding the multifaceted disease process, not all of the types of studies that have been conducted are appropriate, practical, or feasible in the clinical evaluation of patients with Sjögren's, particularly in the current climate of the restricted reimbursement practice of clinical medicine. First a summary of investigations that have provided basic information about disease pathogenesis will be presented. Second, a more practical approach to the neurodiagnostic evaluation of the patient suspected of having CNS involvement will be presented.

Neuroradiological Studies in CNS-SS

Various imaging techniques are used to examine the brain and/or spinal cord to look for evidence of CNS-SS. These include MRI, CT scanning, SPECT (single photon emission computed tomography), and cerebral angiography.

Brain MRI (3 Tesla) commonly demonstrates multiple small regions of increased signal intensity predominantly within white matter, and also gray matter. These MRI abnormalities are observed in patients with focal CNS disease as well as a subset of patients with nonfocal disease. Approximately 80% of Sjögren's patients with progressive focal neurological dysfunction have brain MRI scans with multiple small regions of increased signal intensity on T2 and hypointense regions on T1 proton-density-weighted images, predominantly in subcortical and periventricular white matter.

In our experience, Sjögren's patients (less than 60 years old) without clinical evidence of CNS disease have a very low frequency of abnormal standard MRI scans with more than one region of increased signal intensity. Others, however, have described small regions of increased signal intensity on brain MRI scans within the basal ganglia and white matter of cerebral hemispheres in up to 60% of Sjögren's patients without clinical evidence of CNS disease. These abnormalities may be secondary to more sensitive techniques or subclinical disease.

Evidence to date suggests that regions of increased signal intensity on brain MRI/CT scans in CNS-SS almost invariably are fixed and usually do not resolve with therapy. Unlike the situation in MS, regions of increased signal intensity in CNS-SS usually are not enhanced by contrast agents (i.e., double/triple-dose gadolinium). This observation would suggest that the blood–brain barrier (BBB) in Sjögren's is intact for the most part, although brain biopsy/autopsy may show small breaches of that barrier. In CNS-SS patients, multiple regions of increased signal intensity on brain MRI are probably related to the underlying pathophysiological process affecting predominantly the small blood vessels of the brain.

In the future (based on preliminary results), more sophisticated, higher-resolution MRI technology may be used to detect brain abnormalities in Sjögren's patients with mild/subtle cognitive impairment, early, and subclinical disease.

Spinal cord MRI studies may identify abnormalities in patients with clinical features consistent with spinal cord involvement such as transverse myelopathy or chronic progressive myelopathy. One or more regions of increased signal intensity consistent with ischemia, infarction, or demyelination have been observed.

Brain CT scans are relatively insensitive in documenting neuroanatomical abnormalities in CNS-SS. Brain CT scans (double-dose enhanced studies with delayed imaging) detect neuroanatomical abnormalities in fewer than 20% of CNS-SS cases. The abnormalities observed on brain CT include large infarcts, intracerebral hemorrhages, and, rarely, subarachnoid hemorrhage. The large infarcts on brain CT scans correspond to large regions of increased signal intensity on brain MRI scans in a subset of CNS-SS patients who have one or more larger (10 mm) regions of increased signal intensity on MRI (also visualized on CT scans), and these patients almost invariably have antibodies to Ro (SS-A) protein.

SPECT measures regional cerebral blood flow/metabolism. Preliminary studies of Technetium-99mHMPAO brain SPECT scans demonstrate a very high frequency of regional cortical hypoperfusion abnormalities in Sjögren's patients with both focal and nonfocal CNS disease. Some CNS-SS patients with normal brain MRI scans may have abnormal SPECT studies. These observational studies suggest that alterations in cerebral blood flow may be an early marker of CNS involvement in CNS-SS.

Cerebral angiography is performed for two main reasons in CNS-SS: to exclude other causes of CNS disease (i.e., arteriosclerosis, cerebrovascular disease, arteriovenous malformations, other vascular abnormalities, and congenital aneurysms), and to establish a potential diagnosis of CNS vasculopathy/vasculitis. Cerebral angiography in CNS-SS detects abnormalities of small cerebral arteries consistent with but is not diagnostic of small vessel angiitis in approximately 20% of highly selected cases of CNS-SS patients.

In a few cases, medium-sized or large vessels are affected. CNS-SS patients with small to medium-sized artery abnormalities on cerebral angiography have a significantly increased frequency of severe focal CNS disease, multiple and large regions of increased signal intensity in brain MRI imaging, and anti-Ro (SS-A) antibodies.

A normal brain MRI scan and/or cerebral angiogram does not exclude the presence of active CNS-SS. The presence of an inflammatory meningeal/cerebral vasculopathy in several CNS-SS patients with normal brain MRIs and cerebral angiograms has been documented at autopsy or brain biopsy. This observation raises the issue of indications for meningeal/brain biopsy in the evaluation of CNS-SS. There are several situations in which a meningeal/brain biopsy could be considered: to establish a definitive diagnosis in cases in which the diagnosis is unknown; to distinguish CNS-SS from other CNS disease, such as MS or Alzheimer's disease; to exclude other etiologies, including infection, malignancy, and lymphoma; to evaluate individuals who have an immunologically reactive cerebrospinal fluid (CSF) analysis (protein elevation, moderate to marked pleocytosis, elevated IgG index, and oligoclonal bands); and to evaluate patients who have a rapid deterioration in their clinical status and who will need aggressive therapeutic intervention.

Electrophysiologic Studies in CNS-SS

Electrophysiologic studies, including MMER (multimodality evoked response) testing, EEG (electroencephalogram), and blink reflex, may be clinically useful in evaluating and following patients with CNS-SS. MMER testing may provide information about brain function in CNS-SS. Evoked potentials are the CNS electrical events generated by peripheral stimulation of a sensory organ (visual, auditory/brain stem, and peripheral nerve) and are used to detect abnormal CNS function that may be clinically undetectable. The blink reflex detects abnormalities of the fifth nerve (peripheral or central), reflected clinically in trigeminal neuropathy. Abnormalities of any one of these MMERs indicate a functional interruption of the involved neuroanatomical pathway. One or more MMER studies are abnormal in approximately one half to two thirds of Sjögren's patients with progressive, recurrent focal CNS disease.

The EEG measures electrical activity of the brain and can identify seizures. EEGs are abnormal in approximately one third of CNS-SS patients with severe progressive disease. Patients with focal neurological deficits may show focal slow wave activity, decreased amplitude, or spikes (sharp waves). In patients with petit mal or temporal lobe epilepsy, EEGs, including sleep studies, may show seizure discharges. In patients with encephalopathy or progressive dementia, there may be diffuse slowing.

MMERs and EEGs may detect subclinical abnormalities in CNS-SS that antedate the development of clinical manifestations or regions of increased signal intensity on brain MRI scans. Therefore, these studies may be useful in diagnosing early CNS involvement and in objectively following patients and monitoring response to therapy.

CSF Analysis Shows Evidence for Brain Inflammation

CSF analysis provides important information on the immunopathogenesis of CNS-SS and reflects the presence of an active immune response within the brain. The CSF IgG/total protein ratio is often mildly elevated. More importantly, the IgG index, indicative of synthesis of IgG within the brain, is elevated in approximately 50% of patients with active focal disease. One or more oligoclonal bands are observed in a similar proportion of patients. Most commonly, there are one or two bands, but multiple bands (up to seven) have been observed. It is not yet known against which antigen(s) these antibodies are directed, but antibodies to Ro (SSA) have been detected in the CSF of Sjögren's patients with active CNS disease, indicating that B/plasma cells making anti-Ro (SS-A) antibodies are present within the nervous system.

The CSF may show evidence for active inflammation in CNS-SS. Mononuclear, polymorphic CSF pleocytosis, usually mild, occurs in a subset of Sjögren's patients with CNS disease. In the case of aseptic meningitis, a larger number of mononuclear cells (i.e., similar in type to those observed in the CNS-SS patients with a mild mononuclear pleocytosis) are present within the CSF.

Cytologic examination of the inflammatory cells demonstrates small round lymphocytes, reactive lymphoid cells, plasma cells, and atypical mononuclear cells with distinctive cleft/reniform nuclei and scant pale cytoplasm. Very importantly, these latter mononuclear cells appear identical morphologically (by light and electron microscopy) to a type of lymphocyte classified as a monocytoid B cell. Monocytoid B lymphocytes normally reside in the region of the gastrointestinal tract termed mucosa-associated lymphoid tissue (MALT). Monocytoid B lymphocytes have the capacity for transformation into non-Hodgkin's B-cell lymphoma, both in Sjögren's and in other disorders, including AIDS. The spectrum of mononuclear inflammatory cells described in the CSF in CNS-SS, including the atypical mononuclear cells, is also observed on histopathological examination of brain tissue (see below) within inflammatory infiltrates in the meninges, in and around blood vessels. Thus, there may be an important immunopathological link between non-Hodgkin's lymphoma and CNS disease in the lymphoproliferative disorder Sjögren's syndrome.

Pathology and Immunopathogenesis of CNS Disease in Sjögren's

The understanding of the immunopathogenesis of neurological disease occurring in Sjögren's has been greatly advanced by pathological observations by our group and other investigators. Abnormalities are consistent with a cerebral vasculopathy characterized as a mononuclear inflammatory ischemic/hemorrhagic small vessel (predominantly venous) cerebral vasculopathy. The vasculopathy is accompanied by pleomorphic mononuclear inflammatory infiltrates within the meninges and choroid plexus (i.e., chronic meningoencephalitis). In some patients, who are positive for the anti-Ro antibody, there also is frank vasculitis (i.e., angiitis) Although some observations are similar to those in MS (perivascular myelin pallor and disorganization), classical demyelinating lesions (i.e., plaques) characteristic of MS are not observed. Sjögren's patients with isolated chronic encephalopathy may resemble Alzheimer's dementia clinically but do not have the characteristic Alzheimer's amyloid brain pathology and may respond to immunosuppressive therapy.

The cerebral inflammatory vasculopathy has several distinctive features. Small cerebral blood vessels are more commonly involved than medium- or large-caliber cerebral blood vessels. The venous system (post-capillary venules, venules, and veins) is involved invariably. Less commonly, the arterial system (usually small arteries or arterioles) also may be involved. There is a striking predilection for inflammatory cells to infiltrate blood vessels within the white matter, particularly in the subcortical periventricular regions. Gray (cortical and basal ganglia) matter involvement also occurs but is always accompanied by vessel abnormalities within the white matter. Mononuclear inflammatory infiltrates surround and in some cases directly invade the vessel wall. Inflammatory infiltrates can extend into the surrounding brain parenchyma. These histopathological features are characteristic of cerebral vasculopathy rather than frank vasculitis/angiitis. In fact, these mononuclear inflammatory infiltrates are dismissed by some as having no pathophysiological significance.

The pleomorphic inflammatory infiltrates are composed predominantly of lymphocytes and plasma cells. Some of the morphology of the atypical mononuclear cells is identical to that of monocytoid B cells derived from MALT. Monocytoid B cells infiltrate salivary glands in Sjögren's and occur in non-Hodgkin's B-cell lymphoma in Sjögren's. Lymphocyte phenotyping studies indicate that the infiltrating lymphocytes are predominantly T cells, with some B cells and plasma cells. Monocytes/macrophages, often containing hemosiderin, are commonly present at the site of subarachnoid or intracerebral microhemorrhages (see below). These observations suggest that in CNS-SS chronic inflammation is associated with microhemorrhages in the meninges (the membrane that covers the brain and spinal cord) and brain tissue.

The cerebral vascular endothelial cell appears to be a target of injury in CNS-SS. The perivascular/vascular inflammatory infiltrates and endothelial cell damage may result in two main pathologic processes in CNS-SS: leaky or occluded blood vessels. In the former case, blood vessels may be leaky to intravascular fluid or erythrocytes. Fluid leaking out of the blood vessels (known as extravasation) results in perivascular edema with myelin pallor and disorganization. Extravasation of erythrocytes results in microhemorrhage. In the second case, occlusion of small blood vessels results in ischemia or infarcts. In CNS-SS, the meningeal and perivascular/vascular mononuclear inflammatory cerebral infiltrates are often associated with micro- and, less commonly, with macro-ischemic infarcts. Microhemorrhages within the meninges are very common but are less common within the brain parenchyma. Rarely, major subarachnoid or intracerebral hemorrhage occurs, almost always in individuals positive for anti-Ro (SSA) antibodies.

These observations strongly suggest that mononuclear inflammatory cells and anti-Ro (SSA) autoantibodies may participate in the immunopathogenesis of inflammatory vascular damage in CNS-SS (see below). Although we do not understand why mononuclear inflammatory cells traffic to the nervous system or know the immunologic events or mechanisms that initiate and perpetuate cerebral vascular inflammation and damage in CNS-SS, the complement pathway is activated in CNS-SS. Furthermore, class II restricted inducible tumor necrosis factor alpha (TNFα) synthesis is associated with CNS-SS. Local TNFα (and potentially other cytokine) synthesis may play a role in mediating vascular permeability, as well as endothelial cell and blood vessel damage, in CNS-SS.

Association of CNS-SS with Peripheral Inflammatory Vascular Disease

An association of CNS disease with coexistent or antecedent peripheral (i.e., skin, nerve, muscle) inflammatory vascular disease (IVD) (i.e., small vessel vasculopathy) has been observed and provides supportive evidence for the importance of small vessel inflammation in the pathogenesis of CNS-SS. A substantial proportion of Sjögren's patients with chronic or recurrent peripheral inflammatory vascular disease (biopsy-documented) have, or subsequently develop, focal or nonfocal CNS disease. Peripheral vascular disease may be of two histopathologic types: mononuclear (MIVD) (i.e., lymphocytic) or neutrophilic (NIVD) (i.e., leukocytoclastic). Patients with recurrent IVD tend to have the same histopathological type of IVD recurring over time.

The two histopathological types of peripheral IVD have consistent differential serological associations. Patients with NIVD are usually seropositive for multiple autoantibodies, including anti-Ro (SS-A) and, less commonly, anti-La (SS-B) antibodies. Patients with MIVD are usually seronegative for these autoantibodies. Patients with NIVD also have higher levels of circulating immune complexes and decreased serum complement levels compared to patients with MIVD. Both histopathological types of peripheral VD have elevated levels of SC5b9, suggesting that the complement pathway is activated.

Anti-Ro (SS-A) antibodies also are present in increased frequency in Sjögren's patients with systemic vasculitis. Both histopathological types (i.e., NIVD and MIVD) of peripheral or systemic IVD are associated with peripheral nervous system and CNS disease in Sjögren's. These observations has led to the recommendation that Sjögren's patients with peripheral or systemic IVD should be assessed carefully for clinical evidence of concomitant CNS disease and, if clinically indicated, evaluated by appropriate neurodiagnostic studies.

Potential Role of Autoantibodies in the Inmunopathogenesis of CNS-SS

Several observations strongly implicate anti-Ro (SS-A) antibodies in the immunopathogenesis of vascular injury and neurological damage observed in CNS-SS. The presence of anti-Ro (SS-A) antibodies is highly associated with: (1) serious focal progressive CNS complications; (2) large "lesions" on brain MRI/CT scans consistent with infarcts or ischemia; (3) abnormal cerebral angiography consistent with small vessel angiitis; (4) histopathology indicative of frank angiitis (in addition to diffuse small vessel mononuclear inflammatory vasculopathy); and (5) the coexistence of necrotizing peripheral and/or systemic IVD in Sjögren's patients with active CNS disease.

Several pieces of experimental evidence support the hypothesis that anti-Ro (SS-A) antibodies may be involved in mediating vascular damage in CNS-SS. Vascular endothelial cells appear to express Ro (SS-A)/La (SS-B) antigens. In *in vitro* studies, we have demonstrated that anti-Ro (SS-A) antibodies preferentially stain the plasma membranes and cytoplasm of proliferating cultured human umbilical vein and bovine retinal endothelial cells. Furthermore, anti-Ro (SS-A) antibody-positive sera from CNS-SS patients have shown 60-kDa and 50-kDa proteins in Western blots of cultured endothelial cells. The molecular weight of these proteins is similar to the 60-kDa proteins that have been cloned and sequenced. The CNS-SS sera also detect the 60-kDa (Ro (SS-A)) and 52-kDa (La (SS-B)) cloned peptides. These observations strongly suggest that endothelial cells may express Ro (SS-A) or closely related antigens. It is attractive to speculate that anti-Ro (SS-A) antibodies may mediate or potentiate endothelial cell injury, perhaps by antibody-complement-mediated damage or by antibody-dependent cellular cytotoxicity (ADCC) and affect endothelial cell proliferation and vessel regeneration in response to injury.

How to Evaluate the Sjögren's Patient Presenting with Neurological Manifestations

The general clinical approach to the evaluation of Sjögren's patients with potential neurological manifestations is presented in Table 10–1.

The general neurodiagnostic approach to the evaluation of Sjögren's patients with neurological manifestations is presented in Table 10–2.

The three most useful and practical noninvasive neurodiagnostic studies in evaluating Sjögren's patients suspected of having active CNS involvement (either focal, nonfocal, or both) are brain (spinal cord as indicated) MRI scans, electrophysiological studies, and CSF analyses (Table 10–3). These diagnostic modalities provide anatomical and functional evidence, on the one hand, for multifocal neurological involvement and, on the other hand, for active

TABLE 10–1

A General Neurodiagnostic Approach to Sjögren's Patients with Neurological Manifestations

- If the patient's internist or rheumatologist feels comfortable and competent in initiating a neurodiagnostic evaluation, the primary physician should proceed with a basic neurodiagnostic evaluation (Table 10–2).
- This initial neurodiagnostic assessment will form the baseline for comparisons with serial, subsequent assessments.
- If abnormalities are present on neurodiagnostic assessments, the studies should be repeated within a responsible time frame (3 to 6 months), depending on the nature and severity of the observed abnormalities.
- The following scenarios are reason for concern:
  - Multiple abnormalities consistent with involvement of more than one area of the nervous system
  - The neuroanatomical location, size, and number of abnormalities
  - Increasing severity or degree of abnormality
  - Evidence for active inflammatory neurological disease
- At this juncture:
  - A neurological consultation should be obtained.
  - A working relationship/partnership between primary physician and neurologist should be solidified.
  - A dialogue should be established, with appropriate additional consultation, to determine the extent and severity of disease and criteria and timing for potential therapeutic intervention.
  - Careful serial monitoring is crucial.

Do not overtreat!
Know what you are treating.
Have criteria/goals for therapy and duration.
Select the best regimen (clinically efficacious, safe, well tolerated, benign side effect profile, cost effective).
Continue to follow for relapse, recurrence.

TABLE 10–2

A General Clinical Approach to Sjögren's Patients with Potential Neurological Manifestations

- Newly diagnosed Sjögren's patients, new referrals, and patients presenting with symptoms and/or signs consistent with central or peripheral nervous system involvement should have a baseline history and neurological examination (in addition to the evaluation for Sjögren's in general) by an internist or rheumatologist competent in clinical neurological assessment.
- This assessment will form the baseline for subsequent longitudinal comparisons.
- If abnormalities are found, the patient should be re-evaluated within a responsible time frame (3 to 6 months), depending on the clinical setting and issues.
- The next step(s) would depend on the evolving clinical picture:
  - Resolved: 1 year re-evaluation
  - Stable (no change): 6 month re-evaluation
  - Progressing: 3 month re-evaluation
- Neurological features that may prompt neurodiagnostic workup are development of:
  - Serious neurological complications
  - Clinical symptoms that suggest the involvement of more than one region of the brain, spinal cord, or optic nerves over time
  - Increasing severity of presenting signs and symptoms
  - Signs and symptoms not managed by appropriate, conservative medical care

TABLE 10–3

A Practical/Feasible Neurodiagnostic Assessment of Sjögren's Patients Suspected of Having Neurological Disease

- Three neurodiagnostic evaluations have proven most clinically useful and feasible in the assessment of the Sjögren's patient suspected of having CNS disease:
  - Neuroimaging: 3 Tesla MRI
  - Electrophysiology: multimodality sensory evoked responses (MMER)
  - CSF analysis: evidence for active inflammatory neurological disease
- The greater number of abnormal results in the three neurodiagnostic studies is associated with the confirmation of neurological disease in Sjögren's.
- Additional neurodiagnostic tests, dependent on the clinical presentation, should be performed as clinically indicated.
- At this juncture:
  - If there are neurodiagnostic test abnormalities at this point of evaluation, the primary physician or rheumatologist might consider consulting with a neurologist, particularly one with expertise in the presenting neurological issues, to assist in the further evaluation of the patient and the interpretation of the neurodiagnostic results.
  - Patients with nonfocal manifestations suspected of having neurocognitive impairment should, in addition, have neurocognitive testing.

cerebral inflammation. At the present time, the use of all three of these modalities is recommended, as each provides different and complementary types of information about the neuroanatomical basis of brain lesions, extent of functional impairment, and severity of disease activity. All are available within community- and university-based facilities and are used routinely to evaluate patients suspected of having MS. A complete panel of autoantibodies, including anti-Ro (SS-A), immmunoglobulins, cryoglobulins, and complement assays also should be obtained and assessed serially.

Summing Up

If the reader answered "yes" to the questions at the beginning of the chapter, we hope this chapter has been informative and has provided a conceptual approach to the recognition, evaluation, management, and potential treatment of the Sjögren's patient with neurological complications. The reader also should recognize that our understanding of the multifaceted manifestations of Sjögren's syndrome, including neurological disease, is in its infancy and evolving. In the case of neurological complications, much has been learned and much remains to be discovered. There are emerging consistencies between neuroimaging studies, electrophysiologic studies, CSF analyses, and histopathology of brain, spinal cord, and peripheral nerves pointing to a role for inflammation in the immunopathogenesis of neurological disease in Sjögren's.

Fundamentally, Sjögren's is a disease of abnormal trafficking of predominantly mononuclear cells preferentially across small blood vessels into organs where they induce dysfunction and damage. This is true for the organs involved as the cornerstone organs of the disease (exocrine glands), other affected organs (extra-glandular), as well as the nervous system (central and peripheral). The small blood vessels of the nervous system appear to be a major focus of a multi-pronged immunological attack by a mononuclear inflammatory vasculopathy. Evidence exists for the participation of multiple, and cascading, inflammatory or immunological insults to the nervous system, including:

1. Abnormal trafficking of mononuclear cells (predominantly lymphocytes, and less commonly plasma cells and macrophages/ monocytes) across the endothelium with breach of the blood–brain and blood–nerve barriers
2. Direct infiltration of mononuclear cells into perivascular spaces and surrounding nervous system tissue, with attendant damage to surrounding cells and tissue
3. Synthesis of molecules (e.g., cytokines and excitatory neurotoxins) by infiltrating inflammatory cells that mediate tissue damage
4. Vascular endothelial cell and vessel wall damage
5. Complement pathway activation

The association of certain autoantibodies (i.e., anti-Ro (SS-A); anti-endothelial cell) with vascular pathology suggests these autoantibodies may play a role in disease pathogenesis in some Sjögren's patients.

The key essentials to the clinical approach to the patient are:

1. Listen, observe, carefully evaluate, record, and document.
2. Follow longitudinally.
3. Create a longitudinal electronic database.
4. Seek consultation and communication with neurologists in the community and at academic centers.
5. Obtain relevant neurodiagnostic testing.
6. Make therapeutic decisions on documented data over time.
7. Objectively monitor response to therapy.

Patients and their families can help build this interactive and communicative team network.

FOR FURTHER READING

Alexander EL. Neurologic disease in Sjogren's syndrome, in *Handbook of Clinical Neurology, Vol. 27 (71): Systemic Diseases, Part III*, MJ Aminoff, CG Goetz eds., Elsevier Science B.V., 1998, 59–98.

Alexander EL. Neurologic disease in Sjogren's syndrome: mononuclear inflammatory vasculopathy affecting central/peripheral nervous system and muscle. *Rheum Dis Clin North Am.* 1993; 19(4): 869–908.

Alexander EL, Malinow K, Lijewski IE. Primary Sjögren's syndrome with central nervous system disease mimicking multiple sclerosis. *Ann Intern Med.* 1986; 104(3): 323–30.

Alexander EL, Beall SS, Gordon B, et al. Magnetic resonance imaging of cerebral lesions in patients with the Sjögren syndrome. *Ann Intern Med.* 1988; 108(6): 815–23.

Alexander EL, Ranzenbach MR, Kumar AJ, et al. Anti-Ro(SS-A) autoantibodies in central nervous system disease associated with Sjögren's syndrome (CNS-SS): clinical, neuro-imaging, and angiographic correlates. *Neurology.* 1994; 44(5): 899–908.

Cai FZ, Lester S, Lu T, et al. Mild autonomic dysfunction in primary Sjögren's syndrome: a controlled study. *Arthritis Res Ther.* 2008; 10(2): R31.

Harboe E, Tjensvoll AB, Maroni S, et al. Neuropsychiatric syndromes in patients with systemic lupus erythematosus and primary Sjögren syndrome: a comparative population-based study. *Ann Rheum Dis.* 2009; 68(10): 1541–6.

Jennings T, Vivino F, Mandel S, et al. Neuropsychological impairments in females with primary Sjögren's syndrome: new insights. *Pract Neurol.* 2010 June.

Mandl T, Granberg V, Apelqvist J, et al. Autonomic nervous symptoms in primary Sjögren's syndrome. *Rheumatology (Oxford).* 2008; 47(6): 914–9.

Morgen K, McFarland HF, Pillemer SR. Central nervous system disease in primary Sjögren's syndrome: the role of magnetic resonance imaging. *Semin Arthritis Rheum.* 2004; 34(3): 623–30.

Segal B, Carpenter A, Walk D. Involvement of nervous system pathways in primary Sjögren's syndrome. *Rheum Dis Clin North Am.* 2008; 34(4): 885–906.

Segal BM, Mueller BA, Zhu X, et al. Disruption of brain white matter microstructure in primary Sjögren's syndrome: evidence from diffusion tensor imaging. *Rheumatology (Oxford).* 2010; 49(8): 1530–9.

Segal BM, Mueller BA. Cognitive disorders and brain MRI correlations in primary Sjögren's syndrome: unlocking the secret of cognitive symptoms. *Int J Clin Rheumatol.* 2011; 6(1).

Small G. *The Memory Bible: An Innovative Strategy for Keeping Your Brain Young.* Hyperion, 2002.

Tzioufas AG, Tsonis J, Moutsopoulos HM. Neuroendocrine dysfunction in Sjögren's syndrome. *Neuroimmunomodulation.* 2008; 15(1): 37–45.

11

The Gastrointestinal Tract
Matthew Nichols, MD

In addition to the classic presentation of xerophthalmia (dry eyes) and xerostomia (dry mouth), Sjögren's syndrome can present with symptoms related to the gastrointestinal (GI) tract and liver. GI and liver manifestations of Sjögren's are typically related to either the decreased secretions related to exocrine gland involvement or to the same underlying autoimmune process that led to salivary and lacrimal gland damage (Table 11–1).

TABLE 11–1
Sjögren's Syndrome and the Gastrointestinal Tract

Esophagus		
	Dysphagia (difficulty swallowing)	Relatively common; usually due to lack of saliva and esophageal lubrication
	Esophageal dysmotility	Muscular incoordination of the esophagus. May affect up to 1/3 of Sjögren's patients with dysphagia.
	GERD	Exacerbated by Sjögren's due to lack of salivary flow to rinse the esophagus of acid
Stomach		
	Atrophic gastritis	Autoimmune destruction of acid-producing parietal cells of the stomach. May lead to vitamin B_{12} deficiency and pernicious anemia. Up to 20% of Sjögren's patients may have antibodies against parietal cells.
	H. pylori infection	Associated with increased risk of GI (MALT) lymphoma
Small intestine		
	Celiac sprue	Also known as gluten enteropathy. May be 10 times more prevalent in Sjögren's patients than in general population.
Pancreas		
	Autoimmune pancreatitis	Rare complication of Sjögren's. Associated with elevated levels of IgG4.
Liver		
	Primary biliary cirrhosis (PBC)	Autoimmune inflammation of small bile ducts. An uncommon complication of Sjögren's. May present with sicca symptoms mimicking Sjögren's.
	Autoimmune hepatitis	Rare complication of Sjögren's. Autoimmune inflammation of liver cells.
	Hepatitis C virus	Not associated with Sjögren's syndrome but can present with sicca symptoms mimicking Sjögren's.

Esophagus

Normal salivary production is a key component in the swallowing mechanism. Difficulty swallowing, or dysphagia, is relatively common in Sjögren's and usually related to the lack of saliva. One of the earliest presentations of the classic dry mouth associated with Sjögren's may be a sense of difficulty initiating the swallowing process, known as pharyngeal dysphagia. Once the swallowing mechanism is initiated in the throat, both normal esophageal lubrication and normal coordination of esophageal contractions are necessary. In addition to a decrease in salivary gland secretions, the mucus-producing cells lining the esophagus can be affected, leading to a dry esophagus and a sense of food passing slowly through the esophagus.

Difficulty swallowing may also be a sign of lack of coordination of the contraction wave that passes food down the esophagus, known as esophageal dysmotility. While more frequently seen in other connective tissue and autoimmune conditions such as scleroderma, esophageal dysmotility may affect up to one third of patients with Sjögren's.

The evaluation of complaints of difficulty swallowing typically includes either endoscopic or radiographic barium evaluation of the upper GI anatomy to rule out strictures, esophagitis, and esophageal webs. If esophageal dysmotility is suspected, esophageal manometry can be obtained to assess the strength and coordination of esophageal contractions.

Reflux of gastric contents and acids in to the esophagus, known as gastroesophageal reflux disease (GERD), is very common, affecting up to 20% of Americans, and may lead to symptoms of heartburn, chest pain, and dysphagia. Chronic or prolonged GERD can lead to irritation and injury of the esophagus (esophagitis), stricture formation, or premalignant changes (Barrett's esophagus). Laryngopharyngeal reflux, or reflux of gastric contents and acids to the level of the throat, can lead to symptoms of hoarseness, chronic cough, throat clearing, mild pharyngeal dysphagia, or globus sensations (sensation of a lump or foreign body in the throat). A small amount of reflux is normal in all individuals. Normal salivary flow is important in washing the esophagus and buffering any residual gastric acid. Reduction of salivary flow and lack of coordination of the esophageal contraction wave are important factors contributing to the development of GERD and laryngopharyngeal reflux in Sjögren's.

GERD may be initially treated with lifestyle modification, including weight loss, elevation of the head of the bed, smoking cessation, avoidance of excessive alcohol intake, and avoidance of large meals or eating within 3 hours of lying down. While mild, intermittent heartburn can be controlled with antacids, chronic or complicated GERD may require the use of medications that reduce the amount of acid produced by the stomach, such as H2-blockers or proton pump inhibitors.

Stomach

Nausea, epigastric discomfort, and dyspepsia are relatively common complaints in individuals with Sjögren's. While heartburn, GERD, and acid dyspepsia are typically treated with acid-blocking medications, some individuals with Sjögren's already have underlying reduced acid secretion by the stomach. Up to 20% of individuals with Sjögren's have antibodies against parietal cells, the acid-secreting cell of the stomach. Destruction of parietal cells, a condition known as chronic atrophic gastritis, can lead to hypochlorhydria (reduced acid secretion) and malabsorption of vitamin B_{12} due to lack of intrinsic factor. Vitamin B_{12} is important for production of red blood cells, and its deficiency may lead to pernicious anemia or peripheral neuropathy. While there is no treatment for atrophic gastritis, vitamin B_{12} deficiency is easily treated with intramuscular cyanocobalamin injections. Diagnosis of atrophic gastritis is made on direct biopsy of the stomach lining during an endoscopy.

Any individual with gastritis or dyspeptic symptoms should be evaluated for *Helicobacter pylori*, a common chronic bacterial infection of the stomach. Diagnosis of *H. pylori* can be made via blood serology tests, breath tests, stool tests, or direct biopsy looking for the organism. A course of antibiotics is effective in eradicating the bacteria in 80% or more individuals; however, for unclear reasons, *H. pylori* may be more difficult to eradicate in individuals with Sjögren's. As Sjögren's is associated with an increased risk of lymphoma above the general population and *H. pylori* infection has been associated with an increased risk of GI (MALT) lymphomas, follow-up testing after treatment is recommended to ensure eradication.

Small Intestine

Celiac disease, also known as celiac sprue or gluten enteropathy, is a condition where the immune system responds abnormally to gluten, a protein found in wheat, rye, barley, and other prepared foods, leading to damage of the small intestinal lining. Celiac disease may affect up to 1 in every 2 to 300 individuals but may be up to 10 times more prevalent in Sjögren's than in the general population. This increased prevalence of celiac disease is seen in other conditions mediated by the immune system, such as autoimmune thyroiditis or type I diabetes. Symptoms of celiac disease include diarrhea, fatigue, weight loss, gas and bloating, and abdominal discomfort. Conditions associated with vitamin and nutrient deficiency (such as iron deficiency anemia or osteoporosis) may also be seen.

While celiac disease is difficult to diagnose based on symptoms alone, simple antibody tests are available to screen for the disease and should be considered in Sjögren's patients with any GI symptoms or nutritional deficiencies.

In individuals with elevated antibody levels suggestive of celiac disease, small intestinal biopsy during an endoscopy of the upper GI tract can confirm the diagnosis. The classic microscopic features seen on biopsy include flattening of the finger-like villi of the intestinal lining. The mainstay of treatment is elimination of gluten from the diet, which typically leads to complete resolution of the small intestinal damage, blood test abnormalities, and symptoms.

Pancreas

Inflammation of the pancreas, known as pancreatitis, can be a consequence of the same autoimmune inflammation that affects the salivary and lacrimal glands. Autoimmune pancreatitis, a rare complication of Sjögren's, is characterized by diffuse swelling of the pancreas and narrowing of the pancreatic duct, leading to abdominal pain, nausea, and vomiting. It has been described as both a primary pancreatic disorder and in association with other conditions of presumed autoimmune cause. Elevated levels of serum IgG4 help to confirm the diagnosis of autoimmune pancreatitis. Patients with Sjögren's and IgG4-related autoimmune pancreatitis may actually have a systemic IgG4-related systemic disease associated with sclerosing sialadenitis, sclerosis cholangitis, or noninfectious aortitis. Early diagnosis and treatment of autoimmune pancreatitis with anti-inflammatory glucocorticoids (prednisone) can prevent the development of chronic pancreatitis and pancreatic insufficiency.

Liver

The liver, one of the largest and most important organs in the body, functions to synthesize proteins and nutrients, detoxify the body, break down medications, and aid in digestion. Inflammation of the liver, usually detected through blood tests showing elevated liver enzymes, can be due to a variety of causes, including viral infections, medication toxicity, and autoimmune inflammation.

Up to 7% of Sjögren's patients may have some degree of liver involvement, usually presenting as subclinical and asymptomatic elevations of liver enzymes. Rarely, a more clinically significant presentation is seen. In these individuals, biopsy of the liver may reveal features of primary biliary cirrhosis (PBC) or autoimmune hepatitis.

PBC is an autoimmune disease of the liver associated with Sjögren's in which the small bile ducts within the liver are attacked and destroyed by the immune system. Continued inflammation and damage of these bile ducts can lead to advanced scarring (cirrhosis) and liver failure. In Sjögren's patients with elevated liver function tests, detection of anti-mitochondrial antibodies suggests a diagnosis of PBC. Approximately 40% to 65% of patients with PBC will have sicca symptoms mimicking Sjögren's, including dry eyes and/or dry mouth. These clinical features typically precede those directly associated with PBC, resulting in an initial diagnosis of Sjögren's rather than PBC. Conversely, PBC is an uncommon complication in patients with primary Sjögren's.

Pruritus, or itching of the skin, is one of the most common symptoms associated with PBC. The exact cause of PBC-related pruritus is unknown. In very mild cases, pruritus can be controlled by such nonspecific measures as emollient lotions or warm baths. In more severe situations, addition of nonabsorbable resins such as cholestyramine or colestipol may aid in management. These resins bind many substances in the GI tract and inhibit the reabsorption of bile acids. Unfortunately, these medications can interfere with absorption of other medications, can cause constipation, and are somewhat unpalatable. If these measures fail, the addition of rifampin (Rifadin), colchicines, or methotrexate may be considered.

Other symptoms and complications of PBC include skin hyperpigmentation, arthritis and joint pain, metabolic bone disease (osteoporosis or osteomalacia), and deficiencies of fat-soluble vitamins (vitamins A, D, E, and K). In late stages, features of advanced scarring and cirrhosis may be seen, including jaundice, edema, portal hypertension (increased pressure in the portal venous system), and ascites (fluid in the abdomen). Classic laboratory features of PBC include the presence of anti-mitochondrial antibodies, elevated liver blood tests (especially alkaline phosphatase and/or bilirubin), and antinuclear antibodies (ANA). A strikingly elevated cholesterol panel may be seen in PBC but is typically not associated with an increased risk of atherosclerosis.

The only treatment proven to modify the natural history and progression of PBC is administration of ursodeoxycholic acid (UDCA) (Actigall), a naturally occurring bile acid. UDCA (13–15 mg/kg daily in divided doses) is a well-tolerated therapy that may improve liver function test abnormalities, delay progression to end-stage liver disease, and improve survival. Addition of colchicine or methotrexate may be considered if significant improvement is not seen with UDCA. If advanced disease, cirrhosis, and liver failure develop, liver transplantation may be required.

Autoimmune hepatitis, also known as chronic active hepatitis, is characterized by continuous attack on the cells of the liver by the body's immune system. This inflammation can eventually lead to chronic injury and scarring of the liver, eventually leading to advanced scarring, or cirrhosis. Most patients with autoimmune hepatitis will present with asymptomatic disease or with nonspecific symptoms such as fatigue, lethargy, poor appetite, and arthralgias. Rarely, autoimmune hepatitis will present with acute hepatitis and jaundice. Autoimmune hepatitis is suspected in individuals with Sjögren's who develop new elevations of liver enzymes without another explanation, such as due to a new medication. Autoimmune hepatitis is diagnosed through a combination of elevated autoimmune antibodies and characteristic features on liver biopsy. Not all individuals with autoimmune hepatitis need to begin treatment immediately. The decision to initiate treatment is based on the severity of symptoms, the severity of the disease (as seen on blood work and biopsy), and the risk of treatment side effects. Treatment of autoimmune hepatitis includes anti-inflammatory glucocorticoids such as prednisone or immunomodulating medications such as azathioprine (Imuran, Azasan) or 6-mercaptopurine.

Individuals with abnormal liver function tests should be evaluated for underlying viral hepatitis infection. While infection with hepatitis C virus (HCV) is no more common in individuals with Sjögren's than in the general population, it can present with a Sjögren's-like syndrome and should be ruled out in anyone presenting with sicca (dry eye/dry mouth) symptoms. In addition to elevated liver enzyme levels, hepatitis C infection can cause xerophthalmia, xerostomia, arthralgias, and lymphocytic sialadenitis, mimicking the classic presentation of Sjögren's. While HCV can cause elevations of autoantibodies such as ANA and rheumatoid factor (RF), anti-Ro (SS-A) and anti-La (SS-B) antibodies are typically absent, thus differentiating it from the classic presentation of Sjögren's.

Summing Up

Any part of the GI tract can be affected in Sjögren's. The possible roles of medication, infection, diet and nutrition, or tumors should be considered. The most common features found include those related to dysmotility, GERD, or atrophic gastritis. Celiac sprue is far more common than previously realized. Up to 15% of patients with Sjögren's may have involvement of the biliary tree, such as biliary cirrhosis or hepatitis. These more serious complications can be suspected in those with positive autoimmune laboratory testing and can be diagnosed by tissue obtained at biopsy. The management of these manifestations is personalized on the basis of symptom severity and systemic inflammatory activity.

FOR FURTHER READING

Belafsky PC, Postma GN. The laryngeal and esophageal manifestations of Sjögren's syndrome. *Curr Rheumatol Rep.* 2003; 5(4): 297–303.

Hatzis GS, Fragoulis GE, Karatzaferis A, et al. Prevalence and long-term course of primary biliary cirrhosis in primary Sjögren's syndrome. *J Rheumatol.* 2008; 35(10): 2012–6.

Iltanen S, Collin P, Korpela M, et al. Celiac disease and markers of celiac disease latency in patients with primary Sjögren's syndrome. *Am J Gastroenterol.* 1999; 94(4): 1042–6.

Kamisawa T, Tu Y, Egawa N, et al. Salivary gland involvement in chronic pancreatitis of various etiologies. *Am J Gastroenterol.* 2003; 98(2): 323–6.

Kogawa H, Migita K, Ito M, et al. Idiopathic portal hypertension associated with systemic sclerosis and Sjögren's syndrome. *Clin Rheumatol.* 2005; 24(5): 544–7.

Matsuda M, Hamano H, Yoshida T, et al. Seronegative Sjogren syndrome with asymptomatic autoimmune sclerosing pancreatitis. *Clin Rheumatol.* 2007; 26(1): 117–9.

Maury CP, Tornroth T, Teppo AM. Atrophic gastritis in Sjögren's syndrome: Morphologic, biochemical, and immunologic findings. *Arthritis Rheum.* 1985; 28(4): 388–94.

Palma R, Freire A, Freitas J, et al. Esophageal motility disorders in patients with Sjögren's syndrome. *Dig Dis Sci.* 1994; 39(4): 758–61.

Skopouli FN, Barbatis C, Moutsopoulos HM. Liver involvement in primary Sjögren's syndrome. *Br J Rheumatol.* 1994; 33(8): 745–8.

Szodoray P, Barta Z, Lakos G, et al. Coeliac disease in Sjögren's syndrome. *Rheumatol Int.* 2004; 24(5): 278–82.

Teufel A, Weinmann A, Kahaly GJ, et al. Concurrent autoimmune diseases in patients with autoimmune hepatitis. *J Clin Gastroenterol.* 2010; 44(3): 208–13.

Tsianos EV, Hoofnagle JH, Fox PC, et al. Sjögren's syndrome in patients with primary biliary cirrhosis. *Hepatology.* 1990; 11(5): 730–4.

Türk T, Pirildar T, Tunç E, et al. Manometric assessment of esophageal motility in patients with primary Sjögren's syndrome. *Rheumatol Int.* 2005; 25(4): 246–9.

12

Gynecological Issues, Including Pregnancy
Thomas R. Allan, MD, and Ann Parke, MD

Sjögren's syndrome affects about 4 million Americans, or about one person in 70. It is nine times more common in women and approximately evenly divided between primary and secondary Sjögren's. Patients with secondary Sjögren's also have an additional connective autoimmune disease such as systemic lupus erythematosus (SLE), rheumatoid arthritis (RA), or scleroderma. These autoimmune diseases also have a similar greater predominance in women.

The symptoms of Sjögren's often are present for many years before recognition and diagnosis. Associated organ involvement and secondary Sjögren's, with the problems and effects of a secondary autoimmune disease, may cause significant complications and comorbidity. The prevalence of primary and secondary Sjögren's in women and the special concerns of pregnancy emphasize the importance of primary care providers and obstetrician/gynecologists in the care of these patients.

Patients with Sjögren's often experience fatigue, chronic pain problems, and increased symptoms of depression. These same symptoms have been found in epidemiological studies to be the most common chief complaints in primary care patients in the general population. Fatigue has been reported to be the most common complaint in primary care and gynecological offices, and it has also been found in about 50% of Sjögren's patients. Pain symptoms, especially myalgia (muscle ache) and arthralgia (joint discomfort and pain), are present in almost half of patients, and symptoms of depression have been reported in one third of women with primary Sjögren's. Primary care physicians and OB/GYNs are essential providers for the diagnosis and care of primary Sjögren's and associated autoimmune diseases. For all women, including patients with Sjögren's, recognition, diagnosis, and treatment of common complaints such as fatigue, pain, and depression are most frequently provided by primary care physicians.

Medical journals and textbooks in primary care and especially in obstetrics and gynecology may only briefly, if at all, discuss Sjögren's, even though it is a relatively common disease of, almost exclusively, women. It is also a connective tissue autoimmune disease that may have significant effects in pregnancy.

Sjögren's also occurs most often when women at middle age are seeing their gynecologists and primary care providers for perimenopause and menopause symptoms. Some of the symptoms of Sjögren's, perimenopause, and menopause significantly overlap, such as hot flashes, symptoms of dryness, fatigue, sleep difficulties, depression, and pain with sexual intercourse. Medical references also often may not provide physicians with up-to-date information on Sjögren's. For example, *The Comprehensive Textbook of Gynecology* (Katz) does not mention Sjögren's. This would appear to be a significant omission, since this illness is primarily a disease of women, and Sjögren's patients, compared to the general population, often experience more troublesome gynecological symptoms, such as vaginal dryness and pain with sexual intercourse (dyspareunia). Similarly, textbooks of obstetrics, including the universally recognized American reference *Williams Obstetrics*, also does not mention Sjögren's, even though in pregnancy it is the most common cause of fetal heart block.

Additionally, secondary Sjögren's is frequently associated with SLE, which may cause significant fetal loss in both early and late pregnancy. Severe SLE may also increase morbidity and mortality for pregnant women. Blood clots (venous thromboses), primarily in the veins of the lower extremities and less frequently the lungs (pulmonary embolism), occur more frequently in patients with SLE, which is often associated with Sjögren's. Blood clots may occur in women who are not pregnant, but they are more common during pregnancy or the postpartum period. Thorough evaluation and preventive treatments, ideally before pregnancy and during preconceptual counseling, are essential in these patients who are at higher risk for complications in pregnancy.

Sex Steroids

The relation of sex steroid hormones, primarily estrogens and androgens, would be expected to be a substantial factor in Sjögren's, considering its predominance in women. For example, one basic science study in laboratory mice showed an association of estrogen deficiency and an autoimmune disease resembling Sjögren's; however, other basic science studies have not clarified the role of sex steroids in this disease. Much further research is needed on basic hormonal processes and their importance in Sjögren's.

Menopause is defined as the permanent cessation of menstruation due to the normal failure of ovarian follicle development and the subsequent marked decrease in estrogen production and other ovarian hormones. Perimenopause is a variable time of irregular menses beginning a few years before the menopause. The average duration of perimenopause is 4 years. The average age of menopause or the last menstrual period is 51 to 52 years but ranges from 40 to 60 years. This age range is very similar to the average age range of the onset of Sjögren's. One large study revealed that the average age of the onset of symptoms in patients with primary Sjögren's was 53 years. Also, the severity of Sjögren's, like RA, often increases after menopause.

There are sex steroid differences reported in some but not all studies of Sjögren's patients compared to the general population. Reduced levels of the androgen dehydroepiandrosterone (DHEA) have been reported with active Sjögren's, and similar findings have been reported in patients with SLE and RA. More severe symptoms were reported with lower androgen levels, and more severe dry eyes were associated with low estrogen levels. The presence of more active disease and higher levels of Sjögren's antibodies (anti-SS-A (Ro) and/or anti-SS-B (La) antibodies) has been associated with low estradiol levels.

Estradiol, estrone, and estriol are the three principal estrogens. Estradiol is the most biologically potent naturally occurring estrogen. These estrogens, which can be synthesized in the laboratory from plant precursors, are identical to the natural human estrogens.

One large study, using local application of estradiol drops in Sjögren's patients, showed improved ocular dryness. The authors of this study suggested that further investigation of estrogen treatment, including systemic (oral or transdermal) administration, is warranted. However, the research in this area is confusing as studies have revealed conflicting results. For example, in another study of dry eyes in postmenopausal women without Sjögren's, combined hormone therapy replacement therapy (HRT) with both estrogen and also with the addition of another sex steroid hormone, a synthetic progestin, was associated with a higher incidence of difficulty with eye dryness. Progestins also have anti-estrogen effects (see *The New Sjögren's Handbook*, 3rd ed.).

Hormone Replacement Therapy

HRT with estrogen and progesterone is commonly used in menopause for severe hot flashes, disrupted sleep, and in some cases mild depressive symptoms. Some of these often-disabling problems are more common in patients with Sjögren's. Many postmenopausal women with severe hot flashes choose to use HRT, the most effective treatment. Use of HRT requires informed patient counseling and a thorough knowledge of recent studies. Complete discussion of this subject is beyond the limitations of this review, but a summary is necessary to aid in the care of Sjögren's patients.

The Women's Health Initiative (WHI) study, published in 2002, should be discussed with all patients considering HRT. The results of this controversial study differed from the reassuring results of multiple previous observational and prospective studies. The WHI study initiated significant concern about the risks of HRT. The use of hormone therapy dropped in a large proportion of postmenopausal women after the release of the initial incomplete results and the sensationalized reports in the public media. This study specifically used conjugated equine (horse) estrogens in combination with medroxyprogesterone, a potent synthetic progestin. The main outcome was a very slight increased risk, primarily in older women, of coronary heart disease, stroke, blood clots (venous thromboembolism), and breast cancer. The risk per year for each of these risks was less than one person per thousand. The beneficial outcomes were significantly less osteoporotic fractures, including the spine and hip, and significantly less colorectal cancer.

The WHI study has subsequently been extensively criticized by many researchers, particularly because of its enrollment, primarily of older women. The average age of patients was 63 years. A minority of patients were in their fifties and no patients were in their forties. The normal range of menopause is, as previously noted, from age 40 to 60, with an average age of 51 to 52. These are the younger patients who often experience severe hot flashes. Half of the patients in the WHI study were in their middle to late 60s and 70s; this is not the age when most patients have hot flashes. The researchers in this study, surprisingly, excluded from the study all patients with hot flashes at any age, including patients in their 50s. These again are the very women who have symptomatic need for HRT and who need accurate information on HRT. Further analysis indicates that the potent synthetic progestin, medroxyprogesterone, NOT estrogen, was the principal cause of the major adverse findings in the WHI study.

More recent research studies of HRT have been more reassuring, especially for younger postmenopausal women. Some of the more recent recommendations by some researchers in this field are (1) lower doses of HRT; (2) use of transdermal estrogen; (3) consideration of bio-identical estrogens such as estradiol; (4) substitution of progesterone for progestins; and (5) alternative methods of progesterone administration. Continuing research and review of recent studies indicates that some of these modifications would result in minimal, if any, increase in most of the adverse events reported by the initial incomplete WHI study, particularly for younger menopausal women. Recent analysis of these studies indicates that the incidence of coronary heart disease, the most common cause of overall mortality in women, would be significantly reduced with the use of estrogen replacement without a progestin for women in their 50s. It is also important to note that observational studies of estrogen replacement without a progestin did not show an increase in breast cancer for up to 10 to 15 years of use. The overall mortality for these younger women from all causes was also decreased. A review of recent additional studies also shows a lower incidence of Alzheimer's disease with use of estrogen without a progestin in the early years of menopause, which also is consistent with the earlier studies.

The current recommendation of most academic and practicing physicians, however, is that estrogen with or without progesterone should at the present time primarily be used at the lowest effective dose for severe hot flashes for the shortest time necessary. Patients who have had a hysterectomy should be prescribed estrogen without progesterone.

In other areas of research with sex steroids in both Sjögren's patients and the general population, DHEA, an androgen, may be helpful for symptoms of fatigue and depression. This medication, although available over the counter in pharmacies, cannot be routinely recommended without further research. Transdermal testosterone, another sex steroid, has also been shown in several research studies to have significant benefit for many patients for low sexual desire or libido. This steroid is available by prescription through compounding pharmacies but also cannot be recommended at this time in this review without FDA approval.

Vaginal Dryness and Sexual Problems

Many women with Sjögren's experience vaginal dryness and discomfort or pain with sexual intercourse (dyspareunia). In one study, 40% of women with Sjögren's experienced dyspareunia, compared to 3% of the normal control group. In the years after menopause, vulvovaginal dryness and atrophy due to estrogen deficiency is common in the general population. Patients with Sjögren's may have more severe symptoms. Decreased estrogen in postmenopausal women results in a thin vaginal mucosa with minimal moisture content, vaginal inflammation, and vulvovaginal atrophy.

A number of water-soluble over-the-counter products such as K-Y jelly, Sylk, and Astroglide are commonly used with sexual intercourse for increased lubrication. K-Y Liquibeads is a convenient, longer-acting product that is preferred by many women with dyspareunia. It may be used 1 hour before sexual intercourse or may be used twice a week for maintenance of vaginal moisture. For postmenopausal atrophic vulvovaginal atrophy, locally acting vaginal estrogen as a cream (Estrace or Premarin) or suppository (Vagifem) or as a longer-acting 3-month ring (Estring) usually reverses vaginal atrophy and dryness in postmenopausal women and also is helpful in Sjögren's patients. Vagifem and Estring have been designed to produce minimal, if any, vaginal absorption of estrogen. Systemic estrogen replacement, as previously discussed for hot flashes, will also be very beneficial for postmenopausal vulovaginal atrophy. Systemic replacement, however, is generally prescribed for severe hot flashes, but most postmenopausal patients who use HRT for hot flashes generally also note reversal of vaginal atrophy and dryness, and relief of discomfort and dyspareunia.

Candida Vaginitis

Vaginal discharge and vulvar burning and itching due to Candida is one of the most common, often recurrent, gynecological problems. Candida vaginitis ("yeast infection") is caused by a ubiquitous airborne fungus. Candida vaginitis is more common with antibiotic use, uncontrolled diabetes, obesity, depressed immune function, and the use of corticosteroids. It is more common in women with Sjögren's. Diagnosis is confirmed by microscopic examination of vaginal discharge in the physician's office. Multiple vaginal antifungal treatments are available, either by prescription or over the counter, such as miconazole (Monistat), clotrimazole (Gyne-Lotrimin), teraconazole (Terazol), or an oral antifungal drug, fluconazole (Diflucan).

Interstitial Cystitis

Interstitial cystitis is a chronic, severely debilitating, inflammatory condition of the bladder of unknown cause. It is characterized by urinary frequency, urgency, a need to pass urine at night (nocturia), and pelvic pain. Interstitial cystitis is also primarily a disease in women and is found in about 1% of all women and 4% to 10% of women with Sjögren's. Since interstitial cystitis is a complex disease, it is best treated by a urogynecologist or urologist with expertise in this often disabling and chronic disease. Usually multiple interventions are necessary, with a combination of pelvic floor physical therapy, medications, and bladder instillations. Interstitial cystitis has similarities to other pain disorders. Central sensitization or a neurogenic-increased perception of pain (hyperalgesia) may be a common pathophysiological mechanism in these poorly understood disorders. Newer medications, such as duloxetine (Cymbalta) and milnaciprin (Savella), which are used to treat fibromyalgia and depression, are promising new medications that may be beneficial for interstitial cystitis and many other pain disorders.

Endometriosis

The literature on endometriosis suggests that it may be an autoimmune disease. One recent controlled study evaluating reproduction and gynecological manifestations in women with primary Sjögren's demonstrated that endometriosis occurs more commonly in patients with Sjögren's than in controls (8.5% vs. 2.1%, a significant difference [$p = 0.03$]).

Pregnancy and Fetal Heart Block

The concerns for any woman with a connective tissue disease who wishes to become pregnant include (1) risks to the mother; (2) risks to the fetus; and (3) safe management of the disease during pregnancy.

Since the incidence of Sjögren's peaks between 40 and 60, the disease is less common in women who are pregnant at younger ages. Therefore, the literature on pregnancy in patients with primary Sjögren's is limited, and clinical manifestations during pregnancy in mothers with primary Sjögren's have not been studied adequately for reasonable conclusions to be drawn. Mothers with secondary Sjögren's can anticipate clinical disease activity based on their other connective tissue disease.

MATERNAL RISKS

Rheumatoid arthritis remits during pregnancy in up to 80% of patients. This benefit is not just a consequence of the hormonal changes that occur with pregnancy, as it may continue for several months after the pregnancy is finished. It is considered to be related to the immune switching that must occur for a mother to stay pregnant and not to reject the growing fetus, as she would with any other foreign tissue transplant. Unfortunately, RA always returns, although this may take several months in some patients.

Patients with SLE can improve, deteriorate, or stay the same during pregnancy. It is difficult to predict which patients will respond in which way, although the changes seen in one pregnancy are usually copied in subsequent pregnancies. One of the most important factors determining pregnancy outcome in patients with SLE is disease activity, and this means that the patient must be seen regularly and followed closely. The presence of phospholipid antibodies can also influence maternal and fetal health, with the mother being at risk for clinical blood clots (thrombotic events) during pregnancy and the pregnancy at increased risk for fetal loss, primarily because of placental insufficiency.

Patients with systemic sclerosis can also have a change in clinical disease activity during pregnancy. Studies have shown that approximately 20% improve, 20% deteriorate, and 60% remain stable. New onset of systemic sclerosis during pregnancy is rare, as is renal crisis. Raynaud's phenomenon, however, generally improves during pregnancy.

PREGNANCY RISKS

Pregnancy outcome in patients with connective tissue diseases may be complicated due to the nature of the underlying pathology—for example, vasculitis (inflammation in blood vessels) or the presence of specific antibodies. The presence of some antibodies may result in impaired development of the placenta, leading to placental failure. Other maternal antibodies may cross the placenta to produce end-organ damage in the fetus. The antibodies that are most frequently associated with end-organ damage in the fetus are antibodies to SS-A (Ro) and/or SS-B (La), antibodies that are most commonly found in patients with SLE and patients with Sjögren's.

One recent study comparing pregnancy outcome in patients with primary Sjögren's and controls determined that pregnancy outcome was no different in patients compared to control subjects, except for the development of congenital heart block in two infants. However, other studies have produced conflicting results, with one study documenting an increased rate of early fetal loss (miscarriage) in patients with primary Sjögren's, whereas several other studies failed to demonstrate any difference in fetal wastage, prematurity, or growth restriction.

It is the risk for fetal congenital heart block that is the major cause for concern for the pregnant Sjögren's patient. This is one feature of the neonatal lupus syndrome, a syndrome that is known to be a consequence of the transplacental passage of maternal antibodies, in particular antibodies to Ro and/or La. The other features of this syndrome include a transient skin rash, which is therefore less troubling. Complete third-degree heart block, which results in a very slow heart beat, however, is permanent, and third-degree heart block is unresponsive to steroids and other treatment modalities. Lesser degrees of heart block may respond to therapeutic maneuvers, and this is why these patients are considered high-risk pregnancy patients and must have fetal echocardiography performed weekly from week 16 to 26 and then every 2 weeks from week 26 to 34. Heart block can start and progress rapidly, but lesser degrees of heart block can be reversed by steroids that cross the placenta. These mothers will require steroids for the rest of their pregnancy. In a study from Israel, 70 fetuses of mothers positive for Ro and/or La antibodies were monitored for early first-degree heart block. In six fetuses, first-degree block developed at 21 to 34 weeks, and maternal steroid treatment was associated with normalization of heart conduction in all fetuses within 3 to 14 days. There were no recurrences, and the infants were all well at a median follow-up of 4 years.

Generally, complete third-degree heart block does not respond to steroid treatment. Patients with a fetus with complete heart block that does not respond to 6 weeks of steroids will have this therapy discontinued unless there is significant other heart or end-organ pathology that is responding to the steroid therapy. These newborns generally require a pacemaker soon after birth.

The good news is that only 2% of mothers with Ro/La antibodies will produce a child with heart block, and the risk of recurrence of fetal heart block in a subsequent pregnancy is approximately 20%. These figures indicate that there must be other fetal factors that dictate disease expression.

Even though the mother still carries the offending antibody, previous studies have suggested that it is safe for these mothers to breastfeed. All babies with any degree of heart block must be followed closely for at least 1 year after birth, as lesser degrees of heart block may progress after birth.

Patients with either primary or secondary Sjögren's, especially if the associated disease is SLE, require special care and monitoring during pregnancy, watching for several possible complications, including complete congenital heart block, clinically active disease, and a propensity to develop blood clots, as is found in patients with the antiphospholipid syndrome.

SAFE MANAGEMENT OF THE DISEASE DURING PREGNANCY

Many medications are contraindicated in the pregnant patient. This is because they cross the placenta and pose a significant risk to the developing fetus. Prednisone is a very good anti-inflammatory agent that crosses the placenta only in miniscule amounts, and therefore it is considered to be comparatively safe for use in pregnancy when the mother is experiencing a flare of disease. In the situation of a fetus developing the neonatal lupus syndrome, where there is significant fetal end-organ damage considered to be a consequence of the transplacental passage of maternal antibody, other steroids that can cross the placenta need to be used so that they may be of benefit to the fetus.

Blood thinners that are taken by mouth (warfarin [Coumadin]) should not be used after 6 weeks' gestation. Patients who have had previous blood clots or have the phospholipid antibodies will need to be treated with heparin, which is given by injection; this should be continued for at least 6 weeks postpartum as the risk for clotting is still increased for several weeks after delivery.

Some other drugs can be used in pregnancy, but patients should plan for pregnancy and discuss the pros and cons of various medications with their physicians prior to attempting to become pregnant. This may take several months of planning, as the effects and half-lives of some drugs are very prolonged.

The other reason for planning for pregnancy is to ensure that the disease is inactive, as disease activity is known to affect pregnancy outcome. We prefer our patients to have inactive disease before attempting pregnancy, and in the case of SLE we prefer that the disease is inactive for at least 6 months prior to conception. Pregnant patients with connective tissue diseases need to be seen regularly and followed closely. Major advances in maternal-fetal and neonatal medicine, improved monitoring of the fetus, and newer treatments over the past several decades have fortunately resulted in vastly improved outcomes and well-being for both the pregnant woman and her baby.

Summing Up

The Sjögren's patient is at increased risk for a variety of unique gynecological and pregnancy complications. As may be expected, the lack of secretions leads to vaginal dryness, dyspareunia, and probably vaginal candidiasis. The increased prevalence of endometriosis and interstitial cystitis found in patients with Sjögren's is not well understood. The relationship of sex hormones and the postmenopausal state predisposing patients to develop this syndrome deserves further study.

Pregnancy poses its own unique problems. As the majority of patients with Sjögren's are older and generally postmenopausal, pregnancy in patients with primary Sjögren's is comparatively uncommon. However, some autoantibodies, in particular those directed towards nuclear antigens Ro and/or La, are known to be associated with the risk for developing the neonatal lupus syndrome. These antibodies are most commonly found in patients with SLE and patients with Sjögren's. Sometimes they may occur in seemingly normal individuals, and an abnormal pregnancy producing a child with congenital complete heart block may be the earliest presentation of an underlying autoimmune diathesis. This syndrome has taught us that the clinical manifestations of autoimmune rheumatic diseases may extend beyond the usual rheumatic disease complaints and that the presence of certain autoantibodies may dictate the development of specific clinical complaints and syndromes.

FOR FURTHER READING

Abeles M, Solitar BM, Pillinger MH, Abeles AM. Update on fibromyalgia therapy. *Am J Med.* 2008; 121(7): 555–61.

Brucato A, Frassi M, et al. Risk of congenital complete heart block in newborns of mothers with anti-Ro/SSA antibodies detected by counterimmunoelectrophoresis: a prospective study of 100 women. *Arthritis Rheum.* 2001; 44(8): 1832–5.

Cunningham FG, Leveno, KJ, Bloom SL, et al., eds. *Williams Obstetrics*, 23rd ed. New York: McGraw Hill Medical, 2010.

Friedman DM, Kim MY, Copel JA, et al. Utility of cardiac monitoring in fetuses at risk for congenital heart block: the PR Interval and Dexamethasone Evaluation (PRIDE) prospective study. *Circulation.* 2008; 117(4): 485–93.

Haga HJ, Gjesdal CG, Irgens LM, Ostensen M. Reproduction and gynaecological manifestations in women with primary Sjögren's: a case-control study. *Scand J Rheumatol.* 2005; 34(1): 45–8.

Haga HJ, Gjesdal CG, Koksvik HS, et al. Pregnancy outcome in patients with primary Sjögren's: a case-control study. *J Rheumatol.* 2005; 32(9): 1734–6.

Izmirly PM, Rivera TL, Buyon JP. Neonatal lupus syndromes. *Rheum Dis Clin North Am.* 2007; 33(2): 267–85.

Katz VL, Lentz GM, Lobo RA, Gershenson DM, eds. *Comprehensive Gynecology*, 5th ed. Philadelphia: Mosby Elsevier, 2007.

Leppilahti M, Tammela TL, Huhtala H, et al. Interstitial cystitis-like urinary symptoms among patients with Sjögren's: a population-based study in Finland. *Am J Med.* 2003; 115(1): 62–5.

Mulherin DM, Sheeran TP, Kumararatne DS, et al. Sjögren's in women presenting with chronic dyspareunia. *Br J Obstet Gynaecol.* 1997; 104(9): 1019–23.

Ostensen M, Khamashta M, Lockshin M., et al. Anti-inflammatory and immunosuppressive drugs and reproduction. *Arthritis Res Ther.* 2006; 8(3): 209.

Rihl M, Ulbricht K, Schmidt RE, Witte T. Treatment of sicca symptoms with hydroxychloroquine in patients with Sjögren's. *Rheumatology (Oxford)*. 2009: 48(7): 796–9.

Tincani A, Bompane D, Danieli E, Doria A. Pregnancy, lupus and antiphospholipid syndrome (Hughes syndrome). *Lupus*. 2006; 15(3): 156–60.

Tincani A, Nuzzo M, Motta M, et al. Autoimmunity and pregnancy: autoantibodies and pregnancy in rheumatic diseases. *Ann NY Acad Sci* 2006; 1069: 346–52.

Walker J, Gordon T, Lester S, et al. Increased severity of lower urinary tract symptoms and daytime somnolence in primary Sjögren's. *J Rheumatol*. 2003; 30(11): 2406–12.

13

Lymphoma

Elke Theander, MD, PhD, and Eva Baecklund, MD, PhD

Upon learning that the incidence of developing lymphoma is higher than the norm in patients with Sjögren's syndrome, a common question arises: "Am I (or, is this patient) at risk?" The answer is that few Sjögren's patients will develop this complication. However, both patient and physician are wise to be aware of this potential development, know the risk factors, and remember that new treatments are being used in lymphoma now and others are under investigation. Our understanding of the potential progression to lymphoma is rapidly changing and knowledge is continually increasing about diagnosis, assessment of risk, and treatment.

Chronic inflammation and stimulation of the immune system, from various causes, may increase the potential for development of lymphoma. Among all autoimmune diseases, the clearest link of development from autoimmunity to lymphoma is established in Sjögren's syndrome. However, the increased risk for lymphoma in Sjögren's is shared with patients who have other rheumatic/autoimmune diseases, such as rheumatoid arthritis (RA) and systemic lupus erythematosus (SLE). It has been estimated that about 5-10% of patients with primary Sjögren's syndrome develop lymphoma. The most common type of lymphoma to develop in Sjögren's is a B-cell non-Hodgkin's lymphoma of mucosa-associated lymphoid tissue (MALT), meaning that it most often develops in the mucosa, the moist lining of some organs and body cavities.

Lymphoma Facts

Lymphomas are a type of cancer occurring in the immune system. Our immune system consists of many different cell types that normally defend us from foreign invaders such as bacteria and viruses. Sometimes a malignant transformation may start in one of these cells and give rise to a process that eventually results in a tumor. Such a transformation is due to a number of contributing events, which so far are not fully understood.

Two common types of white blood cells in the immune system are the B and T lymphocytes. From these cells, the two major groups of lymphomas, called B- and T-cell lymphomas, evolve. B-cell lymphomas are the more common, representing about 90% of all lymphomas. B- and T-cell lymphomas are in turn divided into many subtypes, and each subtype is regarded as a separate disease with different clinical features, localization, prognosis, and treatment options. There is a span from indolent, low-grade lymphomas, which sometimes do not require treatment at all, to the so-called aggressive, high-grade lymphomas, which may cause severe symptoms and are treated with chemotherapy, radiation, and sometimes bone marrow transplantation. The separation of lymphoma into subtypes is based on microscopic examination of lymphoma tissue.

Signs of Lymphoma

The most common first sign of a lymphoma is a painless swelling or enlargement of one or more lymph nodes. In primary Sjögren's, the lymphoma may be located in the salivary glands and is often noted as an increasing firm swelling of the parotid gland. It may sometimes be difficult to distinguish if the swollen gland is due to inflammation caused by Sjögren's or an evolving lymphoma. Typically inflammation causes a tender swelling that comes and goes in both parotid glands. If the reason for the swelling is unclear, it may be wise to take a biopsy from the gland and have it examined by a pathologist.

Lymphoma also may arise in other parts of the body, and varying symptoms may occur depending on the organ involved (e.g., stomach pain from a lymphoma in the stomach). In lymphoma patients with more extensive and later-stage disease, systemic symptoms may arise. These typically include weight loss, fever, and severe night sweats.

Workup for Lymphoma

If lymphoma is suspected, the first step is to find and remove lymphoma tissue for histologic examination under the microscope. Depending on the localization, the biopsy or removal (extirpation) of the swelling may be performed under local anesthesia, but sometimes surgery with general anesthesia is required.

The potential spread of the lymphoma in other parts of the body will be determined. A number of methods can detect a mass in different parts of the body, such as x-ray, CT scan, MRI, and PET scan. Sometimes a bone marrow biopsy is needed. The workup also includes blood tests to analyze blood cells and function of different organs. Increased lactate dehydrogenase (LDH) levels may indicate a more widespread lymphoma or larger mass, but blood tests may also be normal even if a lymphoma is present.

Based on the imaging results, a staging of the lymphoma will be performed to describe the spread of lymphoma in the body. The most favorable stage is when the lymphoma is localized to one site or organ. Together, the information about the lymphoma subtype from the pathologist and results from the staging form the basis for treatment decisions.

Treatment for Lymphoma

The most common therapy for lymphoma is chemotherapy in different combinations. Chemotherapy for B-cell lymphomas is often combined with rituximab (Rituxan), a monoclonal antibody directed against B cells that is also used to treat some of the rheumatic diseases. Rituximab is currently being evaluated as therapy for patients with Sjögren's without lymphoma. Chemotherapy is often given intravenously, and the length of treatment depends on the effect on the lymphoma. This will be evaluated by, for instance, CT or PET scan.

Localized extranodal marginal zone lymphoma of MALT is often treated and cured by radiation given on repeated occasions. An indolent MALT lymphoma may sometimes transform into a more aggressive lymphoma subtype and then needs to be treated by chemotherapy. After treatment patients are usually followed for 5 years by the oncologist or hematologist before the lymphoma can be considered as cured.

Lymphoma in Sjögren's

Typical for lymphoma in primary Sjögren's is the occurrence of MALT lymphoma in the salivary glands. MALT lymphoma is one of the indolent lymphoma subtypes with a good prognosis. Some Sjögren's patients may develop diffuse large B-cell lymphoma, a more aggressive lymphoma subtype that may evolve in and spread to different organs in the body.

Prognosis

Lymphoma in primary Sjögren's is often associated with a good prognosis (i.e., the indolent MALT lymphomas), and even in patients with more aggressive lymphoma subtypes, about 50% are cured by chemotherapy.

Risk Factors for Lymphoma in Patients with Primary Sjögren's

Several studies have tried to identify risk factors for lymphoma development in Sjögren's. Such factors may help the physician to follow high-risk patients more closely and take prompt action if symptoms that could indicate lymphoma occur. This is important as prognosis in case of an aggressive lymphoma depends on early diagnosis and treatment.

The risk factors that have been identified are associated with other more severe complications in Sjögren's. Risk factors for development of an indolent lymphoma versus an aggressive lymphoma have not been determined. Clinical signs predicting lymphoma found in most of the studies are:

1. Recurrently or persistently swollen salivary glands (Fig. 13–1)
2. Swollen lymph nodes
3. Skin vasculitis, which causes a typical rash
4. Peripheral neuropathy

Laboratory parameters that may predict lymphoma are:

1. Cryoglobulinemia
2. Low complement factor C4 levels
3. Low complement factor C3 levels
4. Cytopenias such as lymphopenia or neutropenia or lack of certain subtypes of blood cells
5. Serum or urine monoclonal bands
6. High serum beta2-microglobulin

Certain findings in a salivary gland or lip biopsy performed at diagnosis of Sjögren's may indicate risk of future lymphoma development. Such findings

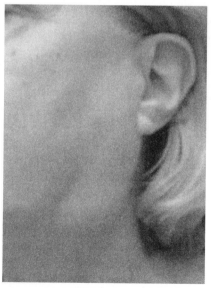

FIGURE 13–1 **Persistently Swollen Parotid Gland in a Patient with Primary Sjögren's as a Risk Factor for Lymphoma Development (Published with Permission).**

include the presence of focal inflammation with activated B, T, and other immune cells in the salivary tissue forming germinal center-like structures.

Summing Up

Although lymphoma can be a serious complication in some Sjögren's patients, it should be emphasized that the knowledge about lymphoma in rheumatic diseases is quickly expanding and is a field of much research. More knowledge about risk factors and biomarkers for lymphoma and better therapies for Sjögren's and for lymphoma will improve the prognosis for this subgroup of patients. Of particular interest will be to evaluate if treatment for Sjögren's with rituximab (Rituxan) or other new targeted therapies can decrease the risk for lymphoma in high-risk patients.

FOR FURTHER READING

Baimpa E, Dahabreh IJ, Voulgarelis M, Moutsopoulos HM. Hematologic manifestations and predictors of lymphoma development in primary Sjögren syndrome: clinical and pathophysiologic aspects. *Medicine (Baltimore).* 2009; 88(5): 284–93.

Brito-Zerón P, Ramos-Casals M, Bove A, et al. Predicting adverse outcomes in primary Sjögren's syndrome: identification of prognostic factors. *Rheumatology (Oxford).* 2007; 46(8) :1359–62.

Ekström Smedby K, Vajdic CM, Falster M, et al. Autoimmune disorders and risk of non-Hodgkin lymphoma subtypes: a pooled analysis within the InterLymph Consortium. *Blood.* 200815; 111(8): 4029–38.

Hammitt KM, Alexander EL. Lymphoma and autoimmune disease. In NR Rose, IR Mackay, eds. *The Autoimmune Diseases,* 4th ed. London/San Diego: Academic Press, Elsevier Ltd., 2006.

Hansen A, Daridon C, Dörner T. What do we know about memory B cells in primary Sjögren's syndrome? *Autoimmun Rev.* 2010; 9(9): 600–3.

Hansen A, Lipsky PE, Dörner T. B-cell lymphoproliferation in chronic inflammatory rheumatic diseases. *Nat Clin Pract Rheumatol.* 2007; 3(10): 561–9.

Jonsson R, Nginamau E, Szyszko E, Brokstad KA. Role of B cells in Sjögren's syndrome—from benign lymphoproliferation to overt malignancy. *Front Biosci.* 2007; 12: 2159–70.

Mackay IR, Rose NR. Autoimmunity and lymphoma: tribulations of B cells. *Nat Immunol.* 2001; 2(9): 793–5.

Mariette X, Gottenberg J, Theander E. Sjögren's syndrome and lymphoproliferations in autoimmune diseases. In Bijlsma, JW, ed. *EULAR Compendium on Rheumatic Diseases.* London: BMJ Publishing Group Ltd; Kilchberg: EULAR, 2009: 314–28.

Pillemer SR. Lymphoma and other malignancies in primary Sjögren's syndrome. *Ann Rheum Dis.* 2006; 65(6): 704–6.

Smedby KE, Baecklund E, Askling J. Malignant lymphomas in autoimmunity and inflammation: a review of risks, risk factors, and lymphoma characteristics. *Cancer Epidemiol Biomarkers Prev.* 2006; 15(11): 2069–77.

Theander E, Baecklund E. Sjögren's syndrome and cancer. In Ramos Casals M, Stone JH, Moutsopoulos HM, eds. *Sjögren's Syndrome: Diagnosis and Therapeutics*. Springer, 2011 (in press).

Theander E, Henriksson G, Ljungberg O, et al. Lymphoma and other malignancies in primary Sjögren's syndrome: a cohort study on cancer incidence and lymphoma predictors. *Ann Rheum Dis.* 2006; 65(6): 796–803.

Voulgarelis M, Moutsopoulos HM. Mucosa-associated lymphoid tissue lymphoma in Sjögren's syndrome: risks, management, and prognosis. *Rheum Dis Clin North Am.* 2008; 34(4): 921–33.

14

Diseases Associated with Sjögren's Syndrome

Frederick B. Vivino, MD, MS, FACR

A variety of disorders may coexist with Sjögren's syndrome and cause further patient morbidity. Early diagnosis is the key to successful management and may improve patient outcomes. The signs, symptoms, and relationship of these disorders to Sjögren's are discussed in the following chapter.

Definitions and Terms

Any disease associated with autoantibodies in the blood (i.e., antibodies directed against one's own cells or tissues) is considered **autoimmune**. The term **connective tissue disorders** or **collagen vascular diseases** refers to a group of chronic, autoimmune, inflammatory diseases that all cause musculoskeletal pain and autoantibodies in the blood and affect the connective tissues (what holds us together). Common symptoms include arthritis (swelling of the joints), joint pain, muscle pain or inflammation, Raynaud's phenomenon (see below), skin rashes, fatigue, interstitial lung disease (scarring of the lungs), esophageal dysmotility (disordered contraction of the esophagus), reflux, and kidney disease. Other internal organs may also be affected.

When a previously healthy person develops dry eyes and dry mouth associated with autoantibodies in the blood or a positive lip biopsy, he or she will be diagnosed with **primary Sjögren's syndrome**. When a person already has a known connective tissue disease (e.g., rheumatoid arthritis [RA] for 5 years) and then later develops dry eyes and dry mouth as a further complication, we call it **secondary Sjögren's syndrome** (i.e., secondary to the underlying disease). The ratio of patients with primary and secondary Sjögren's is roughly 1:1. These categories are currently defined according to the American European Consensus Group classification criteria (Table 14-1).

TABLE 14–1
Classification Criteria for Sjögren's Syndrome

1. **Ocular symptoms** (any 1 of 3)
   Dry eyes more than 3 months
   Tear use more than three times/day
   Foreign body sensation in eyes
2. **Oral symptoms** (1 of 3)
   Dry mouth more than 3 months
   Swollen salivary glands
   Need liquids to swallow
3. **Ocular signs** (1 of 2)
   Unanesthetized Schirmer's 5 mm/5 min or less O.U.
   Positive vital dye staining (Rose Bengal, fluorescein, lissamine green)
4. **Oral signs** (1of 3)
   Abnormal salivary gland scan
   Abnormal parotid sialography
   Abnormal salivary flow (unstimulated salivary flow 0.1 mL/min or less)
5. **Positive lip biopsy**
   Focal lymphocytic sialadenitis (focus score 1/4 mm^2 or more)
6. **Positive Anti-SSA and/or SSB antibodies**
   (Exclusions: hepatitis C, graft-versus-host disease, anticholinergic medications, etc.)
   Diagnosis of primary Sjögren's requires **4 of 6 criteria, including # 5 or 6.**
   Diagnosis of secondary Sjögren's requires established connective tissue disease, plus one
     sicca symptom (#1 or 2) plus 2 of 3 objective tests for dry eyes and mouth (#3–5).

Modified from Vitali et al. *Annals of Rheumatic Disease*, 2002.

Connective Tissue Disorders

The most important connective tissue disorders besides Sjögren's include RA, systemic lupus erythematosus (SLE), scleroderma, polymyositis, dermatomyositis, mixed connective tissue disease, undifferentiated connective tissue disease, and vasculitis.

RHEUMATOID ARTHRITIS

RA is the most common autoimmune rheumatic disease and may affect up to 1% to 1.5% of the North American population. It occurs most often in people 40 to 60 years old but may develop at any age, even in children. The female-to-male ratio is 2.5 to 1. As the name implies, the target organ for inflammation in RA is the joint, particularly the joint lining or synovium. RA patients typically develop painful swelling of small and large joints over a period of weeks to months (Table 14–2). A symmetrical polyarthritis develops over time. In rare cases this process occurs more acutely. The proximal interphalangeal and

TABLE 14–2
Criteria for the Classification of Rheumatoid Arthritis

1. Morning stiffness for more than 1 hour
2. Arthritis of more than three joint areas
3. Arthritis of hand joints (proximal interphalangeal and metacarpophalangeal) or wrists
4. Symmetrical arthritis
5. Rheumatoid nodules
6. Serum rheumatoid factor
7. Radiographic changes (erosions, periarticular demineralization)

Note: Criteria 1–4 must be present for at least 6 weeks. Classification or diagnosis as RA requires 4 of 7 criteria. Modified from *Arthritis Rheum* 1988;31:315–324.

metacarpophalangeal joints (the knuckles closest to the wrist) of the hands, wrists, elbows, shoulders, hips, knees, ankles, and feet are usually affected. The arthritis is associated with fatigue and generalized morning stiffness that can limit mobility and lasts 45 to 60 minutes or longer before maximal improvement. In some cases, subcutaneous nodules (rheumatoid nodules) develop around the elbows or at pressure points in the extremities.

The diagnosis of RA is based on clinical findings, laboratory studies, x-rays, and joint fluid analysis. The latter test is performed by taking a small sample of synovial fluid from a swollen joint to look for inflammation (i.e., white blood cell count >2,000/mm^3) and exclude infections and other causes of arthritis. The diagnosis of RA requires the presence of symptoms and signs for at least 6 weeks. Serum rheumatoid factor is positive in 70% to 80% of patients at onset and 90% of patients in advanced cases. Although helpful in diagnosis, serum rheumatoid factor is not specific for the disease and may occur in primary Sjögren's syndrome and other connective tissue diseases. X-rays in chronic cases show symmetrical narrowing of joint spaces due to cartilage loss, thinning of bone around inflamed joints (periarticular demineralization), and erosions. Erosions (little holes at the edges of the bone ends) develop as early as 1 year after onset and exemplify the destructive nature of RA. In a subset of patients the inflammation spreads to other organs and causes secondary Sjögren's syndrome and other problems. Patients with primary Sjögren's can also develop an inflammatory polyarthritis that resembles RA but erosions are not typically observed.

Most cases of RA require aggressive treatment, including multiple medications and physical therapy to prevent disability, deformity, and other complications. Nonsteroidal anti-inflammatory drugs (NSAIDs) (e.g., ibuprofen), oral and intra-articular steroids, hydroxychloroquine (Plaquenil), methotrexate, and the TNFα inhibitors etanercept (Enbrel), infliximab (Remicade), and adalimumab (Humira) are the most commonly used treatments. Rituximab (Rituxan) and abatacept (Orencia) are also used. Patients who fail to respond to medical therapy eventually may require joint replacement surgery.

SYSTEMIC LUPUS ERYTHEMATOSUS

SLE is a chronic autoimmune rheumatic disorder characterized by immune complex (antigen–antibody complex) deposition in various tissues, causing multiple organ disease and/or failure in association with antinuclear antibody (ANA) production in the blood. In North America, lupus affects approximately 0.05% of the general population and preferentially strikes young women (female-to-male ratio is 8:1) in the 15- to 40-year-old age group, especially African Americans. Less commonly, SLE occurs among men, children, older adults, and other ethnic/racial groups. Lupus can run in families.

Because lupus patients may manifest a myriad of medical problems, diagnosis can be challenging. However, the American College of Rheumatology has devised a set of research classification criteria that also provide a useful framework for diagnosis (Table 14–3).

The criteria recognize the high prevalence of mucocutaneous manifestations and autoantibody production in the disease. Four of 11 criteria must be satisfied either simultaneously or sequentially for classification as SLE. Since some patients don't exhibit the full-blown syndrome at disease onset, the diagnosis of lupus is sometimes suspected but not unequivocally confirmed until months to years later.

Lupus causes a variety of skin rashes, including hives, blisters, a measles-like rash, and a rash that resembles psoriasis. The most characteristic skin and mucous membrane abnormalities, however, include the malar rash, discoid rash, skin photosensitivity, oral ulcers, or nasal ulcers. The malar or butterfly rash looks like a red patch over the nasal bridge, nose, and cheeks in the shape of a butterfly and heals without scarring. In contrast, discoid lupus causes raised, red plaques on the head and extremities. These plaques are often associated with scaling and follicular plugging (skin pores/hair follicles develop

TABLE 14–3

Criteria for the Classification of Systemic Lupus Erythematosus

1. Malar rash
2. Discoid rash
3. Photosensitivity
4. Oral ulcers
5. Arthritis
6. Serositis
7. Renal disorder
8. Neurological disorder
9. Hematological disorder
10. Abnormal immunology test
11. Antinuclear antibody positivity

Note: Classification as SLE requires that 4 of 11 criteria be met. Modified from *Arthritis Rheum.* 1982;25;1271–7.

dark spots) and heal with loss of pigmentation, scarring, and/or loss of hair. In some instances patients with lupus develop severe skin rashes in sun-exposed areas (photosensitive rashes) following brief exposure to the sun or ultraviolet light. Painless or painful oral and nasal ulcers can also occur, especially in individuals with active skin disease.

The diagnostic hallmark of SLE is the presence of ANAs, found in up to 95% of patients when tested by indirect immunofluorescence using the Hep-2 cell substrate. Cases of ANA-negative lupus (i.e., patients with clinical lupus but a negative test) can be diagnosed by testing for anti-SSA and anti-SSB using a different assay system. Thus, the marker autoantibodies for Sjögren's, anti-SSB and anti-SSA, are also found in 15% to 45% of SLE patients. Anti-Sm antibodies are most specific for SLE but are found in less than 30% of patients. Anti–double-stranded-DNA antibodies occur in less than 60% of patients and correlate best with disease activity, especially lupus kidney disease. Titers tend to rise with disease flares and fall toward normal with improvement. In contrast, levels of complement (immune mediator proteins) C3, C4, and CH50 tend to fall with disease exacerbations (as immune complexes are formed and bind complement) but rise with remissions.

Constitutional symptoms in lupus include fevers, weight loss, malaise, and fatigue. Internal organ involvement in SLE also causes serious and sometimes life-threatening complications. Interstitial lung disease, pleurisy (inflammation of the lining around the lung), pleural effusions, inflammatory pneumonitis (pneumonia), and pulmonary hemorrhage all cause shortness of breath and, in the most severe cases, lead to respiratory failure. Pericarditis (inflammation of the heart lining) and pericardial effusions cause chest pain and shortness of breath. Heart failure, valvular heart disease, and accelerated coronary atherosclerosis also occur. Acute or chronic kidney inflammation (lupus nephritis) due to glomerulonephritis (inflammation of the kidney filtration units) or interstitial nephritis (inflammation of the tissues surrounding the glomeruli) leads to loss of kidney function and the appearance of protein, cells, and/or casts in the urine. In the most severe cases lupus nephritis may rapidly progress and necessitate prompt diagnosis and treatment to prevent dialysis and patient demise.

Critical complications can also develop with central nervous system involvement. Lupus can cause seizures, psychosis, coma, stroke, mini-stroke, mood disorders, confusion, cognitive dysfunction, chorea (movement disorders), transverse myelitis (spinal cord damage due to inflammation), and abnormalities of the cranial nerves. Peripheral neuropathies also occur. The musculoskeletal manifestations of lupus include arthralgias and myalgias (joint and muscle pain) along with polyarthritis. The arthritis of SLE can cause deformities similar to those seen in RA but rarely causes erosions. Hematological abnormalities in lupus include autoimmune hemolytic anemia and thrombocytopenia (low platelets). In these conditions the body forms antibodies against its own red blood cells or platelets, and patients develop fatigue, shortness of breath, or bleeding.

The 10-year survival rate in lupus is approximately 90%, and many patients have mild cases (e.g., skin rashes, joint pain) that do not require treatment with toxic drugs. Skin rashes, hair loss, and oral ulcers can be effectively managed with hydroxychloroquine, other antimalarial drugs, and/or topical steroids. Hydroxychloroquine and NSAIDs alleviate arthritis and joint or muscle pain. Use of oral steroids (e.g., prednisone), intravenous steroids, and/or more toxic immunosuppressives (e.g., azathioprine [Imuran], cyclophosphamide [Cytoxan]) is indicated in patients who fail to respond to more conservative measures or develop life-threatening problems such as hemolytic anemia, severe thrombocytopenia, or disease of the heart, lungs, kidneys, or central nervous system.

SCLERODERMA

As the name implies, scleroderma is an autoimmune rheumatic disease characterized by progressive thickening and induration of the skin in association with fibrosis (scarring) of the internal organs and thickening of small blood vessels. It affects a small percentage of the general population (0.02% to 0.075%), with peak occurrence at ages 35 to 65 years and a female preponderance. In early stages it causes puffiness of the hands, later followed by skin thickening on the fingers and toes. The skin on the digits becomes tight and shiny, like leather (sclerodactyly), and this process gradually spreads up the arms and legs to involve the face and, occasionally, the trunk as well. Diagnosis can be made by skin biopsy or documentation of skin involvement and typical features by an experienced clinician. Classification of a patient as having scleroderma requires the presence of one major and two minor criteria (Table 14–4).

Patients are classified into disease subsets and prognostic categories according to the degree of skin involvement and autoantibody profile. People with **limited scleroderma** have cutaneous thickening of the distal limbs

TABLE 14–4
Criteria for the Classification of Scleroderma

A. Major: Symmetrical thickening, tightening, and induration of skin above the metacarpophalangeal joints (where the fingers join the hands) <u>or</u> metatarsophalangeal joints (where the toes join the feet)

B. Minor
1. Sclerodactyly
2. Scarring of fingertips or loss of finger pads
3. Chest x-ray that shows scarring at the base of both lungs

Note: Classification of scleroderma requires one major or two minor criteria. Modified from *Arthritis Rheum.* 1980; 23: 581–90.

(below the elbows and knees) without truncal involvement and are typically anti-centromere antibody-positive (40% to 50%). Involvement of the face may occur but is not considered in this classification scheme. The CREST syndrome (calcinosis, Raynaud's, esophageal dysmotility, sclerodactyly, telangiectasias) falls within the classification scheme of limited systemic sclerosis. People with **diffuse scleroderma** have skin thickening above and below the elbows, knees, and/or trunk. They are typically anti-scleroderma or anti-Scl 70 antibody-positive (20% to 30%) and carry a worse prognosis due to greater internal organ disease.

Raynaud's phenomenon (cold-induced color changes in the fingers) is discussed further below and may predate the onset of scleroderma by months to years. When the skin thickening begins, patients can also develop itching, malaise, fatigue, arthritis, and musculoskeletal pain. Involvement of the gastrointestinal tract causes difficulty swallowing due to esophageal dysmotility (disordered contractions of the esophagus) and severe gastroesophageal reflux disease (GERD). Interstitial fibrosis and pulmonary hypertension (high blood pressure in the lungs) lead to progressive shortness of breath, especially during exertion. Pericarditis, pericardial effusions, heart rhythm abnormalities, and heart failure result from inflammation and scarring of cardiac tissue. Hypertension associated with acute renal failure, also called scleroderma renal crisis, is a medical emergency that may necessitate dialysis or cause patient demise. Muscle weakness due to myositis (muscle inflammation) can also occur.

Symptomatic treatments are available and used according to organ involvement. Some patients will note spontaneous improvement of skin thickening over time or following use of medications such as D-penicillamine, methotrexate or mycophenolate mofetil. Reflux is treated by diet and use of proton pump inhibitors (e.g., omeprazole [Prilosec]). Angiotensin-converting enzyme (ACE) inhibitors (e.g., captopril) can control blood pressure and preserve kidney function if initiated early in scleroderma renal crisis.

RAYNAUD'S PHENOMENON

Raynaud's phenomenon is defined as cold-induced color changes of the fingers, toes, nose, or earlobes that result from spasm and/or thickening of small arteries at involved sites. It can exist as an isolated problem (primary Raynaud's disease) or in association with any of the connective tissue disorders, including Sjögren's (secondary Raynaud's). It causes the worst problems among individuals with scleroderma. Patients typically develop blanching of part of the fingers or involved areas after exposure to cold, followed by cyanosis (bluing) and later erythema (redness) upon rewarming. Occasionally, episodes can be induced by nicotine from cigarette smoke or emotional stress. Primary Raynaud's disease usually affects young women and may be annoying to the patient but seldom causes significant discomfort or permanent damage. In contrast, secondary Raynaud's may cause ischemic pain and/or numbness followed eventually by complications such as digital ulcers, infections, loss of the fingertip pads or bone, and digital gangrene (blackening of the fingers). Patients are counseled to avoid the cold and other precipitating factors. Patients are also treated with calcium channel blockers such as nifedipine (Procardia) to relax the blood vessels and with antiplatelet agents, such as aspirin, to prevent clots. Phosphodiesterase inhibitors that are used to treat erectile dysfunction (e.g., sildenafil [Viagra]) may also provide relief. The most severe cases require use of intravenous medications, nerve blocks, or surgical amputation.

POLYMYOSITIS AND DERMATOMYOSITIS

Polymyositis and dermatomyositis represent a group of autoimmune rheumatic diseases that cause skeletal muscle weakness and inflammation (myositis). Dermatomyositis also causes a characteristic rash. These disorders affect 0.05% to 0.08% of the population, with peak age at onset of 10 to 15 years in children and 45 to 60 years in adults. The female-to-male ratio is 2:1. Polymyositis is more common than dermatomyositis in adults, and the reverse is true for children.

Patients insidiously develop symmetrical weakness of proximal muscles around the shoulders and hips over weeks to months. This may cause difficulty getting up from a chair, climbing stairs, walking, or raising an arm to comb the hair or hang up a coat. The myositis may spread to muscles that control breathing or swallowing and cause shortness of breath or dysphagia (difficulty swallowing). Other problems include fatigue, arthritis, joint and muscle pain, Raynaud's, interstitial lung disease, GERD, esophageal dysmotility, and heart failure. Secondary Sjögren's can also complicate polymyositis and dermatomyositis, and myositis can occasionally be a manifestation of primary Sjögren's.

People with dermatomyositis exhibit one or more of several characteristics rashes. These include the heliotrope rash (lilac discoloration of the eyelids), Gottron's sign (a scaly, red rash over the knuckles), shawl sign (redness of the posterior shoulders and neck), and the V-sign (redness of the anterior neck and upper chest). Children with dermatomyositis often develop ectopic calcifications (painful calcium deposits of the skeletal muscle and subcutaneous tissues). The diagnosis of polymyositis and dermatomyositis is suspected when the skeletal muscle enzymes creatine phosphokinase (CPK) and aldolase are elevated in the blood of a patient who is weak. An electromyographic (EMG) study will demonstrate abnormal electrical activity of the muscles and will help eliminate a neuropathy as the cause of the weakness. The diagnosis is confirmed by biopsy of an involved muscle that shows damage and infiltration of muscle fibers by lymphocytes and other inflammatory cells.

Most patients with polymyositis and dermatomyositis respond to treatment with high-dose oral and/or intravenous steroids followed by physical therapy for gait training and muscle strengthening. Patients who fail to respond to steroids or develop unacceptable side effects may be treated with other immunosuppressive agents, including methotrexate, azathioprine, cyclosporine, and intravenous gamma globulin.

MIXED CONNECTIVE TISSUE DISEASE

Mixed connective tissue disease, as originally described, denotes a subset of connective tissue disease patients whose blood contains high titers of anti-RNP (ribonucleoprotein) antibodies. Antinuclear antibodies and rheumatoid factor are also observed. Patients typically manifest features of several different connective tissue diseases, including RA, SLE, scleroderma, and polymyositis and dermatomyositis. Secondary Sjögren's may also occur. The most common signs and symptoms include puffy hands, sclerodactyly, Raynaud's, skin rashes, pleurisy, polyarthritis, dysphagia, reflux, myalgias, and myositis. Most patients evolve into classic lupus or scleroderma over time, and autoantibody profiles may change. When patients meet diagnostic criteria for only two different collagen vascular diseases at the time of diagnosis, the term **overlap syndrome** is preferred.

Secondary Sjögren's Syndrome: Clinical Manifestations, Diagnosis, and Prevalence

The onset of secondary Sjögren's syndrome among connective tissue disease patients is highly variable (1 to 40 years after diagnosis of the primary underlying disorder) but occurs in the majority of people about 5 to 10 years after diagnosis of the underlying connective tissue disease. Sicca symptoms in secondary Sjögren's are generally milder than those of primary Sjögren's. It remains unclear whether this phenomenon reflects lesser severity or earlier diagnosis facilitated as a benefit of regular rheumatological care for other problems. Clearly, however, the prevalence of salivary gland swelling, adenopathy (swelling of the lymph nodes), and lymphomas in secondary Sjögren's is diminished compared to its primary counterpart.

Some studies suggest that dry eye occurs more commonly than dry mouth in lupus and RA patients with secondary Sjögren's, while in patients with scleroderma and secondary Sjögren's, the reverse seems true. Interestingly, in scleroderma, secondary Sjögren's occurs more commonly among the limited variant than the diffuse form of the disease. Treatments for these patient groups are typically directed toward the underlying disease. However, symptomatic patients with secondary Sjögren's may also benefit from therapy with secretagogues and other measures for dryness.

The prevalence of secondary Sjögren's in other collagen vascular disorders is variable and depends on how this diagnosis is made. When older diagnostic criteria were applied to large patient populations, prevalence figures for secondary Sjögren's of 31%, 20%, and 20% were reported in patients with RA, SLE, and scleroderma, respectively. According to one survey, anti-SSA and anti-SSB are normally present in primary Sjögren's and SLE, as described above, but become more prevalent in all patient groups with the development of secondary Sjögren's: RA (24%/6%), SLE (73%/46%), and scleroderma (33%/18%). Studies of positive lip biopsies in the same patient groups suggest prevalence figures that are even higher: RA 35%, SLE 18% to 90%, and scleroderma 17% to 51%). Interestingly, the proportion of patients with positive biopsies in these studies was always substantially higher than the number of patients with symptoms. Future studies of prevalence using the new classification criteria will provide more precise information on prevalence.

How Sjögren's Syndrome May Influence the Expression of Other Connective Tissue Diseases

Little information is available regarding the influence of secondary Sjögren's on the course of other connective tissue diseases. In RA patients the coexistence of secondary Sjögren's reportedly has little effect on the course of arthritis or other clinical manifestations. However, dryness of the gastrointestinal tract from Sjögren's could potentially exacerbate a variety of problems common to these disorders, including reflux, dysphagia, dyspepsia (upset stomach), and constipation. Respiratory dryness from Sjögren's could not only aggravate chronic cough due to interstitial lung disease but also predispose to recurrent respiratory infections. In lupus, two studies suggest that secondary Sjögren's is associated with an increased incidence of erosive polyarthritis, an uncommon complication of SLE. In scleroderma, a study of over 800 people reported that patients with systemic sclerosis and secondary Sjögren's (particularly the CREST variant) were at increased risk of developing vasculitis. Another study reported that autoimmune liver disease, particularly primary biliary cirrhosis, was more prevalent in scleroderma patients with secondary Sjögren's compared to scleroderma patients alone. Further studies will shed additional light on these observations.

Antiphospholipid Antibody Syndrome (APS)

APS is an autoimmune disorder characterized by recurrent arterial and venous thromboses (blood clots) and/or recurrent spontaneous abortions (miscarriages) associated with the presence of antibodies to phospholipids in the blood.

It can occur by itself as a primary disorder (primary APS) or in association with connective tissue diseases (secondary APS), most notably SLE. Its occurrence in primary Sjögren's syndrome is infrequent. It most commonly causes deep venous thromboses (blood clots) in the arms and legs, pulmonary emboli (clots in the lungs), strokes, mini-strokes, or recurrent miscarriages (usually in the second or third trimester). Blood clots must be documented by objective medical testing, and antibody presence is demonstrated when one or more of the following blood tests is positive: anticardiolipin antibodies, lupus anticoagulant, or anti-B$_2$ glycoprotein I. Platelet counts may be low in APS, but this doesn't prevent clots.

The major treatment is lifelong anticoagulation with blood thinners such as heparin or warfarin. Other causes of blood clots and pregnancy loss must always be excluded in the diagnostic evaluation. The antibodies may occasionally occur in normal people and don't always cause clots when present.

Vasculitis

Vasculitis is a broad term that describes a heterogeneous group of about 30 collagen vascular disorders that cause blood vessel inflammation with subsequent damage to the vessel wall, tissue necrosis from ischemia (poor blood supply), and in some cases eventual organ failure. Clinical manifestations vary according to the site of involvement. It can be localized to a single organ or cause systemic disease. Vasculitis can exist as a primary disorder (e.g., polyarteritis nodosa) or occur as a complication of another connective tissue disease, including Sjögren's. It can sometimes be precipitated by infections or medications. Vasculitic disorders are grouped according to (1) the size and type of vessel involved, (2) the type of cells that cause the vessel inflammation, (3) etiology, and (4) affected organs.

The subset of Sjögren's patients with extra-glandular manifestations (i.e., serious internal organ disease) seem to be at greatest risk to develop vasculitis. Laboratory clues may include the appearance of cryoglobulins in the blood (proteins that precipitate out in the cold); high titers of anti-SSA antibodies; elevation of serum IgG, gamma globulins, or the erythrocyte sedimentation rate; low levels of complement C3 or C4; or positive anti-neutrophil cytoplasmic (ANCA) antibodies. However, like other patient groups, the definitive diagnosis of vasculitis in Sjögren's can only be made by biopsy of an involved organ or by doing an arteriogram. The biopsy should show invasion and/or damage of blood vessel walls by inflammatory cells. The arteriogram is performed by injecting radiopaque contrast dye into an artery to look for abnormalities of vessel shape, including aneurysms, segmental narrowing, or dilatation.

The skin is the most frequent site of vasculitis in Sjögren's syndrome. Cutaneous vasculitis affects small vessels (arterioles, capillaries, venules) and typically causes raised reddish-purple spots on the legs, called palpable purpura. These lesions may be painful or pruritic. Other vasculitic rashes in Sjögren's include urticaria (hives), skin ulcers, or erythema multiforme (red spots of variable size and shape). Vasculitic involvement of small to medium-sized arteries in Sjögren's syndrome will occasionally affect the nervous system and cause strokes, mini-strokes, or peripheral neuropathies. A particular type of peripheral neuropathy, mononeuritis multiplex, is highly suggestive of vasculitis and is suspected when the patient develops foot drop associated with patchy loss of sensation in the lower extremities. The diagnosis is confirmed by performing an EMG/nerve conduction study of the legs followed by biopsy of the sural nerve. Vasculitis of the medium-sized arteries of abdominal organs is rare in Sjögren's but can cause life-threatening complications. The diagnosis is proven by arteriogram or examination of tissue specimens obtained during emergency surgery.

Treatments for vasculitis vary with the organs involved but in some cases prove to be long, difficult, and extremely toxic. Therefore, every effort should be made to obtain a proper diagnosis at the time of initial presentation and exclude other disorders that cause similar symptoms but require different treatments.

Undifferentiated Connective Tissue Disease

This term describes a group of individuals who exhibit signs and symptoms of connective tissue disease as described above and are ANA-positive but anti-RNP-negative. These patients fail to meet the diagnostic criteria for any one specific disorder. They may complain of sicca symptoms, but lip biopsies are typically negative. In some cases, a change over time in clinical features or autoantibody profile may yield a specific diagnosis. Treatments vary according to major symptoms.

Evolution of Sjögren's into Other Disorders

As alluded to previously, patients with various connective tissue disorders, including Sjögren's syndrome, share overlapping clinical and laboratory features and are sometimes difficult to tell apart. RA, for example, may be complicated by secondary Sjögren's, and the initial manifestations of primary Sjögren's can include a rheumatoid-like polyarthritis with rheumatoid factor in the blood. Sjögren's was once thought to be a benign variant of lupus, and the presence of anti-SSA and anti-SSB antibodies in both diseases suggests a common pathogenic mechanism. Reports also exist in the medical literature of patients who met criteria for both diseases at the time of presentation and were therefore felt to have an SLE/Sjögren's overlap syndrome. Not surprisingly, there are even reports of individuals who started with one disease and evolved into another.

One study from France described 55 patients who presented with sicca symptoms, anti-SSA or anti-SSB, and other manifestations of connective tissue disease and who fulfilled the European diagnostic criteria for primary Sjögren's. Other autoantibodies tested negative. During a subsequent period of 12 to 14 years, four patients developed new signs and symptoms (malar rash, pleuropericarditis, glomerulonephritis) thought to be atypical for Sjögren's. Follow-up testing revealed the presence of anti-Sm (two patients) and anti–double-stranded DNA (two patients) antibodies. These patients were eventually diagnosed with SLE according to the American College of Rheumatology criteria. In another report a patient with primary Sjögren's (dry eye, dry mouth, anti-SSA/anti-SSB) turned anti-centromere-positive about 3 years after he developed parotid swelling and renal tubular acidosis (failure of the kidneys to excrete acid form the blood). He was eventually diagnosed with the CREST variant of scleroderma following the onset of Raynaud's phenomenon, digital ischemia, nail fold capillary dropout, and telangiectasias (dilated small vessels in the skin that cause red spots). Thus, in clinical situations where new symptoms cannot be explained by an established diagnosis of Sjögren's, further evaluation and consideration of a new diagnosis may be necessary.

Other Autoimmune Disorders Associated with Sjögren's

Other autoimmune disorders that primarily affect a single organ system may coexist with primary Sjögren's but are not strictly classed among the connective tissue diseases (Table 14–5).

Any patient with known autoimmune disease is at increased risk for developing a second autoimmune disorder. Autoimmune disorders (but not always the same disease) typically run in families. This phenomenon occurs due to common inheritance of immune response genes that predispose to one or more of these disorders. A second autoimmune disease can be difficult to diagnose in

TABLE 14–5
Autoimmune Diseases Associated with Sjögren's Syndrome

Hashimoto's thyroiditis	Celiac sprue
Graves disease	Multiple sclerosis
Primary biliary cirrhosis	Myasthenia gravis
Chronic active autoimmune hepatitis	Pernicious anemia
Addison's disease	Interstitial cystitis

Sjögren's because symptoms often begin insidiously and overlap with those of primary Sjögren's. Some of these disorders are discussed below.

HASHIMOTO'S THYROIDITIS

This autoimmune disease can be associated with Sjögren's and cause thyroid enlargement (goiter), thyroid nodules, and most commonly hypothyroidism. Hypothyroidism can also result from other etiologies and causes fatigue, dry skin, coarse hair, constipation, headaches, arthralgias, myalgias, facial swelling, cognitive dysfunction, and hoarseness. Hypothyroidism is diagnosed by blood tests (high TSH, low or normal free T4). Hashimoto's is confirmed by the presence of one or more thyroid autoantibodies in the blood, including anti-microsomal and anti-thyroid peroxidase antibodies. It is treated with thyroid hormone replacement. Frequent monitoring of thyroid function tests is required.

CELIAC DISEASE

Celiac disease (a.k.a. celiac sprue, nontropicial sprue, or gluten-sensitive enteropathy) is a common autoimmune disease that targets the small intestine and may cause multiple organ problems. It can present in children and adults and is now thought to affect as many as 1:132 people in the United States. It often runs in families. Celiac can be an isolated problem or coexist with other diseases, including Sjögren's. Studies suggest that up to 97% of celiacs share the same genes (HLA-DQ2 and/or HLA DQ8), which are found in only 40% of the normal population. Celiac is caused by an abnormal immune response to gluten, a protein found in wheat, barley, rye, oats, and many other foods. Repeated exposure to dietary gluten stimulates an inflammatory reaction (genetically controlled) in the small intestine that leads to malabsorption, nutrient deficiencies, and other heath problems.

Symptoms may include weight loss, abdominal pain, diarrhea, bloating, anemia (especially iron deficiency anemia), vitamin D deficiency, osteoporosis, fatigue, headaches, neurological problems, dermatitis herpetiformis (shingles-like skin rash), and other symptoms. Celiac is most often diagnosed by blood tests or a biopsy of the small intestine. Serum IgA anti-tissue transglutaminase and IgA anti-endomyseal antibodies have the highest sensitivity and specificity. For patients who are IgA-deficient (up to 1:500 individuals), an IgG anti-tissue transglutaminase and IgG anti-endomysial antibody test should be done. An intestinal biopsy will show lymphocyte infiltration of epithelial cells or the lamina propria (inflammation of the intestinal lining cells or layer below) and shrinkage/flattening of intestinal villi (finger-like projections of intestinal surface that absorb nutrients). Genetic testing can be helpful in doubtful cases.

Currently, the major treatment is to follow a life-long gluten-free diet. Consultation with a registered dietitian can be extremely helpful. Other resources are available (see below). In most cases, strict adherence to the diet will lead to complete resolution of symptoms over weeks to months. Some diagnostic tests may also improve or normalize. Therefore, all diagnostic testing should ideally be completed before initiation of the diet. Several drugs that change or interfere with the body's handling of gluten or the subsequent immune response are under development and could provide a greater variety of therapeutic options in the future.

INTERSTITIAL CYSTITIS

The term **interstitial cystitis** (a.k.a. bladder pain syndrome) refers to a family of conditions that all cause bladder or pelvic pain, urinary frequency, and urinary urgency in the absence of infection. The majority of affected patients are female (ratio 9:1), and symptoms typically worsen during menstruation or when under stress. This condition also causes pain during vaginal intercourse and frequent nighttime urination. Interstitial cystitis can be associated with autoimmune diseases like SLE and Sjögren's.

Diagnostic evaluation usually includes a urinalysis and culture, cystoscopy (insertion of a small scope in the bladder), biopsy of the bladder wall, and distention of the bladder under anesthesia. Cystoscopy may show glomerulations (areas of pinpoint bleeding) or Hunner's ulcers (patches of eroded lining on the bladder wall). A biopsy of the bladder wall will demonstrate inflammation and is also performed to rule out cancer. A variety of treatments may alleviate symptoms and include dietary modification, pelvic floor exercises, bladder training techniques, instillation of dimethyl sulfoxide (DMSO) into the bladder, smoking cessation, electrical stimulation using TENS or devices (InterStim System), and analgesics or other medications such as pentosan (Elmiron) or amitriptyline (Elavil).

FIBROMYALGIA

Fibromyalgia is not considered an autoimmune disease but nevertheless represents an important comorbidity in Sjögren's that can exacerbate pain, fatigue, and cognitive dysfunction. Fibromyalgia may be due to an abnormality of pain processing in the central nervous system or related to problems with sleep. In Sjögren's, sleep abnormalities are common and may result from nighttime dryness of the eyes and mouth or occur for other reasons. One study also observed an increased incidence of restless leg syndrome in Sjögren's at bedtime compared to other groups. Besides disturbed sleep, patients also note whole body pain, morning stiffness, fatigue, and modulation of symptoms by the weather (symptoms usually worst on cold, damp days). Patients frequently have trouble falling asleep or staying asleep or admit to nonrestorative sleep (i.e., waking up tired). Other symptoms can include joint swelling, numbness and tingling of the extremities, dry eyes, dry mouth, and "brain fog" (memory loss, difficulty with concentration).

Fibromyalgia can be easily misdiagnosed as Sjögren's or vice versa or can coexist with Sjögren's. It can be found in 47% to 55% patients with Sjögren's, depending on the study. Fibromyalgia may be associated with a variety of other disorders, including irritable bowel syndrome (spastic colon), bladder pain syndrome, temporomandibular joint syndrome (TMJ), migraines, depression, and costochondritis.

The diagnosis is based on clinical findings. On physical examination numerous "tender points" (localized areas of muscular tenderness) are found in the characteristic areas (Fig. 14–1) when 4 kg of local pressure (enough to blanch your thumbnail) is applied. It is not necessary to have all 18 tender points in order to make this diagnosis. Patients with fibromyalgia may have tenderness in other areas as well. Despite patient complaints of joint swelling and tingling of the extremities, no objective abnormalities of the joints or nervous system are typically observed on physical examination.

Blood tests are usually done to rule out other causes of muscle pain (e.g., hypothyroidism, vitamin D deficiency). In certain individuals sleep studies are performed to look for potentially treatable causes of disturbed sleep such as sleep apnea, upper airway resistance syndrome, restless leg syndrome, or periodic limb movement disorder of sleep. In fibromyalgia, the most commonly

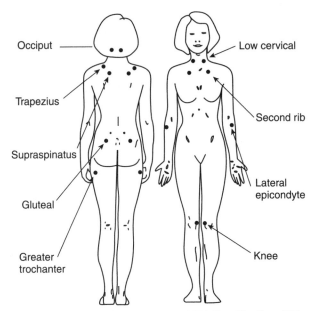

FIGURE 14–1 **The American College of Rheumatology 1990 Classification of Fibromyalgia: Distribution of Tender Points.**

observed sleep study pattern is termed "alpha wave intrusion in delta non-REM sleep." A similar pattern may also be observed in other patients with chronic pain syndromes. Specific treatments are generally directed at finding ways to promote restful sleep, palliate pain, and improve patient function.

Summing Up

A variety of connective tissue diseases and other disorders (both autoimmune and non-autoimmune) can coexist with Sjögren's syndrome and add to the patient's burden of illness. Each of these conditions presents unique challenges that affect the diagnosis and management of Sjögren's.

FOR FURTHER READING

Fassano A. Surprises from celiac disease: part I and II. *The Moisture Seekers*. Sjögren's Syndrome Foundation, December 2009–January 2010.

Klippel J, Crofford L, Stone J, Weyland C, eds. *Primer on the Rheumatic Diseases*, 13th ed. Atlanta: Arthritis Foundation, 2008.

Libonati C. *Recognizing Celiac Disease*. Fort Washington, PA: Gluten Free Works Publishing, 2007.

Lowell JP. *The Gluten Free Bible*. New York: Henry Holt and Co., 2005.

Wallace D, Wallace J. *All About Fibromyalgia: A Guide for Patients and Their Families*. New York: Oxford University Press, 2002.

15

The Dry Eye
Abha Gulati, MD, Reza Dana, MD, MPH, M.Sc., and
Gary N. Foulks, MD, FACS

Dry eye, also called keratoconjunctivitis sicca (KCS), is a component of the dryness (sicca) that characterizes Sjögren's syndrome. A recent survey of the members of the Sjögren's Syndrome Foundation determined that dry eye is the most bothersome symptom to many patients with Sjögren's. Since the tears serve to protect the front of the eye and provide a smooth surface that maintains clear vision and comfort, the tear film is an important feature of the healthy eye. Disruption of the tear film produces discomfort and disturbance of vision as well as possible damage to the ocular surface. The ocular surface consists of the conjunctiva (the mucous membrane covering the outside of the eyeball and the inner lining of the eyelids) and the cornea (the central transparent part of the eyeball that helps focus the entering light rays). Dry eye syndrome includes a variety of disorders that affect the ocular surface, both conjunctiva and cornea.

> Dry eye is a multifactorial disease of the tears and ocular surface that results in symptoms of discomfort, visual disturbance, and tear film instability with potential damage to the ocular surface. It is accompanied by increased osmolarity of the tear film and inflammation of the ocular surface.

There are greater than 20 million dry eye sufferers in the United States and approximately 4 million of these people also have Sjögren's syndrome. The dry eye associated with Sjögren's syndrome (KCS) is generally more severe and requires more intensive therapy.

What Causes Dry Eye?

The tear film that covers the surface of the eye is normally uniformly spread across the eye in a very stable layer. The tear film has been described as consisting of three layers: (1) a superficial lipid layer, (2) a middle aqueous layer, and

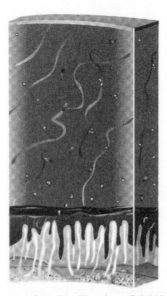

Superficial lipid layer
~ 0.1 – 0.2 microns thick

Aqueous layer
~ 7 – 8 microns thick

Adsorbed mucin layer
over 1 micron thick

Microvilli of epithelium
extend into and stabilize
mucin layer

FIGURE 15–1 **Layers of the Tear Film: Superficial Lipid Layer, Middle Aqueous Layer, and Deeper Mucin Layer.**
Interactions of lipids with proteins do occur within the aqueous layer.

(3) a deep mucin layer (Fig. 15–1), but recent studies suggest that there is significant interaction between the proteins and lipids in the aqueous layer. The aqueous layer forms the greatest bulk of the tear film and is secreted by the lacrimal (tear-producing) glands (Fig. 15–2). The aqueous layer contains water-soluble factors and electrolytes that wet the ocular surface and provide nutrition to the cornea as well as mechanical clearing of debris and microorganisms. The proteins contained in the aqueous layer inhibit growth of organisms and contain growth factors for the ocular surface cells. Disruption of the tear film either because of inadequate secretion of tears (aqueous deficient dry eye) or excess evaporation of the tear fluid (evaporative dry eye) can result in dry spots and damage to the ocular surface. One of the most common causes of evaporative dry eye is obstruction of the lipid-producing glands in the eyelid (meibomian glands) (Fig. 15–2). Both aqueous-deficient and evaporative dry eye occur frequently in patients with Sjögren's, and they can occur together.

What Damage Can Occur to the Surface of the Eye from Dry Eye?

When the tear film is unstable or too concentrated, it can damage the surface of the eye. Loss of the lubricating ability of the tear film results in greater blink-induced shear force of the eyelid against the ocular surface. This increased shear force can cause changes in the cells of the ocular surface. The normal tear

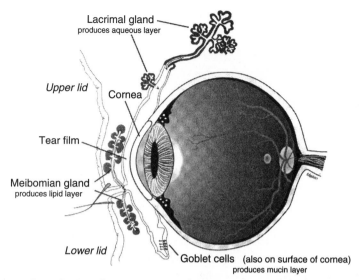

Lacrimal gland
produces aqueous layer

Upper lid

Cornea

Tear film

Meibomian gland
produces lipid layer

Lower lid

Goblet cells (also on surface of cornea)
produces mucin layer

FIGURE 15–2 **Cross-Section of the Eye Showing Tear Film-Producing Structures.**
Lacrimal glands produce aqueous tears. Meibomian glands produce lipids. Goblet cells produce mucin.

film also contains essential growth factors that are required for surface cell healing; deficiency of these factors contributes to impaired healing of the damaged surface in dry eye patients.

The corneal epithelium (the most superficial cell layer) provides a protective barrier between the environment and the underlying structures of the eye. In moderate to severe dry eye there is increasing loss of corneal epithelial cells, which are replaced by smaller epithelial cells, or there may be loss of cells to cause persistent epithelial defects since the normal healing process is impaired. In severe cases of dry eye, corneal defects may enlarge and deepen to produce corneal ulcers that lead to thinning of the cornea. Such ulcers, although usually sterile, may become secondarily infected. In the most severe cases, the cornea can thin considerably (melt) and even perforate. Melting of the cornea is most often seen in patients who have rheumatoid arthritis.

The dry eye tear film has a higher concentration of electrolytes and molecules that increase the osmolarity of the tears. This elevated osmolarity can stimulate inflammation in the ocular surface, which releases chemicals that can also damage the corneal surface and produce symptoms of irritation in the eye. In time, the combined damaging effects on the cornea lead to decreased sensation of the surface of the eye, which further retards normal healing.

Paralleling the decrease in tear secretion from the lacrimal glands is a decrease in certain enzymes in the tears (lysozyme, lactoferrin, and others) as well as normally secreted antibodies that protect the eye against infection. Absence of these protective agents results in decreased resistance to infection.

Dry eye patients who wear contact lenses are at higher risk of developing infections of the cornea, presumably due to increased adherence of bacteria to the contact lens and the ocular surface.

How Does One Recognize Dry Eye?

The patient history is extremely important in diagnosing dry eye. Most symptoms in patients with KCS result from instability of the tear film, producing discomfort and fluctuation of vision for prolonged reading or near tasks. Further symptoms occur because the lubrication of the surface is inadequate, resulting in reduced ability of the ocular surface to respond normally to environmental challenges. Symptoms vary from one patient to another depending upon the severity of the dryness and the patient's tolerance for ocular discomfort. Patients often use the term "dryness" to describe their symptoms but may have difficulty defining exactly what it means. Burning, itching, a sensation of a foreign object in the eye, a sandy sensation, and light sensitivity also may be reported. Some patients describe their discomfort as fatigue of the eye.

The principal function of the tear film is to maintain a smooth, clear refractive corneal surface in a hostile external environment. Any adverse effect on the corneal regularity and clarity will interfere with vision; instability of the tear film is such an adverse event. Thus, blurred vision, particularly for near tasks or prolonged reading, may also be one of the initial complaints in a dry eye patient. It is somewhat like looking through a dirty windshield. If the dry eye is due to evaporation, then the vision may be improved by blinking frequently. Patients may also complain of excess secretion of mucus, heaviness of the eyelids, and inability to produce tears when crying. Associated inflammation of the surface of the eye may cause pain and redness. Pain may also be due to filaments, which are strands of adherent mucus that are covered by epithelial cells on the corneal surface (Fig. 15–3).

Dry eye patients are highly sensitive to winds and drafts. They often volunteer that they are intolerant to air conditioning and riding in a car with the window down. Reading is often difficult for dry eye sufferers, as is prolonged work at a computer. Some patients complain that they have discomfort on awakening, which may be due to further decreased tear production during sleep, but most patients describe increasing discomfort as the day progresses, particularly if they have been doing prolonged computer work or reading. Smoke in the air is almost universally intolerable to tear-deficient patients.

Patients may not be able to produce tears in response to irritant or emotional situations. Inability to cry when peeling onions or when hurt suggests severe compromise of lacrimal gland function. Some patients will report having used artificial tears or ointments for relief of symptoms, and although most patients with dry eye will improve with topical lubricant therapy, excessive use

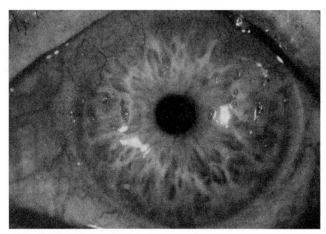

FIGURE 15–3 **Filamentary Keratopathy.**
Strands of mucus adherent to cornea.

of artificial tears containing preservatives may actually worsen the symptoms. Some systemic medications such as antihistamines and antidepressants may worsen symptoms by decreasing tear production.

A history of other associated systemic signs of dryness is important in identifying the sicca condition. Dry mouth or vaginal dryness can be other signs of Sjögren's. Patients with severe dry mouth may have difficulty swallowing crackers, bread, or meat without additional fluids. Such patients are also at risk of dental and gum disease due to lack of saliva. Women may experience a decrease in vaginal secretions, which can lead to sexual dysfunction. It is helpful to know if there is a family history of any blood relative with dry eye, Sjögren's, collagen vascular disease, or other eye disease.

Evaluation of Dry Eye

CLINICAL EXAMINATION

A full clinical examination is advisable as part of the evaluation of dry eye. Facial skin must be inspected for evidence of rosacea, a skin condition commonly associated with meibomian gland dysfunction and evaporative dry eye. Salivary gland enlargement may occur in patients with Sjögren's. The thyroid gland also should be examined for signs of enlargement or presence of nodules, as this may be seen in Sjögren's as well.

Examination of the eye includes evaluation of the lacrimal glands to determine whether there is enlargement or signs of inflammation. Redness of the eyes due to dilated conjunctival blood vessels can be a sign of inflammation of the surface of the eye, which occurs in moderate to severe dry eye.

Detailed examination of the ocular surface, including cornea and conjunctiva, is best done with magnification using the slit-lamp biomicroscope. Distortion of the light reflexes on the cornea indicates disruption of the tear film or damage to the superficial cells of the cornea. There may be excess mucus fragments or debris in the tear film. Sometimes mucus strands stick to the cornea at sites of focal desiccation and surface cells extend onto the strand, making it very adherent to the cornea. Filaments can cause discomfort or even pain when blinking pulls on the strand. This condition is called filamentary keratopathy.

The health of the meibomian glands in the eyelid must be examined to determine if thick, turbid secretions are obstructing the glands. Foam in the tear film suggests meibomian gland dysfunction. The eyelid margins are examined for thickening of the lid margin, increased numbers of blood vessels, broken or missing eyelashes, or other signs of inflammation (blepharitis) in the eyelid.

TEAR FUNCTION TESTING

The Schirmer Test

The Schirmer test is the most traditional test to determine the level of tear production. Small strips of filter paper 35 mm long are placed on the lateral lower eyelid margin of both eyes and left in place for 5 minutes (Fig. 15–4). The amount of wetting of the strip is measured; less than 7 mm of wetting suggests dry eye. There is great variability in this test, however, and it can be affected by environmental conditions of temperature and humidity as well as the level of room illumination.

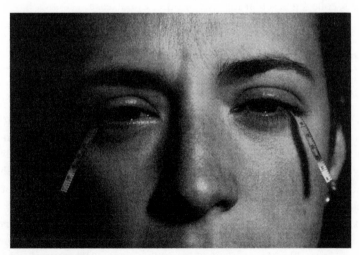

FIGURE 15–4 **Schirmer Test.**
Tear production is measured by length of wetting of the filter strip.

Tear Breakup Test

Measurement of tear breakup time (TBUT) is a standard part of the evaluation of dry eye since instability of the tear film is a characteristic of both forms of dry eye. TBUT is a measure of how well the cornea remains moist between blinks. Typically the test is done by instilling a small amount of fluorescein dye into the tear film and having the patient blink several times. The observer at the slit-lamp will measure the time between when the patient blinks and the first evidence of tear film disruption, seen as a dark spot in the otherwise green-colored tear film, occurs. The normal TBUT is considered more than 10 seconds.

Tear Osmolarity Test

Tear osmolarity testing measures the concentration of the tear film which can be elevated in either aqueous-deficient or evaporative dry eye. In-office testing is now available and provides an easy, rapid, and reliable measure of tear function (Fig. 15–5). Since increased tear osmolarity plays an important role in damage to the ocular surface, this test can be a valuable diagnostic test and a potential monitor of the effectiveness of therapy.

Fluorescein Test

Fluorescein staining of the surface of the eye is an effective way to determine the stability of the tear film and the integrity of the ocular surface. It is an orange dye that fluoresces green when illuminated by a blue light to reveal disruptions of the cells of the surface of the eye. Fluorescein staining is a standard method of demonstrating damage to the surface of the eye (Fig. 15–6).

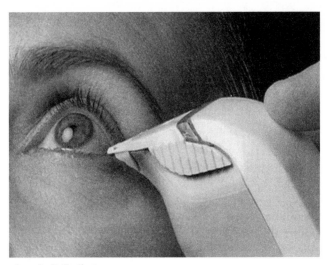

FIGURE 15–5 **Osmolarity Testing.**
The TearLab Osmometer in use.

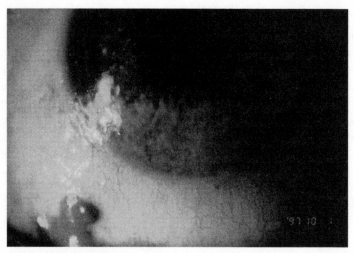

FIGURE 15–6 **Fluorescein Staining of Cornea.**

Rose Bengal and Lissamine Green Test

Rose Bengal and lissamine green dyes are used to determine if surface cells of the eye have lost their normal mucin coating. Both stains demonstrate similar abnormalities, but Rose Bengal provides a more intense pink stain while lissamine green provides a more subtle blue stain of damaged or mucin-deficient cells (Fig. 15–7). Rose Bengal has the disadvantage of stinging on application; lissamine green is less irritating. Since loss of the protective mucin covering of the cells is a feature of dry eye, these dyes help to determine the severity of the dryness and the degree of damage to the surface of the eye.

LABORATORY TESTS

Tear Lysozyme and Lactoferrin

Tear lysozyme and lactoferrin levels can be measured by a number of methods. Normal tear lysozyme levels are between 2 and 4 mg/mL. Normal lactoferrin level is above 0.9 mg/mL. Sjögren's-related dry eye results in decreased levels of these antibacterial enzymes.

Tear Proteins

Tear protein analysis can be performed by several different tests. Electrophoresis is a method to separate various proteins in tears using electric gradients. Enzyme-linked immunosorbent assay (ELISA) testing identifies proteins by using antibodies directed against specific proteins in the tear film. Protein array analysis can measure large numbers of proteins and identify patterns associated with dry eye. Decreased levels of the goblet cell-specific mucin MUC5AC have been demonstrated in tears of patients with Sjögren's.

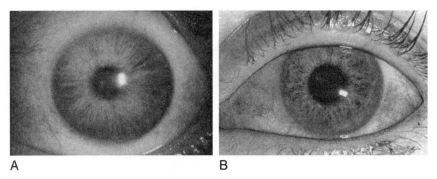

A   B

FIGURE 15–7 **Rose Bengal (A) and Lissamine Green (B) Staining of the Conjunctiva.**

Conjunctival Impression Cytology

Conjunctival impression cytology is a method of sampling superficial cells of the surface of the eye using application of a specific filter paper to the anesthetized surface of the eye. In addition to detecting characteristics of cells of the surface that can indicate the presence of dry eye, the test measures the number of active goblet cells in the conjunctiva that release mucin into the tear film. The number of goblet cells is reduced in dry eye and Sjögren's.

CONDITIONS THAT MIMIC DRY EYE

Certain eye conditions may produce a sensation of dryness. Blepharitis (inflammation of the eyelid) is a very common condition that can mimic dry eye due to the similarity of symptoms. Patients with blepharitis have symptoms of burning and scratchiness of the eye that are worse on awakening and are associated with crusting of the eyelashes. There is only a modest response to use of artificial lubricants, and treatment is more effective with eyelid hygiene that is done on a regular basis. It is important to recognize that blepharitis and dry eye can coexist.

In allergic conjunctivitis, symptoms are primarily itching. A history of hay fever, asthma, or atopic dermatitis can be present. Typically there are fine strands of mucus in the tear film with redness of the eyes. The Schirmer test is normal or high due to reflex tearing and there is usually no fluorescein, Rose Bengal, or lissamine green staining of the surface. Allergy and dry eye often coexist. Also, systemic anti-allergy medications can exacerbate dryness by reducing tear production.

A variety of conditions that disturb the surface of the eye may be perceived as dryness. Such conditions include viral infections, contact lens irritation, and medication-induced irritation. The lack of aqueous tear secretion in KCS results in an inability to dilute or wash away substances that contact the eye either purposely, like medications or lubricants, or inadvertently, like cosmetics to the face and eyelids. Some medications and preservatives in medications or in lubricants can cause tear film and surface epithelial abnormalities. Discontinuing such exposure reduces or reverses the toxic effects to the surface and the symptoms they produce.

Social Aspects of Dry Eye

Dry eye can produce chronic symptoms of ocular dryness and discomfort that can be debilitating. When severe, the symptoms may affect psychological or emotional health and the ability to work. Because of the chronic nature of the problem, many patients experience periods of despondency and depression. Physicians caring for Sjögren's patients must recognize this aspect of the illness and encourage their patients to pursue their normal activities while complying with recommended treatments. Patients need to remain hopeful since new advances in the understanding of dry eye disease and Sjögren's are continually being made. New therapies are forthcoming and the management of the disease is improving.

Summing Up

Dry eye (known as keratoconjunctivitis sicca [KCS]) is one of the most bothersome complaints of Sjögren's patients. It represents the failure of tears to protect the eye and provide a smooth corneal surface. KCS is a consequence of aberrant interactions between proteins and lipids in the aqueous layer of tear film or reduced production of tears. Diagnosis of KCS by clinical examination, tear function testing, and laboratory analysis of tears, requires that other common conditions such as allergies or blepharitis are ruled out, along with the use of drying medication.

FOR FURTHER READING

2007 Report of the International Dry Eye Workshop (DEWS). The Ocular Surface 2007; 5: 65–202.

American Academy of Ophthalmology Preferred Practice Pattern: Dry Eye (2008) Available at: http//www.one.aao.org/CE/PracticeGuidelines/PPP

Burden of illness and general health-related quality of life in a U.S. Sjögren's syndrome population. Survey of the Sjögren's Syndrome Foundation membership, 2007.

Pflugfelder SC, Beuerman RW, Stern ME, eds. Dry Eye and Ocular Surface Disorders. New York: Marcel Dekker, 2004.

16

The Dry Mouth

Ava J. Wu, DDS, and Troy E. Daniels, DDS, MS

Dry mouth is a common complaint, with an estimated 25 million Americans or 15% of adults afflicted. The range of experience varies from a temporary, minor annoyance to a serious, likely irreversible complication of a disease process. The symptom of dry mouth is often referred to as xerostomia. It is usually caused by a gradual decrease in the amount and quality of saliva produced by the salivary glands but paradoxically may be associated with normal salivary gland function. Because it is a subjective perception, the symptom of dry mouth may not be experienced by all patients who have abnormal salivary function. As a result, it is important for patients with Sjögren's syndrome to be professionally examined for clinical signs of decreased salivary function, whether they have dry mouth symptoms or not. Strategies may then be initiated to increase oral comfort and, most importantly, prevent irreversible damage to the teeth. Most Sjögren's patients experience some degree of continuous or long-term dry mouth.

What Is Dry Mouth?

The sensation of dry mouth in any group of individuals is represented by a spectrum of severity. Typically, a complaint of dry mouth will be associated with one or more of the following: a feeling of cotton in the mouth; tongue and cheeks stick to the top of the mouth or the teeth; sores inside the mouth or at the corners of the lip; difficulty with swallowing, eating dry food, or talking; abnormal taste; burning of the tongue or inside of the mouth; and dental cavities occurring at the gum line of teeth despite diligent oral hygiene. At the other end of the spectrum are individuals who did not realize that they had dry mouth until they developed dental problems. It is important to realize that dry mouth is a symptom that usually indicates that the salivary glands are malfunctioning by producing less saliva that is also qualitatively deficient (i.e., missing or altered amounts of proteins or enzymes). As noted later in the chapter, there are various causes of dry mouth, making it important for individuals experiencing it to determine its cause with their physician.

The Salivary Glands and Saliva

Saliva is produced by three major pairs of salivary glands (parotid, submandibular, and sublingual) and hundreds of minor salivary glands located throughout the mouth. All of these glands may be affected in Sjögren's syndrome. The right and left parotid glands are located in the cheek area in front of the ears and are responsible for making a serous or watery saliva. The saliva from the parotid glands enters the mouth at the parotid papillae located on the inner cheek opposite the upper molar teeth. The submandibular and sublingual glands are located underneath the floor of the mouth and tongue. The submandibular and sublingual glands produce a thicker saliva that exits into the mouth underneath the tongue. Saliva is mainly water but contains a complex array of proteins in very small amounts that have important functions, described below.

PROTECTING, LUBRICATING, AND CLEANSING THE ORAL MUCOSA

Saliva coats the tissues of the mouth and ingested food, allowing the mucosa and food to move smoothly over the teeth. This moist coating facilitates chewing and swallowing and acts as a barrier to irritating and harmful substances contained in food. The saliva coating all the oral surfaces greatly facilitates speech.

PROTECTING AGAINST DENTAL CARIES (DECAY)

Dental caries results from the exposure of teeth to acids produced by bacteria attached to the tooth surface. As discussed below, normal saliva has the ability to help wash away the bacteria, counter the effects of the acid produced by the bacteria, and repair the damage produced by the acid.

MAINTAINING A NEUTRAL PH

Normal saliva contains several chemical systems called buffers that can neutralize the potentially damaging acidity from bacteria, foods, beverages, and gastric reflux on the teeth.

DENTAL REMINERALIZATION

Normal saliva is a reservoir of calcium and phosphate ions that replenish these elements, as they are lost from the tooth surface. This is essentially a tooth surface "repair" at a microscopic level.

PROTECTION AGAINST INFECTION BY BACTERIA, YEASTS, AND VIRUSES

There are several protein components in normal saliva (e.g., lactoferrin, peroxidase, histatins, and secretory leukocyte protease) that have antibacterial, antifungal, or antiviral properties. Secretory IgA is a unique antibody found in saliva that can coat many oral bacteria, interfering with their ability to adhere to teeth.

AIDING DIGESTION AND TASTE

The initial stages of digestion occur in the mouth by way of enzymes contained in saliva. Taste buds, which are located in the mouth, can respond only to dissolved substances. Saliva enhances the sense of taste by both dissolving and beginning digestion of solid foods. The solvent and digestive roles of saliva allow the taste buds to convey food flavors and enhance enjoyment of a meal.

Thus, quantitative and qualitative changes in saliva resulting from diminished salivary gland function in Sjögren's lead to a loss of oral protection and oral comfort.

Causes of Dry Mouth

While there are many causes of dry mouth (Table 16–1), the most frequent one is chronic use of prescription medication. Hundreds of medications have been associated with varying degrees of dry mouth (Table 16–2). Clinical experience also suggests that dry mouth may occur as a result of interactions between medications not usually associated with dry mouth alone. In most cases, the drugs causing dry mouth do so through their effect on nerves that regulate salivary function. The use of prescription drugs often exacerbates dry mouth in patients with Sjögren's. Accordingly patients should review with their physicians any prescription drugs they are taking to determine if those medications are contributing to their dry mouth. Often there are alternative or equivalent drugs available. Temporary symptoms of dry mouth, such as when taking over-the-counter medication for cold symptoms, should not be a problem. However, if chronic drug-induced dry mouth persists for many weeks or months, detrimental changes will begin to occur to the teeth and oral function.

Sjögren's is a systemic autoimmune disease that prominently attacks the salivary glands and lacrimal glands, compromising their function. A type of white blood cell (lymphocyte) enters these glands, replaces normal salivary gland cells that produce saliva (acinar cells), and affects the function of the duct cells that deliver the secretion to the mouth. Sjögren's patients may have an antibody in their bloodstream that can affect the nerves controlling salivary function. The onset and progression of dry mouth in patients with Sjögren's is

TABLE 16–1
Causes of Dry Mouth

Temporary Dry Mouth
- Effect of short-term medication use (e.g., antihistamine)
- Viral infection (e.g., mumps)
- Dehydration
- Psychogenic condition (e.g., anxiety)

Chronic Dry Mouth
- Effect of chronically administered drugs (see Table 16–2)
- Chronic diseases
  - Sjögren's syndrome
  - Sarcoidosis
  - HIV or hepatitis C infection
  - Depression
  - Diabetes mellitus, uncontrolled
  - Amyloidosis (primary or secondary)
  - Central nervous system diseases
  - Rarely, an absent or malformed salivary gland
- Other effects of treatment
  - Therapeutic radiation to the head and neck
  - Graft-versus-host disease (following bone marrow transplant)

usually gradual, and most patients cannot determine exactly when it began. It may progress until little or no saliva is produced, but more commonly patients' symptoms and salivary dysfunction progress to some intermediate point and do not progress further.

Radiation to the head and neck for cancer treatment causes direct damage to the salivary glands, greatly reducing their function.

Dry mouth can also be caused by other chronic systemic diseases such as sarcoidosis, HIV or hepatitis C infection, uncontrolled diabetes, or depression. Previous medical treatment such as radiation therapy to the head and neck, bone marrow transplantation (graft-versus-host disease), or chemotherapy for treating malignancies can directly damage the salivary glands and result in decreased salivation (see Table 16–1). The effects of such treatment can be either temporary or permanent, depending on the type and intensity of the treatment.

Oral Problems Associated With Dry Mouth

The importance of saliva in our quality of life is not appreciated until it is reduced or missing. Progressive loss of saliva production and quality correspondingly decreases the protection and comfort afforded by normal saliva,

TABLE 16–2
Medications with Anticholinergic Effects*

Antidepressants: amitryptiline (++++), clomipramine (++++), doxepin (+++), imipramine (+++), desipramine (++), nortryptiline (++), (+), selegiline (0), tranylcypromine (+), mirtazapine (+), nefazodone (0), trazadone (0), bupropion (+), duloxetine (+), venlafaxine (+)

Antipsychotics: thioridazine (++++), clozapine (++++), chlorpromazine (+++), olanzapine (++), perphenazine (++), aripiprazole (+), fluphenazine (+), haloperidol (+), quetiapine (+), risperidone (+), thiothixene (+), ziprasidone (+)

Antihistamines/Antiemetics: brompheniramine (+++), chlorpheniramine (+++), dexchlorpheniramine (+++), carbinoxamine (++++), clemastine (++++), diphenhydramine (++++), pyrilamine (+/0), tripelennamine (+/0), promethazine (++++), cyproheptadine (+++), phenindamine (+++), azelastine (nasal only, +/0), cetrizine (+/0), levocetrizine (+/0), desloratadine (+/0), fexofenadine (+/0), loratadine (+/0)

Antiacne: isoretinoin

Antianxiety: alprazolam, hydroxyzine

Bronchodilator: ipratropium, tiotropium, albuterol

Drugs for Bladder Overactivity: oxybutinin, tolterodine, trospium, solifenacin, darifenacin

Decongestant: pseudoephedrine

Anti-Parkinson's: benztropine, trihexyphenidyl, selegiline

Anxiolytic: hydroxyzine HCl

Opioids: meperidine

Muscle Relaxant: cyclobenzaprine

Rating of anticholinergic (drying) effects: ++++, high; +++, moderate; ++, low; +, very low; 0, absent

*For consistency and clarity, all drugs are listed by their generic names. There are hundreds of drugs associated with dry mouth, but with most of them the symptom is generally mild and occurs in a small minority of patients taking the drug, or the drug is not prescribed for chronic use. This list includes the categories of drugs that most commonly cause significant dry mouth but is not all-inclusive. When questions arise, patients should consult with their physician or a reliable drug information source.

Source: Wells BG, Dipiro JT, Schwinghammer TL, Dipro CV. *Pharmacotherapy Handbook*, 7th ed. McGraw-Hill, 2009. Used with permission.

as listed above. The most severely affected patients do not produce measurable amounts of saliva, even with stimulation, but the majority of patients retain some residual salivary gland function, ranging from a small amount to almost normal. The most common oral problems associated with chronic dry mouth are oral discomfort, dental caries, oral fungal infections, halitosis (bad breath), and in about one quarter of patients enlargement of major salivary glands.

ORAL DISCOMFORT

The sensation of dry mouth does not occur until saliva production drops to about half of that person's normal value. The feeling of oral dryness in Sjögren's often develops over a period of months or years. Sudden-onset oral dryness is rare. Occasionally, an individual with Sjögren's is not aware of being dry until asked if she can eat a cracker without supplemental water to aid swallowing. The severity of oral dryness in Sjögren's may fluctuate, but it usually does not include periods of time during the day where the mouth feels normal.

Normally, little saliva is produced during sleep, so it is common for every-one to feel some oral dryness in the morning or on awakening during the night. However, this symptom may be more severe in patients with Sjögren's and should be managed at night with small amounts of a commercial saliva substitute, instead of water, to avoid sleep disruption caused by the urge to urinate following water intake.

DENTAL CARIES

The process of tooth decay is caused by interactions between several types of bacteria commonly found in the mouth and sugar present in the diet of most individuals. These bacteria form colonies or plaques that coat the teeth so rap-idly that they can be seen by the unaided eye after a day or two without tooth-brushing. Sucrose (common table sugar) and other carbohydrates can be digested by these bacteria, allowing the organisms to proliferate and release acid as a byproduct. The acid progressively erodes the mineral content of the tooth surface, the first stage of dental caries.

For individuals with deficient saliva, dental caries can progress rapidly, even in those with good oral hygiene. The pattern of dry mouth caries is dis-tinctive, occurring in areas typically thought to be accessible to cleaning. These caries are mostly located on the necks of the teeth near the gum line and are called root caries (Fig. 16-1), and also on the cusp tips of back teeth or biting edges of front teeth. Importantly, these caries also occur along the margins between existing crowns or fillings and the tooth, ultimately causing those restorations to fail and need replacement. The location of dry mouth caries dif-fers from dental caries in individuals with normal saliva but inadequate oral hygiene. These caries usually occur between teeth and in the pits and fissures on the chewing surfaces of the back teeth, called interproximal or occlusal caries (Fig. 16-1). Insufficient saliva contributes to caries in several ways: a decreased ability to buffer acid that is produced by bacteria next to the tooth surface; an insufficient reservoir of calcium and phosphate ions to replenish that naturally lost from the tooth surface; a reduction of antimicrobial proteins; and reduced oral cleansing from the lack of saliva flowing across the oral surfaces.

Dental caries typically causes no symptoms until it penetrates through the outer enamel surface of the tooth into the inner dentin layer. Dental enamel is dense and composed almost entirely of non-organic material, like ivory. The inner dentin is like bone with many organic components, including nerves, which can transmit the sensation of pain, heat, and cold. Thus, when decay or the cavity enters the dentin layer, the tooth may become sensitive to heat, cold, and sweets. If untreated, the caries can progress to the tooth interior, the pulp composed of soft tissue, nerves, and blood vessels. Involvement of the pulp is usually associated with spontaneous pain. From the pulp, invading bac-teria can expand into bone surrounding the root tip, causing a painful abscess.

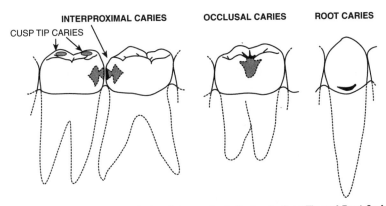

INTERPROXIMAL CARIES   OCCLUSAL CARIES   ROOT CARIES

CUSP TIP CARIES

FIGURE 16-1 **Locations of Dental Caries: Interproximal, Occlusal, Cusp Tip and Root Caries.**

Early dental caries appears as a flat, whitish spot (decalcification) on the tooth's surface. As the process continues, there is progressive loss of tooth structure, and the cavity can appear tan to black in color. It is now believed that the early caries process (white spot) can be significantly slowed or reversed with the preventive strategies of remineralization(e.g., topical fluoride application).

FUNGAL INFECTIONS

About one third of patients with long-term salivary deficiency will develop symptoms of burning on their tongue or elsewhere in their mouth and/or intolerance to acidic or spicy foods. These symptoms are usually caused by localized infection of the lining of the mouth by different species of the fungus *Candida*. This organism is often found normally in the mouth, but susceptible individuals with decreased saliva production may experience an overgrowth of these organisms. When this occurs in dry mouth patients, the affected tissue of the mouth will be red. The tongue may appear red, lose its normal carpet-like texture, and develop grooves. Other affected areas develop well-defined or diffuse red areas caused by thinning of the mucosa (atrophy). These intra-oral changes are often associated with redness or crusting at the corners of the lips, called *angular cheilitis*. This combination of clinical features is called erythematous candidiasis. Effective treatment with antifungal medication will lead to complete restoration of the mucosal color and elimination of the burning despite an ongoing salivary deficiency. However, in a few individuals, this condition will recur or persist, requiring retreatment, which can be repeated as often as necessary.

ORAL FUNCTIONAL PROBLEMS

It is common for patients with Sjögren's to have difficulty swallowing dry foods, when there is insufficient saliva to adequately moisten the food bolus. They may have difficulty speaking because the tongue and lips get stuck to the teeth and palate. This can be overcome temporarily with frequent small sips of water, the use of a secretagogue, or sugar-free hard candy or gum to stimulate saliva production. Sjögren's patients wearing complete dentures often experience problems from the lack of oral lubrication that causes the tongue to continually move the lower denture from its normal position, decreasing its stability. Where it is possible, surgical implants can be considered for the lower jaw as a means to increase denture stability.

PERIODONTAL DISEASE

Because chronic inflammatory periodontal disease is a very common disease worldwide, it is sometimes assumed that patients with Sjögren's will be at increased risk to develop this disease. However, most of the research that has examined this question has not shown that the frequency or severity of periodontal disease is greater in the Sjögren's population than in the general population. Perhaps there is greater awareness of the beneficial effects of good oral hygiene, resulting in the inability of investigators to find periodontal disease of increased severity in patients' with Sjogren's.

HALITOSIS (BAD BREATH)

Halitosis can occur when there is an overgrowth of certain types of odor-causing bacteria in the teeth or oral soft tissue. These bacteria can be the result of active dental caries, active periodontal or gum disease, inadequate oral hygiene, or deficient saliva. The problem is managed by appropriate dental or periodontal treatment to eradicate the underlying infection, along with regular and careful oral hygiene.

SALIVARY GLAND ENLARGEMENT

Salivary gland enlargement or swelling occurs in about one quarter of patients with Sjögren's, while the majority of the general population never experiences this change. The enlargement is usually gradual in onset and without symptoms or with only slight discomfort. It can slowly regress and recur over a period of several months or become chronic. In rare cases, the swelling can rapidly grow if it transforms into a malignant condition, usually lymphoma. In patients experiencing prolonged salivary gland enlargement, it may be appropriate to consider other causes of the enlargement by way of MRI, fine-needle aspiration cytology, and/or salivary gland biopsy.

Diagnostic Testing of Dry Mouth

Dry mouth resulting from Sjögren's and other causes can be evaluated by both dentists or physicians using a combination of methods.

SYMPTOMS AND FOLLOW-UP QUESTIONS

In evaluating oral symptoms experienced by individuals with Sjögren's, it is helpful to ask if the mouth feels dry while eating dry or solid food. A positive answer suggests that the salivary glands are not producing enough saliva to allow for mastication and swallowing to occur smoothly, even while the salivary glands are stimulated by taste and chewing.

SALIVARY AND ORAL EXAMINATION

In examining patients suspected of having Sjögren's, the major salivary glands may exhibit evidence of tenderness, changes in consistency, or enlargement. Saliva expressed from the major gland ducts intraorally may exhibit changes in its clarity, viscosity, and wetting ability. The oral mucosa may exhibit changes in its lubricity (normal wet and slippery vs. dry and sticky) and its color. The tongue may exhibit changes described previously. The pattern and extent of dental caries must be noted, as described above.

SALIVARY FLOW RATE MEASUREMENT

Salivary gland function is most easily assessed by collecting saliva over a specified amount of time. The collection can be made of whole saliva (from all major and minor salivary glands) by simply expectorating (spitting) into a preweighed cup. This can be done to assess the severity of salivary gland dysfunction and monitor the progression of disease severity over time, and the effects of treatment. There is no universally accepted measure that defines normal salivary function, but an unstimulated whole salivary flow rate less than 0.1 mL/min is widely accepted as a threshold of abnormal function. A reduction in salivary flow rate may be caused by many different conditions and is not diagnostically specific for Sjögren's.

SCINTIGRAPHY

This test measures the rate at which a small amount of injected radioactive material is taken up from the blood into the salivary glands and secreted into the mouth. It is another method to measure salivary gland function and is usually done in a hospital setting. All four of the major salivary glands are evaluated at the same time during this test.

SIALOGRAPHY

This technique uses a liquid radiographic contrast medium injected into a salivary duct, followed by an x-ray image of the gland to show the ductal structures.

This technique is useful to explore duct obstructions and distinguish between chronic inflammatory changes and neoplasms but is limited in its ability to provide diagnostically specific information regarding Sjögren's. Sialography in patients with significant salivary hypofunction must be done with a water-based contrast medium to avoid the risk of a chronic foreign body reaction coming from the use of an oil-based contrast medium leaking outside the ducts.

ULTRASOUND AND MRI

These noninvasive imaging techniques can determine structural abnormalities in the salivary glands. Ultrasound examinations may be helpful in identifying vascular or cystic lesions. MRI is an excellent technique for imaging masses or tumors in the salivary glands, particularly as part of a presurgical evaluation. There have been only a few studies examining these techniques in the context of Sjögren's. The possibility of its use for the diagnosis of the salivary component of Sjögren's has been suggested, but evidence of its usefulness remains inconclusive.

SIALOCHEMISTRY

These techniques examine saliva for the presence and amount of particular substances. Sialochemistry has been applied to compare saliva samples from normal individuals to those with Sjögren's with the hope of identifying differences that can be used as diagnostic criteria for Sjögren's. Differences between normal and Sjögren's saliva have been identified but have not yet been tested in large trials.

MINOR SALIVARY GLAND BIOPSY

This test, also known as the lip biopsy, is currently considered the gold standard for diagnosing the salivary component of Sjögren's. Using local anesthesia, a superficial and small incision is made on the inner surface of the lower lip to directly visualize and remove at least five of these small glands. There are hundreds of these minor salivary glands located throughout the mouth; they are between 1/16 and 1/8 inches (1 to 3 mm) in diameter. This technique is preferable to the punch biopsy technique, which is a blind procedure and may not yield a sufficient sample of minor salivary glands and may endanger sensory nerves in the area. A pathologist will examine the glands for the presence of changes characteristic of the salivary component of Sjögren's (focal lymphocytic sialadenitis) or occasionally of other diseases.

Summing Up

Sjögren's syndrome affects the salivary glands, which are responsible for making and secreting a complex fluid that provides a multitude of protective and essential functions. The reduction or loss of saliva results in a decrease of these essential functions and significant oral discomfort and pathology. However, loss of saliva and a complaint of "dry mouth" can be the result of diverse causes (see Table 16–1). Some of these diverse causes require different treatment. Thus, it becomes important to evaluate the cause of a complaint of dry mouth and the severity of salivary dysfunction. With this knowledge, individualized preventive measures may be promptly initiated to reduce symptoms and to minimize the impact of dry mouth on the oral cavity.

FOR FURTHER READING

Daniels TE. Evaluation, differential diagnosis, and treatment of xerostomia. *J Rheumatol [Suppl]*. 2000; 61: 6–10.

Daniels TE, Wu AJ. Xerostomia—clinical evaluation and treatment in general practice. *J Calif Dent Assoc.* 2000; 28(12): 933–41. Accessed May 2011 at: http://www.cda.org/library/cda_member/pubs/journal/jour1200/xero.html

Sreebny LM. A useful source for the drug-dry mouth relationship. *J Dent Educ.* 2004; 68(1): 6–7. Accessed May 2011 at: http://www.jdentaled.org/cgi/reprint/68/1/6

Wells BG, Dipiro JT, Schwinghammer TL, Dipro CV. *Pharmacotherapy Handbook*, 7th ed. McGraw-Hill, 2009.

17

Salivary Glands, Ears, Nose, and Throat
Robert S. Lebovics, MD, FACS

Sjögren's syndrome in its primary form, also known as the sicca syndrome, is a multisystem disease with a multiplicity of target organs and clinical effects. Understanding the otolaryngologic manifestations of this disease can best be appreciated with a brief introduction to the anatomy of the upper airways and alimentary tract (Fig. 17–1).

Anatomy

The lining of the nose, also known as the nasal mucosa, is a moist, fluid-producing organ that is rich in glandular material. In the average adult, the nose and paranasal sinuses secrete about one quart of thin, clear, mucoid fluid a day, which as part of our normal physiology is secreted, passed, and eventually swallowed. In many disease states, Sjögren's being a prime example, this physiology is altered, with several manifestations of clinical presentation. In the simplest sense, treatment is directed at restoring this mucociliary flow and facilitating the cleansing of the inner tubes and passageways of the head and neck.

Upon entering the nasal cavity through the nasal vestibule, a rich network of glandular structures is present on direct examination. Laterally in both sides of the nose are the nasal turbinates (passages), which are rich in glands secreting fluid as well as being actively involved in humidification of the airflow and regulating temperature. The secretions often contain various enzymes such as lactoferrin and lysozyme in addition to several types of immunoglobulins, specifically certain subclasses of the IgG molecule as well as the secretory form of the IgA molecule. In a sense, the paranasal sinuses are a reservoir for producing these secretions as well as acting as a capacitor for the storage of warmth and/or cold as well as humidity. There are probably hundreds of minor salivary glands in the nose as well as the nasopharynx, oral cavity, hypopharynx, and larynx.

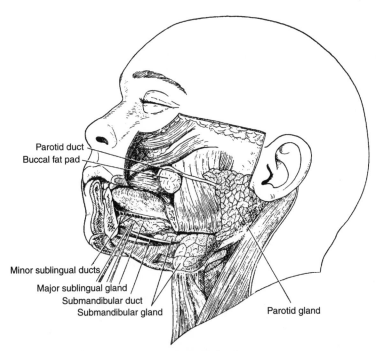

Parotid duct
Buccal fat pad

Minor sublingual ducts
Major sublingual gland
Submandibular duct
Submandibular gland

Parotid gland

FIGURE 17–1 **Salivary Glands Important in Sjögren's Syndrome.**
(Reprinted with permission from Sichel and DuBrul, *Oral Anatomy*. Mosby, 1975.)

As one progresses down the nasopharyngeal tube, one gets to the back of the nose, which in reality is the top of the throat. While the lining here becomes more squamous rather than respiratory in nature, the basic functions of humidification, clearing of particles, and maintenance of immunity are still paramount. Additionally, the eustachian tube orifices exit into the nasopharynx, and this is a conduit for draining the middle ear space and by extension the mastoid air cells. Inflammation or disease at this point may have otologic implications. As one continues back down the nasopharynx, the tongue base can be visualized as well as the larynx, where both vocal cords are easily visualized, and one can often see clear, thin fluid coming up from the tracheobronchial tree, which is the lower-airway equivalent of the secretions that begin in the nose and sinus passages. The hypopharynx also acts as a point or a separate conduit for entering the alimentary tract—that is, the esophagus. A change occurs here, and the lining again is much more squamous and rich in glands such that saliva can be secreted to aid in the early digestion of food particles. Of course, we all know that the oral cavity and the oral tongue are the main inflow point for nutritional support in addition to a bypass mechanism for respiration. A basic understanding of the anatomy therefore is critical to understanding the ear, nose, and throat manifestations of Sjögren's and by extension its treatments.

Nasal Manifestations

As the autoimmune process within the nasal cavity progresses, one may see the clinical consequences of this destructive process. The destructive, crust-like pattern is often referred to as *atrophic rhinitis*. A foul smell, crusts, and even nasal bleeding can be seen. As secretions become thick and occasionally foul-smelling, secondary infection may appear. This can cause further local destruction of the glandular tissue and sometimes even the nasal septum. It is not uncommon to see a perforation of the cartilaginous portion of the nasal septum due to this inflammatory process, with or without secondary bacterial infection.

The paranasal sinuses drain through the various ostia (openings) into the nasal cavity, and with the exception of the sphenoid sinus, they drain from under one of the nasal turbinates. As the inflammatory process proceeds, one may see obstruction of the middle or superior meatus, thus causing secondary outflow problems from the maxillary, ethmoid, and/or frontal sinuses. The narrowest portion of the sinonasal tract in terms of drainage is at the ostiomeatal complex, which is anatomically close to the middle meatus. Even mild local inflammation can cause sinus infections. Symptoms include pain, headache, and occasional fever, in addition to the atrophic symptoms. Many patients will complain of anosmia (loss of smell) and a sense of fullness inside the nose. Secondary infections of the paranasal sinuses need to be treated medically.

My personal bias in treating Sjögren's of the nose and sinus tract revolves around humidification and replacement of what is lost. Specifically, water in all its forms is critical for reversing the atrophic/inflammatory destruction and for allowing the passage of thick, crusty material down into the oral cavity so that it can eventually be swallowed or spit out through the mouth. The over-riding principle here is one of humidification using clean, balanced saline solutions. There are various brands of over-the-counter saline sprays, and I have no preference for any particular one. The critical point here is constant and prophylactic humidification and saline replacement. Recently, a longer-acting form of nasal lubricant is available that is glycol-based (Rhinaris®). It comes both in a mist and a gel, with the latter being particularly useful for longer-term lubrication and hydration, particularly while sleeping at night. The use of topical intranasal steroids is often suggested, although its efficacy has yet to be clearly demonstrated.

Additionally, some people with severe crusting need to irrigate with a WaterPik®, and various nasal attachments exist that facilitate nasal hygiene. Other devices, such as a neti pot, may have value, in addition to hot, steamy showers. For all patients with Sjögren's, the use of concurrent medications that can facilitate dryness needs to be avoided; this particularly is important with respect to antihistamines and systemic decongestants.

How Is the Ear Affected in Sjögren's?

Hearing loss as a result of Sjögren's disease is uncommon but does occur. Some autoimmune diseases have clearly been linked with a sensorineural (nerve-type) deafness; however, this does not appear to be the case here. There are patients, however, who occasionally complain of tinnitus, hearing loss, or otalgia in small degrees; this can be as high as one quarter of all patients. Because the middle-ear fluid needs to drain into the back of the nose through the eustachian tube orifice, disease with severe inflammation in the nasal cavity could potentially block the eustachian tube or cause an inflammatory condition, resulting in a conductive hearing loss. Fortunately, this is easily treated with ventilating tubes, amplification devices, or local hygiene. Sometimes, increased doses of immunosuppressives or steroids may have value.

How Is the Mouth Affected in Sjögren's?

See Chapter 16.

How Is the Larynx Affected in Sjögren's?

The larynx or voice box is involved in protecting the airway from foreign bodies and promoting good airflow into the tracheobronchial tree. It is also involved in diverting food to the alimentary tract (esophagus), and it is the most important organ in terms of our ability to phonate. Laryngeal disorders in Sjögren's are often manifested by coughing and occasionally hoarseness. Voice changes may be present, as the glands below the vocal cords and the trachea are also affected in addition to the minor salivary glands from above. Patients infrequently develop respiratory symptoms attributable to Sjögren's; however, professional singers or people who use their voice frequently during the day are at increased risk for chronic laryngitis and its sequelae. Inspissation (thickening) of mucus and other secretions can cause a foul smell and occasionally a sense of blockage in one's airway. As in treating disease in the mouth, vigorous oral hydration is the primary treatment in addition to systemic immune system modulation with either steroids or glandular stimulation with drugs such as cevimeline (Evoxac®) and pilocarpine (Salagen®). Other treatments include voice rest and occasionally guaifenesin-containing products to help thin mucus, not only in the nasal tract but also in the tracheobronchial tree.

Summing Up

The otolaryngologic (ear, nose, and throat) manifestations of Sjögren's disease are significant and varied. It is critical to remind patients and their physicians to limit drugs that can dry the mucous membranes within the upper airways. Antihistamines and decongestants are but two of a class of medications that have these effects. Oral hydration and replacement with artificial saliva have value, as does replacing sinonasal secretions with saline or glycol-based nose sprays. Guaifenesin is useful in helping the larynx to clear itself.

FOR FURTHER READING

Belafsky PC, Postma GN. The laryngeal and esophageal manifestations of Sjögren's syndrome. *Curr Rheumatol Rep.* 2003 Aug; 5(4): 297–303.

Freeman SR, Sheehan PZ, Thorpe MA, Rutka JA, Ear, nose, and throat manifestations of Sjögren's syndrome: retrospective review of a multidisciplinary clinic. *J Otolaryngol.* 2005 Feb; 34(1): 20–4.

National Institutes of Health, Dry Mouth brochure. View at http://www.nidcr.nih.gov/OralHealth/Topics/DryMouth/DryMouth.htm.

Sharp K, Sjögren's syndrome. In: Krapp K, Longe JL, eds. *Gale Encyclopedia of Alternative Medicine*. Gale, 2001.

Ship, JA. Diagnosing, managing, and preventing salivary gland disorders. *Oral Dis.* 2002 Mar; 8(2): 77–89.

Thomas BL, Brown JE, McGurk M. Salivary gland disease. *Front Oral Biol.* 2010; 14: 129–46.

18

Lab Work
BLOOD TESTS, IMAGING, BIOPSIES, AND BEYOND
Alan N. Baer, MD

The diagnostic evaluation and management of a patient with Sjögren's syndrome involves laboratory tests, imaging studies, and often a biopsy of minor salivary glands from the lower lip. In general, the clinician will use these various testing modalities to establish the correct diagnosis of Sjögren's, to define the extent of disease involvement both in the lacrimal and salivary glands as well as in internal organs, and to monitor disease progression and the appearance of disease complications (Table 18–1). Additionally, scientists may use sophisticated laboratory analyses of blood and tissue specimens from Sjögren's patients to uncover new disease mechanisms. In this chapter, the more common testing modalities used in Sjögren's patients will be reviewed, with an emphasis on how the clinician uses these tests. A brief overview of two new research methods for exploring the pathogenesis of Sjögren's is also provided.

Establishing the Diagnosis of Sjögren's

The diagnosis of primary Sjögren's syndrome requires demonstration of an autoimmune basis for the presence of dry eyes and/or dry mouth. The current classification criteria for Sjögren's mandate that affected individuals have antibodies to distinct small intracellular RNA–protein complexes, termed SS-A or SS-B, or that they have a lip biopsy that shows a characteristic pattern of inflammation, termed focal lymphocytic sialoadenitis. Many Sjögren's patients will have other immunological abnormalities, evident in blood testing, which will lend support to the diagnosis. These include the presence of rheumatoid factor, antinuclear antibodies, an elevated level of serum immunoglobulins (antibody proteins), and occasionally a monoclonal protein. Imaging the salivary glands can define structural or functional alterations that also lend support to a Sjögren's diagnosis.

TABLE 18–1

Diagnostic Testing in Sjögren's

Establishing the Diagnosis of Sjögren's

- Mandatory tests
  - Positive test for anti-SS-A and/or SS-B antibodies

OR

  - Lip biopsy showing focal lymphocytic sialoadenitis with focus score of 1 or greater
- Tests to exclude Sjögren's mimics
  - HIV blood test
  - Hepatitis C blood test
  - Chest x-ray and/or angiotensin-converting enzyme (ACE) level
  - Serum IgG4 level
- Diagnostic test results that support diagnosis of Sjögren's
  - Abnormal parotid scintigraphy or sialography
  - High titer of antinuclear antibodies
  - Positive test for rheumatoid factor
  - Elevated serum IgG levels
  - Low complement C3 and/or C4 levels
  - Low white blood cell count (leukopenia)

Defining internal organ involvement

- Careful history and physical examination
- Blood tests: complete blood counts, urinalysis, blood chemistries
- Additional tests will depend on findings from initial evaluation.

Monitoring disease progression and risk for lymphoma

- Routine blood tests: complete blood counts, urinalysis, blood chemistries
- Parotid scintigraphy and/or sialometrics
- Immunoglobulin quantitation
- Serum protein electrophoresis and/or immunofixation electrophoresis
- Serum cryoglobulins
- Serum C3 and C4 levels

SS-A AND SS-B ANTIBODIES

Antibodies are a large family of proteins in the blood that are capable of binding to molecular targets, termed antigens, on the surfaces of microorganisms, cells, and blood proteins. Each antibody protein has a binding site that can attach to only a very specific molecular target. However, the large array of such antibody proteins in our blood ensures that a diverse and large number of molecular targets can be recognized. Binding of such molecular targets is an essential step in our defense against infections and cancer. Cells that produce antibodies against molecular targets on our own tissues are actively eliminated from our bodies, particularly early in life. If this mechanism goes awry, then we may form antibodies to self material and be susceptible to autoimmune disease.

SS-A and SS-B antibodies are examples of two antibodies that bind molecular targets within our own cells. The SS-A and SS-B targets (also known respectively as Ro and La) are proteins that are attached to a strand of ribonuclear material (RNA). These RNA–protein complexes can be located either in the nucleus or the cytoplasm of the cell. Since they can be found in the nucleus, they are one of the potential targets of antinuclear antibodies, present in patients with systemic autoimmune diseases, such as systemic lupus erythematosus (SLE), Sjögren's, and scleroderma. Since the SS-A and SS-B RNA–protein complexes are normally contained within the cell, they are not accessible to antibodies in the blood. However, these proteins are clustered in packets and brought to the surface of the cell during the process of cellular death. It is hypothesized that this process, termed apoptosis, may allow susceptible individuals to form antibodies to the SS-A and SS-B proteins.

SS-A antibodies are found in approximately 40% to 60% of Sjögren's patients (Table 18–2). SS-B antibodies are less common, being found in approximately 20% to 30% of Sjögren's patients. SS-A antibodies thus occur commonly by themselves; however, it is very uncommon for SS-B antibodies to occur alone. Accordingly, 40% to 60% of Sjögren's patients may lack SS-A and/or SS-B antibodies. The finding of SS-A and/or SS-B antibodies is not specific to Sjögren's patients. These antibodies may also be found in patients with SLE and occasionally in other autoimmune diseases, such as rheumatoid arthritis (RA). Additionally, they may be found in approximately 1 in 200 healthy women.

TABLE 18–2

Features of Primary Sjögren's Patients, Defined by 2002 American-European Criteria, at Three Academic Centers

Feature	Baltimore[1] (N = 214)	Athens[2] (N = 536)	Barcelona[3] (N = 286)
Age (yrs, mean ± SD)	55 ± 14	53 ± 13	55 ± 16
Women (%)	91	92	94
ANA (%)	84	68	84
SS-A antibodies (%)	62	37	65
SS-B antibodies (%)	31	19	
Centromere antibodies (%)	6		
dsDNA antibodies (%)	6		
Rheumatoid factor (%)	47	37	54
Hypergammaglobulinemia (%)	38	26	14
Monoclonal protein (%)	18	4	18
Low C4 (%)	11	4	11
Leukopenia (%)	18	14	19

[1] Patients of the Jerome L. Greene Sjögren's Center at Johns Hopkins, May 2010.
[2] Medicine 2009; 88: 284–93.
[3] Clin Rev Allerg Immunol. 2010; 38: 178–85.

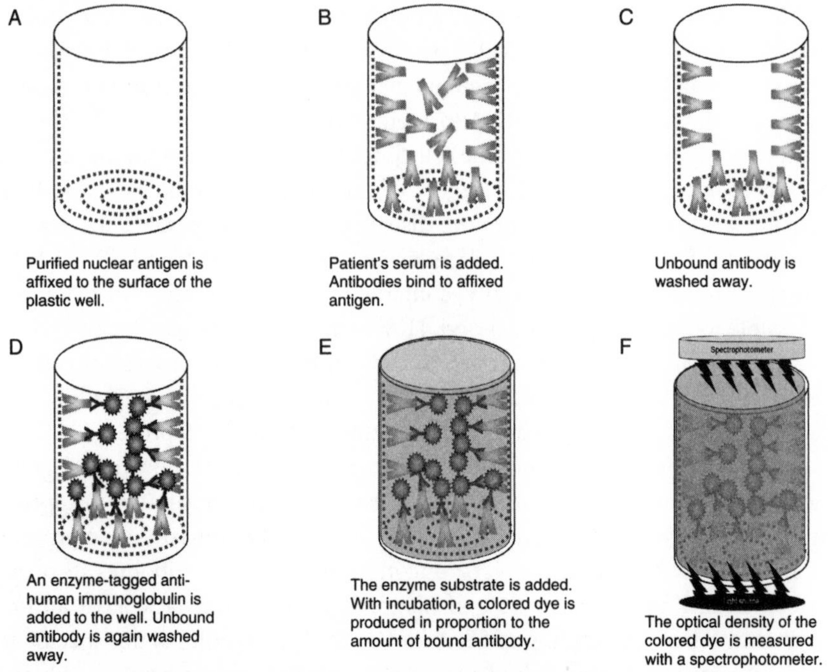

A

Purified nuclear antigen is affixed to the surface of the plastic well.

B

Patient's serum is added. Antibodies bind to affixed antigen.

C

Unbound antibody is washed away.

D

An enzyme-tagged anti-human immunoglobulin is added to the well. Unbound antibody is again washed away.

E

The enzyme substrate is added. With incubation, a colored dye is produced in proportion to the amount of bound antibody.

F

Spectrophotometer

The optical density of the colored dye is measured with a spectrophotometer.

FIGURE 18–1 **Principles of Enzyme-Linked Immunosorbent Assay (ELISA) for Detection of Antinuclear Antibodies.**
The ELISA test is often performed using a plastic plate with 96 wells. One such well is illustrated in the figure. Purified nuclear antigen is affixed to the surface of the plastic well. In a multi-step process, a patient's serum sample can be tested for the presence of antibodies that bind specifically to the nuclear antigen. Detection of this binding requires the use of a commercially available antibody to human immunoglobulin that is generated in an animal (such as a rabbit or goat) and subsequently tagged with an enzyme. Akin to the formation of a sandwich, this commercially available antibody binds to those in the patient's serum that have attached to the nuclear antigen on the surface of the plastic wells. In the next step, the enzyme converts an added colorless substrate (chromogen) to a colored product, and the amount of chromogen produced is an indication of the amount of antibody–antigen binding in the well.

SS-A and SS-B antibodies are most commonly detected using a test called an enzyme-linked immunosorbent assay (ELISA, Fig. 18–1). This assay method measures the binding of serum antibodies to purified SS-A and SS-B proteins that are bound to the surface of plastic wells. Results are typically reported as positive or negative along with an index. The ELISA test is preferred by most large laboratories since it is automated and easily quantifiable. However, it can sometimes detect weak and nonspecific binding of other serum antibodies to the SS-A and SS-B targets, leading to a false-positive test result. It is thus prudent to have the test repeated at a different laboratory if a positive result does not correlate with the clinical findings.

LIP BIOPSY

A biopsy involves the surgical excision of a small amount of tissue for diagnostic purposes. In Sjögren's, the removal of several minor salivary glands from the inner surface of the right or left lower lip is an important diagnostic test. The biopsy is performed by numbing the inner lip on either the left or right side with a local anesthetic and then making a superficial incision. The glands are located just beneath the inner (mucosal) surface of the lip and pop into view when the surgeon opens up the incision. They are then snipped free and placed in fixative. The incision site is typically closed with resorbable sutures. Some numbness may persist in the area of the biopsy site, but this usually resolves in several weeks.

The salivary glands comprise specialized cells that produce a fluid, the precursor of saliva, that contains water, electrolytes, mucus, and enzymes. These cells are clustered together in a ring-like structure termed the acinus (acini, plural) and secrete this fluid into the center of the ring. The fluid then travels down tubular structures, termed collecting ducts, where its composition is gradually altered to that of saliva. It is brought into the mouth via progressively larger ducts. In Sjögren's, the minor salivary glands show a typical pattern of inflammation, termed focal lymphocytic sialoadenitis (Fig. 18–2). Aggregates of inflammatory cells, termed lymphocytes, are typically clustered around the glandular ducts. These aggregates of lymphocytes can interfere with the function of the gland, either by affecting the function of adjacent

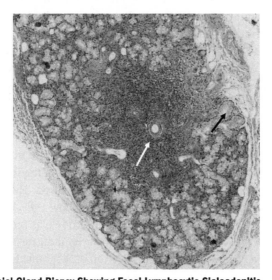

FIGURE 18–2 **Labial Gland Biopsy Showing Focal Lymphocytic Sialoadenitis.**
A duct is seen in the center of this salivary gland lobule (*white arrow*). The duct is surrounded by a large number of small, round dark-staining cells (lymphocytes). The salivary acini (ring-like structures) are seen at the periphery of the lobule (*black arrow*).

nerve fibers that control gland secretion or by gradually destroying normal acini. When these aggregates contain more than 50 lymphocytes in a cross-section of the gland tissue, they are termed lymphocytic foci. The presence of one or more lymphocytic foci in a 4-square-millimeter area of salivary gland tissue (termed a focus score of at least 1) is a feature of Sjögren's. The presence of lymphocytic aggregates around the salivary gland ducts is felt to be an indication of the autoimmune process directly attacking the salivary gland and affecting its function.

The minor salivary gland (i.e., lip) biopsy cannot by itself be used to make the diagnosis of Sjögren's. Focal lymphocytic sialoadenitis can occasionally be found in other autoimmune diseases and in individuals without any symptoms to suggest Sjögren's. Thus, a positive biopsy can be considered indicative of Sjögren's only when other features of the disease are present. The lip biopsy may also reveal other salivary gland diseases, such as sarcoidosis, IgG4 plasmacytic infiltrative disease, or lymphoma, which may mimic Sjögren's.

COMMON BLOOD AND URINE TEST ABNORMALITIES IN SJÖGREN'S PATIENTS

Certain abnormalities in the blood and urine are commonly seen in patients with Sjögren's. Their presence can thus lend support to the diagnosis. The following tests are routinely performed in the evaluation of a patient with suspected Sjögren's:

1. The **complete blood count (CBC)** determines the number of red cells (RBCs), white cells (WBCs), and platelets as well as the level of hemoglobin (oxygen-carrying protein in red cells) in the blood. A low number of WBCs (leukopenia) can be found in approximately 15% to 20% of Sjögren's patients but is usually not associated with an increased risk of infection. Anemia, defined by a low hemoglobin level and low number of RBCs, is less common.

2. The **complete metabolic panel** (i.e., blood chemistries) measures the electrolytes as well as chemicals or proteins in the blood that reflect the function of the kidneys, liver, and immune system. In Sjögren's, the total protein level may be elevated, reflecting the increase in antibody (or immunoglobulin) levels in the blood. The serum bicarbonate or carbon dioxide level may be low, reflecting a disorder of the kidney that may occur in Sjögren's known as renal tubular acidosis. An elevation of the creatinine level indicates the presence of kidney dysfunction, a rare complication of Sjögren's. Elevation of the liver enzymes alkaline phosphatase, aspartate aminotransferase (AST), and alanine aminotransferase (ALT) can be seen in liver diseases, some of which occur more commonly in Sjögren's (e.g., primary biliary cirrhosis).

3. The **antinuclear antibody (ANA) test** is positive in the majority of Sjögren's patients. However, a positive ANA test is also common in healthy individuals. The ANA test is most commonly performed using a technique that involves immunofluorescent staining of human cells grown in tissue culture (Fig. 18–3). With this test, a positive result is listed as the last dilution of serum that results in visible staining of the nucleus of the cultured human cell. Typical dilutions are 1:40, 1:80, 1:160, 1:320, and 1:640. Positive ANA test results of 1:80 and 1:160 may be seen in up to 15% and 5% of healthy individuals, respectively. A negative ANA test does not exclude the diagnosis of Sjögren's; some of these individuals may still have SS-A and/or SS-B antibodies. With the immunofluorescent staining test, the pattern of nuclear

A
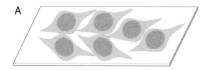

Human tissue culture cells are grown on a glass slide.

B
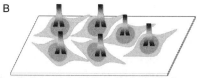

The patient's serum, containing anti-nuclear antibodies, is layered over the cells. After a period of incubation, the serum is washed away. The antinuclear antibodies remain affixed to the nuclei of the cells.

C
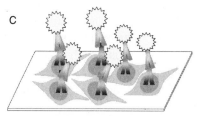

An antibody labeled with a fluorescent chromophore and directed against human immunoglobulin, is layered over the cells. The antibody binds to the human anti-nuclear antibodies. The excess is washed away.

D
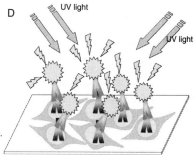

When exposed to ultraviolet light, the chromophore emits yellow-green light, allowing visualization of the antibodies which have bound to the cellular nuclei.

FIGURE 18–3 **Principles of the Immunofluorescent Staining Technique for Detection of Antinuclear Antibodies.**
An immunofluorescent staining technique is commonly used to detect the presence of antinuclear antibodies. In this multi-step process akin to making a sandwich, the patient's diluted serum is layered over human tissue culture cells that have adhered to a glass slide. After a period of incubation, the patient's serum is washed away. Binding of antinuclear antibodies to the cellular nuclei is then detected with the use of a commercially available antibody to human immunoglobulin that is generated in an animal (such as a rabbit or goat) and subsequently tagged with fluorescein, a fluorescent dye. When viewed under a microscope equipped with special lighting, the fluorescent dye can be seen "staining" the cellular nuclei if antinuclear antibodies were present in the patient's serum.

staining is reported. Most Sjögren's patients have either a speckled or homogeneous pattern. However, some patients may have a centromere pattern, denoting staining of centromere proteins in the mitotic spindle of dividing cells.

4. The **rheumatoid factor** test detects immunoglobulins in the blood that bind to other immunoglobulins, resulting in large protein complexes. Rheumatoid factor is a characteristic feature of RA, being found in up to 80% of affected patients. However, it is also common in Sjögren's patients and in this setting does not indicate the presence of or predict the later development of RA.

5. The **erythrocyte sedimentation rate** (ESR) measures the degree to which whole blood, collected in tubes containing a chemical that prevents clotting (anticoagulant), separates into plasma (the upper layer) and packed red cells (the lower layer) over the course of 1 hour. The rate at which red cells settle to the bottom of the tube depends largely on the amount of fibrinogen protein in the blood. Fibrinogen binds to the surface of red cells and decreases their negative electrostatic charges, allowing the cells to aggregate and settle more quickly. The amount of fibrinogen produced by the liver increases with systemic inflammation. Thus, the ESR is a simple test for measuring the degree of inflammation. The ESR can also increase when there are higher levels of immunoglobulins in the blood, as is the case for some Sjögren's patients.

6. The **C-reactive protein** (CRP) test measures systemic inflammation. It is elevated most commonly in the setting of an infection or tissue injury, such as a myocardial infarction (heart attack). In the setting of autoimmune disease, the CRP may be elevated, but usually to a much lesser extent than during an infection.

7. **Urinalysis** detects a variety of abnormalities in the kidney or genitourinary system, including the bladder. Protein in the urine (proteinuria) is an indication of kidney disease, stemming from a disorder of the glomerulus (the filtering structure) or the tubules (the structures within the kidney responsible for reabsorbing filtered salts, water, and acids from the initial blood filtrate). Blood in the urine may arise from a glomerular disease or from a disorder in the urine collecting system or bladder (such as a kidney stone or tumor). WBCs in the urine denote the presence of inflammation or infection anywhere in the kidneys, urine collecting system, bladder, or urethra. The specific gravity is an indirect measure of the concentration of the urine. The pH indicates the extent of urine acidification. In Sjögren's, the most common abnormality is inflammation in the tissue surrounding the tubules (interstitial nephritis), and this may lead to poorly concentrated urine (with a low specific gravity), protein in

the urine, and occasionally a high urine pH. Inflammation or damage in the glomerulus (glomerulonephritis) is a less common form of kidney disease in Sjögren's and is characterized by protein in the urine, occasionally with RBCs and/or WBCs.

8. The **immunoglobulin quantitation** test measures the levels of the most common types of immunoglobulins in the blood, known as IgG, IgM, and IgA. Some patients with Sjögren's have elevated levels of these immunoglobulins, termed hyperglobulinemia, reflecting overactivity of the immune system.

9. The **serum protein electrophoresis** and the **serum immunofixation electrophoresis** tests analyze the types of proteins present in the liquid phase of the blood (serum). These tests rely on an electric field to separate the proteins based on their electrical charge. In the diagnostic evaluation of a patient with Sjögren's, particular attention is paid to the immunoglobulins, proteins produced by plasma cells. Each of these cells creates a unique antibody, with a structure different from that produced by most other plasma cells. In approximately 10% of Sjögren's patients, a clone of plasma cells proliferates and produces increased amounts of one immunoglobulin, with identical structure and specificity. This is called a monoclonal protein. This monoclonal immunoglobulin protein can be detected and characterized with electrophoretic techniques that rely on its distinctive properties in an electrical field.

10. The **complement proteins, C3 and C4,** are part of a group of proteins that mediate tissue inflammation and damage in certain immuno-logical diseases, including Sjögren's. Low levels of these proteins generally reflect the ongoing utilization of these proteins in a process triggered by the binding of immunoglobulins to molecular targets in the serum (thereby forming immune complexes) or to targets on cellular surfaces. Very low levels of C4 can also reflect the genetic absence of this protein.

EXCLUSION OF SJÖGREN'S MIMICS

Certain other diseases can mimic Sjögren's and should be excluded in the diagnostic evaluation of a patient with suspected Sjögren's. Hepatitis C and human immunodeficiency virus (HIV) infections can be excluded with blood tests. IgG4 plasmacytic infiltrative disease is characterized by elevated serum levels of IgG4 (a subclass of the IgG immunoglobulin family) and/or infiltra-tion of the salivary or lacrimal glands with IgG4-producing plasma cells. Thus, a biopsy of the salivary or lacrimal glands may be required. Lymphoma requires biopsy of an enlarged salivary or lacrimal gland or lymph node for definitive diagnosis.

IMAGING MODALITIES USED IN THE EVALUATION OF SJÖGREN'S

Both the structure and function of the major salivary glands can be assessed with currently available imaging techniques. Such tests may be ordered for one of the following reasons: (1) to determine if there is impairment of the function of the salivary glands that might underlie a patient's sensation of a dry mouth; (2) to quantify the function of the major salivary glands, providing an important measure that can be followed over time; (3) to determine the presence of an anatomical defect, such as a blocked salivary duct, as the basis for recurrent salivary gland swelling; (4) to assess whether there is evidence of diffuse alterations in the structure of the salivary glands, indicative of a chronic inflammatory process affecting the glands; and (5) to evaluate whether enlargement of one or more salivary glands is due to a tumor. The usual imaging modalities include parotid scintigraphy (also known as salivary gland function scanning), sialography, MRI, and CT.

1. **Parotid scintigraphy**. This is a nuclear medicine test that evaluates the function of the parotid and submandibular glands. Salivary gland function is assessed by the pattern of uptake and secretion of a radioactive tracer. It is typically performed in a hospital nuclear medicine department or outpatient radiology facility. The patient receives an injection of pertechnetate, a low-level radioactive marker, and is then positioned in front of or under a gamma scintillation camera, which detects the radiation and produces an image (Fig. 18–4). Imaging typically begins immediately after the injection to observe the progressive accumulation of the radioactive tracer in the glands. After 45 minutes, the patient is given a hard lemon candy or similar sour substance to stimulate the emptying of the salivary glands. Another set of images is then made for comparison purposes. The entire process takes about 60 minutes. With the aid of a computer, the uptake and secretion of the radioactive tracer can be quantified for each gland. Salivary gland scans are safe. The level of radioactivity used to obtain the images is low; however, women who are pregnant should not have this test unless necessary.
2. **Contrast sialography**. This test assesses the structure of the major salivary glands. It involves a series of x-rays that are taken immediately after the retrograde injection of a contrast dye into the duct of the parotid (Stensen's duct) or submandibular gland (Wharton's duct). The test requires the insertion of a small tube into the salivary gland duct. The contrast dye may be either water- or oil-based; generally a water-based dye is preferred. The resulting x-rays may show strictures of the ducts, dilatation of the terminal portions of the ducts (sialoectasia), or duct blockages. These anatomical alterations are not specific for Sjögren's, if found.

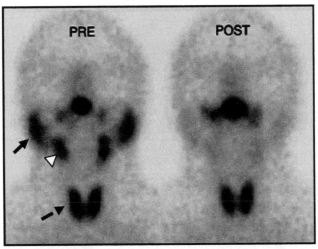

FIGURE 18–4 **Parotid Scintigraphy.**
In the image on the left, the parotid (*black arrow*), submandibular (*white arrowhead*), and thyroid glands (*dashed arrow*) are visualized, as a result of their uptake of the radioactive tracer over the course of 45 minutes. The image on the right was taken shortly after the patient had sucked on a hard lemon candy. The radioactive uptake in the parotid and submandibular glands is no longer evident, reflecting the lemon-stimulated discharge of saliva from these glands.

3. **MRI.** MRI of the salivary glands is an excellent tool to assess the structure of the major salivary glands (Fig. 18–5). This imaging modality uses strong magnetic fields to assess the properties of hydrogen atoms in different tissues within the human body. The human body is composed primarily of hydrogen atoms, found in water. MRI uses a property of atoms called "spin" to distinguish differences between tissues such as muscle, fat, and tendon. With a patient in the magnetic field of the MRI machine, the nuclei of the hydrogen atoms may spin in one of two directions. The MRI machine emits a radiofrequency pulse that causes the nuclei to absorb energy and then transition from one spin orientation to the other. The energy that is then released by the hydrogen molecules as they transition back from their high-energy to their low-energy state is detected by the MRI machine and is used to create the cross-sectional image. This exchange of energy between spin states is called resonance (thus the name magnetic resonance imaging). Since the properties of these atoms vary in the main tissues of the body, such as muscle, fat, brain, and so forth, MRI is an excellent technique for imaging the soft tissues of the body, including the salivary glands. There is no radiation involved. MRI is particularly useful for assessing whether a swollen salivary gland might be related to a tumor. A new MRI technique,

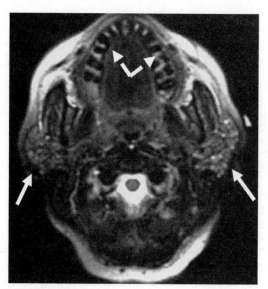

FIGURE 18–5 **MRI of Parotid Glands.**
This cross-sectional image of the head was taken at the level of the parotid glands
(*white arrows*) and the upper teeth (*dashed white arrows*). This is a T2-weighted image
that shows water as an intense (white) signal, such as the cerebrospinal fluid surrounding the
spinal cord in the center of the image. In this patient with Sjögren's, there are a number of small
"dots" of intense signal in the parotid glands, indicative of structure damage.

MR sialography, allows visualization of the larger salivary gland ducts
and may be an alternative to contrast sialography (described above).
4. **CT.** CT is a diagnostic procedure in which special x-ray equipment is
used to obtain cross-sectional images of the body. The CT computer
displays these pictures as detailed images of organs, bones, and other
tissues. CT scans can be used to obtain cross-sectional images of any
portion of the body. Radiation is involved in obtaining the images,
15 to 90 times more than a plain chest x-ray. Such scans of the face
and neck can thus be used to determine the size and structure of the
lacrimal (tear) and salivary glands (Fig. 18–6). This can be particularly
helpful to look for stones within the salivary gland and to determine if
swelling of the gland might be related to a tumor.

Defining the Extent of Disease Involvement

Sjögren's may involve organs other than the salivary and lacrimal glands in up
to 50% of patients. A search for this "extra-glandular involvement" begins with
the history and physical examination and is aided by basic laboratory tests,
including a urinalysis and complete metabolic panel (see above). If there is

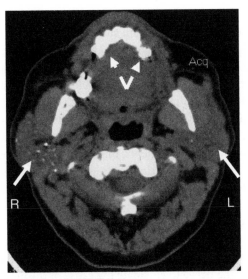

FIGURE 18–6 **CT Scan of the Parotid Glands.**
This cross-sectional image of the head was taken at the level of the parotid glands
(*white arrows*) and the upper teeth (*dashed white arrows*). With this x-ray technique, white
structures in the image are those that block the transmission of the x-rays to the detector. Thus
bone, teeth, and other calcium-containing structures are seen as white. In this patient with
Sjögren's, there are specks of calcium in the right parotid gland, indicative of glandular damage.

concern about the presence of specific organ involvement, different test modalities may be employed. These are described briefly below.

1. **Skin involvement.** Patients with Sjögren's may develop skin rashes,
    usually related to the presence of vasculitis or to the deposition of
    immune complexes at the junction of the epidermis (outer layer of the
    skin) and the subjacent dermis (so-called interface dermatitis). A **skin
    biopsy** may be required for accurate diagnosis of these conditions.
    This is usually performed with a punch technique, in which a 3- to
    4-mm cylindrical plug of previously anesthetized skin is removed and
    sent to the laboratory.

2. **Peripheral nervous system involvement.** Damage of the peripheral
    nerves ("peripheral neuropathies") can occur in Sjögren's as a result of
    diverse autoimmune mechanisms. Symptoms include burning pain or
    numbness of the hands and feet, weakness of the extremities, poor
    balance, and altered gait. The diagnosis of a peripheral neuropathy
    requires **electrodiagnostic testing**, including electromyography
    (EMG) and nerve conduction studies. These tests measure the
    electrical activity of muscles and nerves and are usually done at the
    same time. The nerve conduction study measures how quickly
    electrical impulses move along a nerve and can distinguish between

neuropathies caused by damage to the nerve's axon and those caused by damage to the myelin sheath surrounding the nerve. The EMG measures the electrical activity of a muscle and provides information about the muscle itself and how well it receives stimulation from the nerve. Patients with Sjögren's may develop a peripheral neuropathy that affects only small nerve fibers. In such cases, the EMG and nerve conduction studies may be normal, since these tests detect abnormalities in the large nerve fibers, responsible for vibratory and position sense. In such patients, injury to the small nerve fibers can be assessed with a series of skin biopsies taken from several sites in an arm or a leg. These skin biopsies are examined with special staining techniques to visualize the small nerve fibers that innervate the skin. An absence or decrease in the density of these nerve fibers in the epidermis (outer layer of the skin) is indicative of a small fiber neuropathy. Rarely, patients with a peripheral neuropathy may require a biopsy of the nerve to elucidate the cause of the neuropathy. The sural nerve (in the ankle) and the superficial radial nerve (wrist) are the sites most often used for biopsy.

3. **Central nervous system involvement.** Sjögren's may involve the central nervous system, such as the brain and the spinal cord. The types of involvement are diverse but usually involve focal areas of damage to the coatings of the nerve fibers (demyelination) or strokes. MRI of the brain and lumbar puncture ("spinal tap") are generally required to diagnose such involvement.

4. **Lung involvement.** Inflammation within the lung tissue (interstitial pneumonitis) may occur in Sjögren's and be manifested by shortness of breath and cough. The diagnostic evaluation usually involves a chest x-ray, CT scan of the lung, and pulmonary function testing. A biopsy of lung tissue may be required to differentiate the various types of lung inflammation that can occur in Sjögren's.

5. **Kidney involvement.** Inflammation of either the glomerulus (i.e., glomerulonephritis) or the supporting tissue of the kidney (i.e., interstitial nephritis) occurs in a small minority of patients with Sjögren's. An excess of protein in the urine or impairment of kidney function (i.e., elevated serum creatinine or decrease in glomerular filtration rate) may indicate either form of kidney disease. Interstitial nephritis may lead to a condition called renal tubular acidosis in which the kidney fails to reabsorb bicarbonate from the urine or to secrete hydrogen ions into the urine. Manifestations include a low serum bicarbonate level, a relatively high urine pH, dilute urine, and excess urine concentrations of glucose, uric acid, phosphate, and amino acids. These types of kidney involvement can be detected initially with an analysis of the urine and the serum

chemistries and creatinine. A kidney biopsy may be required for definitive diagnosis.

6. **Liver involvement.** Autoimmune hepatitis occurs in approximately 5% of Sjögren's patients. Symptoms, if present, usually include fatigue, itching, nausea, poor appetite, and abdominal pain. The diagnosis is first suggested by the finding of elevated liver function tests on blood chemistries (particularly the aminotransferases, ALT and AST). The finding of characteristic antibodies, such as anti-mitochondrial and anti-smooth muscle (actin) antibodies, supports the diagnosis. Confirmation requires a liver biopsy.

7. **Gastrointestinal involvement.** Sjögren's can affect the ability to chew, swallow, and digest food through a variety of mechanisms. Difficulty swallowing may relate to lack of saliva, dryness of the esophagus, or poor esophageal contractions. Poor digestion may result from impaired secretion of acid by the stomach or digestive enzymes by the pancreas. Absorption of nutrients can be impaired by the presence of a second autoimmune disease, celiac disease, which may occur in patients with Sjögren's. Testing for gastrointestinal involvement usually requires x-ray studies, endoscopy, and blood tests.

8. **Hematologic involvement.** Abnormalities of the blood counts, including low numbers of RBCs (anemia), WBCs (leukopenia), and platelets (thrombocytopenia), occur in a minority of Sjögren's patients. They may arise from a variety of mechanisms, not all of which are autoimmune. Thus, it is important that these abnormalities be evaluated carefully, since some may reflect nutritional deficiencies (such as low levels of iron, folic acid, vitamin B_{12}) or primary bone marrow disorders. The evaluation usually requires blood tests and occasionally a bone marrow aspiration.

Monitoring Disease Progression and Risk for Lymphoma

Sjögren's is a chronic disease that shows minimal progression over years of follow-up for most patients. Thus, measures of saliva and tear production often do not decline significantly over periods of greater than 5 years. However, it is important that patients with Sjögren's be evaluated on at least an annual basis to assess their oral and ocular health and monitor for the development of internal organ involvement and lymphoma. Additionally, patients taking hydroxychloroquine need to be examined by an ophthalmologist annually to make sure that there is no evidence of retinal damage, a rare complication of this treatment. Laboratory monitoring every 2 to 3 months may also be required for patients taking immunosuppressive treatments for their Sjögren's syndrome.

The periodic evaluation of a patient with Sjögren's generally involves a careful history and physical examination, including specialized examinations of the eyes (preferably by an ophthalmologist) and the mouth (by a dentist). Laboratory testing, such as a CBC, complete metabolic panel, and urinalysis, may serve to screen for internal organ involvement. Certain immunological tests may help define whether there is a high risk for the development of lymphoma. These include the presence of low levels of the C_4 complement protein, a monoclonal immunoglobulin, and serum cryoglobulins (serum proteins, often a mixture of monoclonal and non-monoclonal immunoglobulins, which precipitate in the cold).

Going Beyond: Pathways of Discovery with Genetic Testing

The field of molecular biology has provided two important laboratory tools for uncovering the disease mechanisms underlying Sjögren's. **Gene expression profiling** allows the scientist to measure the activity or expression of thousands of genes at once, thereby creating a global picture of cellular function. Such profiling can be performed on cells felt to be important to the development of Sjögren's, such as salivary gland tissue or blood immune cells. In so doing, the profile of genes that are expressed can be compared with that in control cells (i.e., taken from a healthy donor or from a patient with another autoimmune disease) and specific pathways of cellular function can be identified that may be relevant to the pathogenesis of Sjögren's. With this technique, patients with Sjögren's and SLE have been shown to have increased expression of a number of genes that are "turned on" by interferon, a protein that normally defends the body against viral infections. This has resulted in intense interest in the role of interferon in these autoimmune diseases and opens the possibility that treatments directed at reducing interferon levels may be beneficial for Sjögren's patients.

The **genome-wide association study** (GWAS) allows scientists to rapidly scan the complete set of DNA, or genome, of many individuals to find genetic variations associated with a complex disease, such as Sjögren's. The identification of such genetic variations can uncover molecular pathways important to the development of Sjögren's and help define an individual's risk of developing Sjögren's or certain complications of the disease. A GWAS of Sjögren's would be typically performed on two groups of participants: people with Sjögren's and people of similar ethnicity and gender without Sjögren's. A large number of individuals, carefully characterized with regards to their Sjögren's, is required for a successful GWAS. DNA is obtained from each participant, usually from cells within a blood or saliva sample. Each person's DNA is then purified from the sample, placed on tiny chips, and scanned on automated laboratory machines. The machines quickly survey each participant's genome for strategically selected markers of genetic variation, called single nucleotide polymorphisms (SNPs). If certain genetic variations are found to be significantly more frequent in people with Sjögren's than people without, the variations are said to be "associated" with the disease. The associated genetic variations can point to the region of the human genome that contains genetic alterations important to the development of Sjögren's.

Summing Up

The diagnosis and management of Sjögren's requires a variety of testing modalities, including blood and urine assays, tissue biopsies, and medical imaging. These tests are essential to establish the correct diagnosis, define the extent of disease involvement, and monitor for potential disease complications. Since Sjögren's is a heterogeneous disorder, the clinician must choose diagnostic testing based on the unique features of each patient. Ongoing research holds promise in defining molecular diagnostic tests that may refine the diagnosis of Sjögren's and better define the potential for certain disease complications.

FOR FURTHER READING

Daniels TE, Whitcher JP. Association of patterns of labial salivary gland inflammation with keratoconjunctivitis sicca. Analysis of 618 patients with suspected Sjögren's. *Arthritis Rheum.* 1994; 37(6): 869–77.

Emamian ES, Leon JM, Lessard CJ, et al. Peripheral blood gene expression profiling in Sjögren's. *Genes Immun.* 2009; 10(4): 285–96.

Fritzler MJ, Pauls JD, Kinsella TD, Bowen TJ. Antinuclear, anticytoplasmic, and anti-Sjögren's antigen A (SS-A/Ro) antibodies in female blood donors. *Clin Immunol Immunopathol.* 1985; 36: 120–8.

Garcia-Carrasco M, Ramos-Casals M, Rosas J, et al. Primary Sjogren syndrome: clinical and immunologic disease patterns in a cohort of 400 patients. *Medicine (Baltimore).* 2002; 81(4): 270–80.

Goeb V, Salle V, Duhaut P, et al. Clinical significance of autoantibodies recognizing Sjögren's A (SSA), SSB, calpastatin and alpha-fodrin in primary Sjögren's. *Clin Exp Immunol.* 2007; 148(2): 281–7.

Gottenberg JE, Cagnard N, Lucchesi C, et al. Activation of IFN pathways and plasmacytoid dendritic cell recruitment in target organs of primary Sjögren's. *Proc Natl Acad Sci U S A.* 2006; 103(8): 2770–5.

Ramos-Casals M, Brito-Zerón P, Perez-De-Lis M, et al. Sjögren syndrome or Sjögren disease? The histological and immunological bias caused by the 2002 criteria. *Clin Rev Allergy Immunol.* 2010; 38(2–3): 178–85.

Ramos-Casals M, Font J, Garcia-Carrasco M, et al. Primary Sjogren syndrome: hematologic patterns of disease expression. *Medicine (Baltimore).* 2002; 81(4): 281–92.

Routsias JG, Tzioufas AG. Sjögren's—study of autoantigens and autoantibodies. *Clin Rev Allergy Immunol.* 2007; 32(3): 238–51.

Solomon DH, Kavanaugh AJ, Schur PH, and the American College of Rheumatology Ad Hoc Committee on Immunologic Testing Guidelines. Evidence-based guidelines for the use of immunologic tests: Antinuclear antibody testing. *Arthritis & Rheumatism (Arthritis Care & Research).* 2002; 47(4): 434–44.

Tzioufas AG, Voulgarelis M. Update on Sjögren's autoimmune epithelitis: from classification to increased neoplasias. *Best Pract Res Clin Rheumatol.* 2007; 21(6): 989–1010.

Voulgarelis M, Skopouli FN. Clinical, immunologic, and molecular factors predicting lymphoma development in Sjögren's patients. *Clin Rev Allergy Immunol.* 2007; 32(3): 265–74.

19

Why Is Sjögren's Syndrome So Difficult to Diagnose?

Robert F. Spiera, MD, and Harry Spiera, MD

Diagnosing a medical disorder can be straightforward when a specific feature defines the diagnosis, such as when a specific bacteria is cultured from urine identifying the problem as a urinary tract infection, or when a mass is biopsied, and the tissue reveals cancer cells. In most conditions, however, in particular in autoimmune diseases, establishing a diagnosis can be difficult. No single clinical feature or laboratory finding is usually sufficient to be sure of the diagnosis, and there can be a spectrum of features that might be present in some patients but not others. Despite the title of this chapter, Sjögren's syndrome may be very easy to diagnose when a patient presents with the classic symptoms, physical findings, and autoantibodies associated with Sjögren's. In that scenario, the physician will be able to make a diagnosis with certainty. In other patients in whom symptoms are vaguer or evolve over time, the diagnosis becomes more difficult, particularly when the autoantibodies that are associated with Sjögren's are absent. In that situation, more delving is necessary to establish the diagnosis. At times, even an invasive procedure such as biopsy of the lip may be necessary.

Thus, the physician must keep in mind the other conditions that can present with the same type of complaints and the physical findings that may occur in a patient with Sjögren's. Physicians refer to this as the "differential diagnosis." Moreover, the symptoms of the disease may evolve slowly over many years and it is only after time has gone by that the diagnosis becomes apparent. In this chapter, we will explore some of the symptoms of Sjögren's and compare those seen in other conditions that can mimic Sjögren's, including other autoimmune diseases (Table 19–1).

The most basic defining clinical features of Sjögren's include keratoconjunctivitis sicca (dry eyes) and xerostomia (dry mouth). These symptoms may or may not be accompanied by a myriad of other systemic features, including fatigue, fever, joint pain with or without joint swelling, skin rash, various neurological symptoms, gastrointestinal problems, rarely kidney problems, rashes,

TABLE 19–1

Diagnosis of Sjögren's Syndrome

Diagnosis of Sjögren's Syndrome	
Symptoms	• Dry mouth (xerostomia)
	• Dry eyes (xerophthalmia)
	• Joint pain (with and without swelling)
	• Fatigue
	• Fever
Physical Findings	• Decreased saliva pool
	• Red eyes
	• Swollen salivary and lacrimal glands
	• Swollen lymph nodes
	• Rash
	• Swollen joints
	• Alopecia
Laboratory Findings	• Anemia
	• Decreased white blood count
	• Decreased platelets
	• Increased ESR
	• Increased CRP
	• Rheumatoid factor
	• Antinuclear antibody
	• SS-A (anti-Ro)
	• SS-B (anti-La)
	• Increased gamma globulin
Special Tests	• Schirmer test to measure tears
	• Rose Bengal test
	• Sialography
	• Saliva flow
	• Salivary chemistry
	• Lip biopsy
	• Salivary gland biopsy
	• Lymph node biopsy
Complications	• Candida
	• Caries
	• Pancreatitis
	• Neuropathy
	• Lymphoma
	• Vasculitis
Associated Disorders	• Rheumatoid arthritis
	• Systemic lupus erythematosus
	• Scleroderma
	• Dermatomyositis/polymyositis
	• Biliary cirrhosis

and other less common manifestations. At times, the systemic symptoms may be the most outstanding features of the patient's illness and the sicca complex can be more subtle. Also, Sjögren's can accompany other better-defined auto-immune conditions such as rheumatoid arthritis (RA), systemic lupus erythematosus (SLE), scleroderma, and dermatomyositis/polymyositis. If systemic features are the most pressing clinical feature but sicca features are present, it becomes almost a semantic question as to whether the patient has so-called primary Sjögren's syndrome with systemic features or has so-called secondary Sjögren's, where the Sjögren's is complicating a primary autoimmune disease. From a therapeutic standpoint, that distinction is less pressing; it may have relevance to prognosis and a better understanding of what clinical issues should be anticipated or screened for.

Autoimmune diseases that may be accompanied by Sjögren's include:

1. RA
2. SLE
3. Scleroderma
4. Dermatomyositis and polymyositis
5. Primary biliary cirrhosis

It is important that the physician assessing the patient with those disorders has Sjögren's on his or her "radar screen."

Symptoms

Dry eyes and dry mouth of themselves are very common in the general population. Certain environmental features such as dry heat may result in symptoms of dry mouth and eye. However, it would be unusual for it to result in complications of the dryness such as corneal erosion or dental carries in that scenario. In addition, a variety of medications have so-called anticholinergic side effects with resulting dry eyes and dry mouth. Common examples include the tricyclic antidepressants such as amitryptiline. Many of the medicines used for female urinary incontinence are also anticholinergic agents that can result in severe dryness of the eyes and the mouth. Medications used to treat Parkinson's disease, diuretics, and antihistamines can similarly be drying. Thus, it is incumbent on the physician to thoroughly review the prescription and over-the-counter medications the patient is taking in the evaluation of a patient with dryness of eyes or mouth concerned about Sjögren's.

An important and common symptom of Sjögren's is fatigue, which is often overwhelming. Fatigue, of course, can be caused by a number of conditions both physical and mental, and it is extremely difficult for a physician to quantify. Whereas it would not be unexpected for a woman taking care of a husband and children and who has a full-time job to feel tired, if fatigue is constant and overwhelming and not related to the degree of activity, it may be related to an underlying medical problem such as an underactive thyroid or anemia. Patients with Sjögren's sometimes have fatigue so overwhelming that they can barely function and may be reduced to a sedentary lifestyle. This incidentally is an important and significant feature of SLE as well and can represent an important limitation in other autoimmune conditions such as RA.

Joint pain with or without swelling is also often a feature of Sjögren's but similarly is not specific to the disease. Almost everybody at one time or the other has joint pain. However, the joint pain in Sjögren's is often severe and involves multiple joints, particularly the small joints of the hands and feet. In contrast to the arthritis of RA, where persistent joint swelling and inflammation observed by a physician is present, the joints of a patient with Sjögren's may not show any swelling. Although swollen joints can occur in Sjögren's, the joint deformity and crippling seen in RA is rarely observed. Indeed, usually x-ray findings are unrevealing. When a patient with Sjögren's has joint deformity, erosions on x-ray, and crippling, it is more likely that the Sjögren's is secondary to RA. If a woman has severe pain in the joints without swelling, redness, or objective findings, strong possibilities include both SLE and Sjögren's.

Skin changes can occur in Sjögren's. Rashes, particularly eruptions of small red raised spots called "palpable purpura" on the extremities, can occur. When biopsied, they demonstrate characteristic though not specific histological features. At times, patients have Raynaud's phenomenon, in which the hands turn white, blue, or red on exposure to cold. This can accompany other autoimmune diseases as well, including scleroderma, where it is even more common, or SLE or RA, in which it is less frequently observed.

Neurological symptoms are frequently seen in patients with Sjögren's. The most common of these are sensations of "pins and needles" or numbness of the extremities, particularly of the feet. Patients also may complain of the feet feeling "cold." This is referred to as peripheral neuropathy. The examining physician will often find decreased sensation of the lower extremity when examined with a pin or a tuning fork. Most commonly, the nerve involvement is mainly sensory. More severe peripheral neuropathy can involve motor nerves, resulting in weakness of the extremities or overt foot drops or wrist drops causing significant functional impairment, not just discomfort. This is a serious complication that may require very aggressive treatment but fortunately is not common. A characteristic yet infrequent form of neuropathy seen in Sjögren's results in the loss of sensing one's position and may severely impair balance and function of the hands. If significant neurological problems occur, the patient will often be seen by a neurologist for further workup to help characterize the type of neuropathy and help establish a cause possibly other than Sjögren's. Other conditions can similarly cause neuropathy, including various vitamin deficiencies (particularly B_{12}), diabetes, celiac disease, other autoimmune problems (such as SLE, vasculitis, or RA), and there are even other "idiopathic" neuropathies where no broader systemic process is operable.

Other types of neurological involvement can include cognitive impairment or transverse myelopathy, where signs, symptoms, and even MRI findings may mimic multiple sclerosis, and the distinction can be made only by recognizing the broader clinical context, or possibly through more specific tests of spinal fluid. Cognitive impairment can occur related to Sjögren's, or at times related to medications used to treat the disease (such as steroids), and of course a broad array of other medical problems such as thyroid disease must be considered in the differential diagnosis. Expert opinion from neurologists and psychiatrists is often necessary to better define the problem and tease out other potential causes.

Various gastrointestinal symptoms can occur in Sjögren's. Most symptoms are a result of the dryness itself. For example, if the bolus of food cannot be adequately moisturized, it would be difficult for the patient to propel the bolus of food to the pharynx, resulting in swallowing difficulty. This must be differentiated from the swallowing difficulty (referred to as "dysphagia") that can occur in dermatomyositis/polymyositis where the patient cannot initiate the act of swallowing due to weakness of the pharyngeal muscles. It also must be distinguished from the swallowing difficulty experienced by patients with scleroderma in which food gets stuck in the middle of the esophagus due to loss of smooth muscle or stricture. Often simple questioning may help make the distinction, but at other times further studies such as electrodiagnostic studies or gastrointestinal imaging may be necessary. Complicating the matter is that those latter forms of dysphagia can also occur in Sjögren's, although not as commonly as in those other autoimmune disorders. This speaks to the overlapping features of many of the systemic autoimmune disorders.

A rare gastrointestinal complication of Sjögren's is pancreatitis. The pancreas is at least partially an "exocrine gland," in many ways similar to the lacrimal gland that produces tears and the salivary gland that produces saliva. When pancreatitis occurs acutely, it can cause abdominal pain. When the pancreatitis is chronic, malabsorption may occur, resulting in weight loss despite an adequate or even excessive dietary intact. It is important to make this diagnosis in a patient with Sjögren's who loses weight, as in that situation, re-supplying pancreatic enzymes may help correct the abnormality.

Laboratory Manifestations

Laboratory manifestations in Sjögren's may be specific or nonspecific. The nonspecific manifestations include elevated erythrocyte sedimentation rate (ESR) or C-reactive protein (CRP). Interestingly, whereas in RA the sedimentation rate may correlate with the severity and activity of the disease, this often is not found in Sjögren's. Thus, the ESR may be very elevated and the symptoms may be minimal. Increased gamma globulin is often present.

The anti-Ro (SSA) and anti-La (SSB) antibodies are characteristic of Sjögren's, although by themselves they are not diagnostic, as they may be found in other conditions such as SLE. In general, they occur in about 60% of patients with Sjögren's. If either the SSA or SSB antibody is found in a patient who has a sicca complex, this would be pretty much diagnostic of Sjögren's. At times, patients are seen who have either the SSA or SSB antibodies but do not yet have a dry eye or dry mouth. Even a lip biopsy in that situation may be negative. In some of the patients, the sicca complex may appear after only many years of observation.

Rheumatoid factor and antinuclear antibodies (ANAs) are extremely frequently found in patients with Sjögren's. Rarely, anti-DNA antibodies are found. The presence of anti-DNA antibodies would suggest to the physician to consider the diagnosis of SLE, or at a minimum to be more vigilant about watching for manifestations of that disease; in SLE kidney issues are a much more frequent concern than in Sjögren's, and they usually occur in the absence of symptoms. A decrease in complement proteins C3 and C4 can be seen and similarly may suggest the need for greater vigilance about the development of more significant organ complications than dry eye and mouth.

Pathological Findings

Biopsy of the minor salivary glands of the lips may be helpful when the diagnosis is otherwise uncertain. The surgeon makes a small incision in the inner part of the lip and takes out one of the tiny minor salivary glands, which is then examined under a microscope. If characteristic lymphocytic infiltration of the gland is seen, this is quite characteristic of Sjögren's. At times, biopsy of either the parotid gland or another major salivary gland is done. That is usually done if there is suspicion of some neoplastic process such as lymphoma occurring in those glands. Biopsy of a minor salivary gland is far less invasive than biopsy of a major salivary gland.

As noted in the preceding sections, many of the symptoms of Sjögren's are extremely nonspecific. Fatigue can be seen accompanying many conditions, such as fibromyalgia and depression. Dryness of the mouth and fatigue, of course, can be seen in diabetes. Hypothyroidism can cause muscle and joint pain as well as profound fatigue and must be a consideration. Hypothyroidism is rather common in other autoimmune diseases, and the diagnosis is easy to establish with routine laboratory testing. Other diseases such as sarcoidosis or infections such as mumps can cause swelling of the parotid and other salivary glands. Distinction can usually be made on the basis of clinical, laboratory, and, at times, histological findings.

Since dryness of the eyes and dryness of the mouth are basically subjective complaints, it often becomes necessary to actually quantify whether indeed there is dry eyes or dry mouth. Thus, the ophthalmologist can on the basis of a Schirmer test measure the amount of tear production. Similarly, saliva production can be quantified by various techniques, but this is far less frequently done than Schirmer testing. Patients with suspected Sjögren's can benefit from consultation by ophthalmologists and dentists, and indeed these professionals ultimately are vital components of the ongoing care of patients with Sjögren's.

Summing Up

Sjögren's syndrome is a clinical syndrome that has an autoimmune basis. The cardinal symptoms of Sjögren's, however, can occur with both autoimmune and non-autoimmune disease. With careful history, physical examination, and laboratory testing, the correct diagnosis can usually be established.

There is much overlap between the clinical and laboratory features of the various autoimmune diseases, particularly Sjögren's and SLE. When the specific causes of the various autoimmune diseases are ultimately better defined, distinguishing between the various syndromes will be easier.

Importantly, the treatments of the various autoimmune diseases are relatively nonspecific, and many of the medications are used in the different autoimmune conditions. Treatment is guided by the manifestations being addressed rather than the "label" of the underlying disease. Thus, exact distinction of the various autoimmune syndromes may not be necessary to offer appropriate care.

FOR FURTHER READING

Garcia-Carrasco M, Ramos-Casals M, Rosas J, et al. Primary Sjogren syndrome: clinical and immunologic disease patterns in a cohort of 400 patients. *Medicine (Baltimore).* 2002; 81: 270–80.

Kassan SS, Moutsopoulos HM. Clinical manifestations and early diagnosis of Sjögren syndrome. *Arch Intern Med.* 2004; 164: 1275–84.

Martinez-Lavin M, Vaughan JH, Tan EM. Autoantibodies and the spectrum of Sjögren's syndrome. *Ann Intern Med.* 1979; 91: 185–90.

Pertovaara M, Korpela M, Uusitalo H, et al. Clinical follow up study of 87 patients with sicca symptoms (dryness of eyes or mouth, or both). *Ann Rheum Dis.* 1999; 58: 423–27.

Ramos-Casals M, Tzioufas AG, Font J. Primary Sjögren's syndrome: new clinical and therapeutic concepts. *Ann Rheum Dis.* 2005; 64: 347–54.

Theander E, Jacobsson LT. Relationship of Sjogren's syndrome to other connective tissue and autoimmune disorders. *Rheum Dis Clin North Am.* 2008; 34: 935–47.

Vitali C. Classification criteria for Sjögren's syndrome. *Ann Rheum Dis.* 2003; 62: 94–95.

PART FOUR

THE MANAGEMENT OF SJÖGREN'S

20

Treatment of Dry Mouth

Philip C. Fox, DDS, Mabi L. Singh, DMD, MS, and
Athena S. Papas, DMD, PhD

Dry mouth is a hallmark symptom of Sjögren's syndrome. The term *xerostomia* is used in the medical literature to describe this subjective sensation of dryness of the oral cavity. The cause of dry mouth in Sjögren's is a reduction in the amount of saliva produced by the major and minor salivary glands and changes in the composition of the secretions. This is a result of autoimmune-mediated alterations in the salivary glands that lead to an irreversible loss of fluid-secreting cells and disruption of normal secretion mechanisms.

A Brief Review of Dry Mouth

There are three pairs of major salivary glands—the parotid, submandibular, and sublingual glands—and hundreds of minor salivary glands scattered throughout the oral cavity. These glands produce and secrete into the mouth a complex fluid containing critical protective factors. Saliva helps preserve the dentition, protect the oral soft tissues, and facilitate important oral functions such as chewing, swallowing, and speaking. In the absence of adequate salivation, there are many negative effects in the mouth.

Due to the loss of the antimicrobial, remineralizing, and cleansing properties of saliva, there is a marked increase in dental caries. Caries may appear and progress rapidly even at the non–plaque-retentive areas. There is an inverse relationship between the microbial populations and salivary hypofunction in the mouth, resulting in an increased incidence of bacterial and fungal infections. In particular, *Candida* species fungal infections are frequent and may be resistant to treatment. The oral mucosa may become thinner, reddened, and painful, with sensitivity to spicy foods. Chewing and swallowing become more difficult with less fluid present in the mouth. It may be hard to form a compact food bolus and move it through the oral cavity to the pharynx. Speaking may be compromised due to lack of lubrication of the soft tissues. Even taste may be affected, as tastants must be in solution and delivered to the taste buds to be fully appreciated. Accompanying these changes is a persistent feeling of dryness, not just of the mouth, but also the throat, nose, and pharynx. The salivary gland dysfunction of Sjögren's has profound effects on the oral cavity and oral functions and quality of life.

Treatment of Dry Mouth

Relief of symptoms of oral dryness is desirable but incomplete. There are several goals to treatment of salivary gland dysfunction and xerostomia in Sjögren's: (1) to relieve dryness symptoms; (2) to prevent anticipated oral complications; (3) to stimulate salivary gland function; and (4) to promote repair of salivary gland damage. The ideal therapy would accomplish all of these. At present, however, there is no single treatment that will satisfy all these goals. However, with careful attention, close cooperation between patients and professionals, and a systematic approach to treatment, most aspects of dry mouth in Sjögren's can be managed and improved.

The mainstay of symptomatic treatment is water. The importance of *adequate hydration* of the oral cavity for the Sjögren's patient cannot be overemphasized. Water should always be available, with small sips taken frequently. Water does more than relieve the immediate sense of dryness. It helps hydrate the oral mucosa and cleanse the mouth, partially replacing these functions of saliva. Dehydration causes oral dryness and reduced salivary output, so adequate water intake is important to maintain maximum salivary function. If small amounts of water are used each time, this will limit the total volume consumed and reduce frequent urination, a complaint of many patients. Small sips of water also help with chewing and swallowing.

Increasing the humidity may be helpful as well. During the winter months, humidity can be very low and this will contribute to feelings of oral dryness. This is a particular problem at night, when salivary function normally is reduced and breathing is often through the mouth. The use of a humidifier placed at the bedside can help relieve nighttime dryness, thereby improving sleep. The recommended humidity level is 50%. Humidifiers should be cleaned often and the water in the reservoir replaced daily.

There are many saliva replacement products (the Sjögren's Syndrome Foundation produces a Product Directory that is available to members upon joining in hard copy and online). Patients should try different products to see if any are beneficial. The effects are temporary but may be helpful for those with very dry mouth. In cases where there is no remaining salivary function, saliva replacements may be the only option for symptomatic relief. Some patients use artificial saliva at bedtime and during the night to limit their nighttime water intake and the subsequent need for frequent urination during the night.

There are also numerous *moisturizers, lubricants, rinses, gels, sprays,* and *emollients* that are promoted for relief of dry mouth symptoms. These can be applied to the lips and inside of the mouth. Personal preference should guide the selection of a product. Most will provide temporary relief of dryness and mucosal discomfort. Alcohol, tobacco, and caffeine can have drying effects on the oral cavity and should be avoided or limited. Many carbonated beverages contain caffeine and are quite acidic. They should not be used regularly for relief of dryness symptoms.

Symptoms often can be relieved effectively by stimulating salivary output. Means of doing this are discussed below in the section on stimulation of salivary gland function.

Prevention of Oral Complications

Generation of *dental caries* requires the presence of bacteria and a fermentable carbohydrate source for them to metabolize. Therefore, much of the destruction of the teeth found in Sjögren's patients can be controlled with effective oral hygiene measures and dietary modifications. Meticulous oral hygiene should include flossing at least daily and toothbrushing after each meal. The goal is to remove the bacteria that attach to the teeth (as dental plaque) and their food sources. In the absence of cariogenic bacteria, decay will not occur.

Similarly, if the bacteria are deprived of fermentable carbohydrates, they will not produce acids that can demineralize the tooth surface. Sugar in the diet should be minimized, and sticky sweets, such as cookies and candies that adhere to the teeth, should be avoided. When sugary foods are consumed, the teeth should be brushed—or at least rinsed—immediately. Regular use of acidic beverages, like many soft drinks, should be avoided as well. Acidic fluids, like lemon juice, may stimulate saliva, but that benefit must be balanced against the negative effects of the acid on the tooth surface. If acidic drinks are consumed, those fortified with calcium and fluoride are recommended, followed by rinsing with water or milk or a low-concentration fluoride rinse. Brushing immediately after acidic food consumption is not recommended, as the incidence of abrasion and erosion can be increased.

In addition to oral hygiene and diet, the use of fluoride is an important preventive measure. Fluoride helps to repair early demineralization of the tooth (the first step in dental caries) and strengthens the tooth surface. A fluoride-containing toothpaste should be used, and topical fluoride applications may be indicated. The frequency, type, and mode of application of topical fluoride (daily, weekly, rinse, high-concentration gel, self-applied or professionally applied, brushed on, applied in a custom tray, etc.) should be discussed with the dentist. The determination should be made based on the caries rate and severity of the salivary gland dysfunction. In some cases, a fluoride varnish may be applied to the teeth by the dentist. Experimental studies have shown that early caries can be repaired with solutions containing high concentrations of calcium and phosphate. This is one of the prominent functions of natural saliva. The use of a remineralizing solution may be indicated in Sjögren's patients and should be discussed with the dentist.

Fungal infections, usually caused by *Candida* spp., are common in dry mouth patients. A confusing aspect of diagnosis is that these often do not present in the common white mucocutaneous form (known by most people as "thrush"). Instead, the mucosa may appear red or irritated, the so-called chronic erythematous form of candidiasis. Patients may complain of a burning sensation. The area should be cultured and treatment instituted with a topical therapeutic. Many infections are difficult to manage and resistant to therapy, and treatment may be prolonged. This is a problem, as most topical antifungal preparations (rinses and lozenges) have a very high sugar content. A rinse without sugar should be used or formulated. If a sugar-containing preparation is used, particularly a slowly dissolving lozenge, patients must brush well afterward. Due to a lack of natural antifungal components usually provided in saliva, the infection may recur. Although use of a systemic antifungal agent seems ideal in Sjögren's, if salivary function is low, this approach may also fail, as much of the drug is delivered through salivary secretion and may fail to reach the affected mucosa. Aggressive topical treatment will be successful given sufficient time and may be repeated as often as necessary. Cleaning of the tongue with a brush or scraper may help reduce fungal populations. Removal of the biofilm from a fissured tongue can be done efficiently with sonic brushes. Also, removable prosthetic devices such as partial or full dentures may harbor *Candida* spp. and should be cleaned and disinfected daily.

Stimulation of Salivary Function

There are many ways to stimulate salivary output. They may be divided into topical or local approaches and systemic therapies (Table 20–1). By stimulating remaining salivary gland tissue, a patient will get all the benefits of natural saliva in the oral cavity and relief of dryness symptoms. The success of this is dependent on the amount of secretory function that remains and the efficacy of the stimulation. Even modest increases in salivary output may translate into significant symptomatic improvement. A deficiency in all current therapies is the transitory nature of the stimulation: even systemic parasympathomimetic drugs have a duration of action of only a few hours. However, symptomatic relief of dryness may persist beyond the immediate period of increased salivary output with chronic use of these agents. This is likely due to beneficial effects on the mucosa from the increased amounts of saliva.

TABLE 20–1
Means of Stimulating Salivary Function

Topical/Local Approaches
  Gustatory stimulation
  Masticatory stimulation
  Acupuncture
  Electrical stimulation
Systemic Secretagogues
  Pilocarpine
  Cevimeline
  Bromhexine
  Anetholetrithione
  B-cell–depleting agents
  Epithelial sodium channel blockers

TOPICAL AND LOCAL THERAPIES

Saliva can be stimulated effectively by almost any oral activity. Chewing or sucking on an object will result in a robust increase in saliva output. Salivation is also responsive to taste, particularly sour and bitter. The use of *flavored gums and lozenges* remains a mainstay of palliative therapy of dry mouth. The combination of gustatory and masticatory stimulation can transiently increase salivation and relieve symptoms of dry mouth. Patients with diminished salivation should use sugar-free gums, lozenges, candies, or mints for symptomatic relief of xerostomia. The use of sugar-free and low-acid products must be stressed, as otherwise the addition of sugar bathing the dentition will only increase the caries risk and negate the benefits of increased salivary output. Xylitol is an acceptable sweetener that has been shown to reduce dental caries. Some patients benefit from sucking on a cherry pit, smooth stone, or other non-nutritive object. This may increase salivation without any sugar or calories.

Although not strictly a local therapy, *acupuncture* relies on application of the needles to specific locations, often in close proximity to the oral cavity. There have been a number of clinical studies of acupuncture to treat xerostomia, and the authors reported some benefit for relief of symptoms and improvement in salivary output. One problem with these studies is the difficulty in providing for appropriate placebo controls in clinical trials of acupuncture. One trial that used superficial, non–site-specific acupuncture as a control found that the control group had improvements similar to those of the active acupuncture group. At present, acupuncture remains a possible approach to enhancing salivary function that requires further study. Acupuncture may serve as a useful adjunct to management of dry mouth.

There has been a revival of interest in electrical stimulation within the oral cavity as a means of increasing salivation and relieving dryness symptoms.

A device that can be attached to a tooth or embedded in a removable appliance is in clinical testing, and initial results are encouraging, with improvements in dryness complaints and increased mucosal moisture reported in small studies. Larger, controlled trials are under way.

SYSTEMIC THERAPIES

There are many systemic agents that are capable of stimulating salivary output (Table 20–1). The most extensive clinical evidence has been with the parasympathomimetic agents pilocarpine and cevimeline.

Pilocarpine (Salagen) is a parasympathomimetic agent with mild beta-adrenergic–stimulating properties. It has been proposed as a treatment for dry mouth for over a hundred years. A number of well-designed and well-controlled clinical trials of substantial size have examined the effects of pilocarpine on dry mouth and salivary function in patients with Sjögren's. These clinical trials have consistently demonstrated that at doses of 5 to 10 mg three or four times daily (maximum 30 mg/day), pilocarpine can significantly improve symptoms of dry mouth and increase salivary output. Salivary secretion is maximally stimulated approximately 1 hour after dosing with pilocarpine, and increases over baseline salivary output are found for 3 to 4 hours. No tolerance to the secretagogue effects of pilocarpine has been reported, nor has long-term improvement in baseline salivary function been found. Increased salivary output is transitory, dose-related, and consistent.

Serious adverse events are rare with pilocarpine. While side effects such as sweating, flushing, and urinary frequency are common, they are typically of mild or moderate intensity and of relatively short duration. Side effects may also be alleviated by taking the medication after meals. Use of pilocarpine is contraindicated in individuals with uncontrolled asthma, narrow-angle glaucoma, or acute iritis. Caution is advised with use in patients with cardiovascular disease.

Another parasympathomimetic agent, cevimeline (Evoxac), has also been studied in large, well-controlled trials. At doses of 30 mg three times daily, cevimeline was shown to improve symptoms of dry mouth significantly and increase salivary output in patients with Sjögren's. Cevimeline is similar pharmacologically to pilocarpine, although the onset of increased salivation may be somewhat later and the duration of action longer. The safety and adverse event profiles are very similar to pilocarpine as well, with sweating, light-headedness, and nausea common complaints among patients. Cevimeline has been reported to have a high selective affinity for M3-subtype muscarinic receptors, the predominant receptor subtype in the salivary glands.

Bromhexine, although not FDA approved, has been proposed as a salivary stimulant and treatment for dry mouth in Sjögren's. However, there are no well-controlled studies demonstrating that this agent will increase salivary output or improve dry mouth symptoms. There may be some benefit for dry eye symptoms in Sjögren's, but this has not been shown for the oral cavity.

Anetholetrithione, also not FDA approved, is an agent that has been demonstrated to increase salivation in individuals with mild salivary gland dysfunction. The dose studied was 25 mg three times daily. In more severe cases of secretory hypofunction in Sjögren's patients, however, anetholetrithione was ineffective. Though there has been an interesting report suggesting a synergistic effect between anetholetrithione and pilocarpine, there are inadequate clinical trials of this drug.

Several large clinical trials have been conducted using interferon-alpha (IFN-alpha) (not FDA approved), as a high-dose injectable or a low-dose lozenge, for treatment of dry mouth and decreased salivation in Sjögren's. The low-dose lozenge formulation, at 150 IU three times a day, was found to reduce xerostomia and increase salivary output in some studies. In one study, after 6 months of treatment minor salivary gland inflammation also improved. Side effects and adverse events were minimal. Further clinical trials will be necessary to define appropriate doses and to demonstrate fully the efficacy of this experimental agent.

Infliximab, etanercept, and adalimumab are TNF-alpha blockers used in treatment of rheumatoid arthritis. (TNF-alpha is a cytokine that is felt to be a central component of inflammatory reactions.) Following encouraging results in uncontrolled preliminary studies with infliximab, larger controlled trials failed to show any benefit in a number of clinical and functional oral parameters. TNF-alpha blockers are not recommended for treatment of dry mouth in Sjögren's.

As hyperreactivity of B cells is a prominent feature of Sjögren's, recent studies have examined the efficacy of the B-cell–depleting agent rituximab (Rituxan) for treatment of the syndrome. Rituximab is a chimeric monoclonal antibody against the protein CD20+, found on the surface of B cells in all stages of development. It downregulates the B-cell receptor and induces apoptosis of CD20+ cells, leading to the elimination of B cells. Encouraging results were seen in initial, uncontrolled trials. Recently, a randomized, blinded clinical trial of primary Sjögren's syndrome patients found significant improvements in the rituximab group for stimulated whole saliva flow rate, as well as in a variety of laboratory and subjective parameters and extra-glandular manifestations compared to placebo. The side effects were judged acceptable and the follow-up period was 48 weeks.

In another small study with rituximab, sequential parotid biopsy specimens were obtained before and after treatment. Reduced glandular inflammation and improvement in ductal histopathology were found, as well as some increase in salivary flow and normalization of sialochemistries. Although the trial looked at only 5 subjects, it is one of the few studies to demonstrate histological improvement and the potential for restoration of exocrine function in Sjögren's.

While further and larger studies are necessary to determine appropriate patients and other factors, B-cell depletion appears to be a major advance in the treatment in Sjögren's. Additional studies with rituximab, as well as other biologics of this class, are under way.

There are ongoing clinical trials in Sjögren's looking at a new class of drugs capable of blocking a sodium channel, which is found in most epithelial tissues. Blocking this channel may alter mucosal fluid movement and increase retention of fluid on the mucosa in the oral cavity. Initial, small controlled trials with an oral rinse have reported relief of oral dryness symptoms in a group with primary Sjögren's. Further studies will determine if this is an efficacious potential new treatment approach for dry mouth in Sjögren's.

Repair of Salivary Gland Alterations

There are no agents that have been shown definitively to promote repair of salivary gland damage in Sjögren's. As noted above, IFN-alpha did show improvements in minor salivary gland histopathology and rituximab led to restoration of parotid tissue. However, these studies were in a small number of subjects and should be repeated. These are a significant findings, however, as other agents, including prednisone and a nonsteroidal anti-inflammatory drug, failed to have any effect on salivary pathology in earlier trials.

Future Directions for Management of Dry Mouth in Sjögren's

There is a need for improved secretagogues that will have fewer side effects, an increased duration of stimulatory activity, and greater potency. Current therapies are restricted to agents that act primarily via the muscarinic receptor. Future drugs may be directed to other receptors known to stimulate salivary cells. It is also possible that small-molecule drugs may be developed that target salivary receptors with greater specificity and consequently have fewer adverse effects.

Novel approaches will have to be found for individuals with too little remaining salivary function to be helped by approaches directed at increasing salivary output. In these individuals, directed cell growth and repair may be possible, perhaps using gene therapy techniques. This will be feasible with improved knowledge of salivary cell growth control. The goal would be natural repair of the salivary gland. There is also the possibility of salivary transplantation or creation of a biocompatible artificial salivary gland. It is likely that a combination of these approaches will result in many more therapeutic options in the future.

Summing Up

The current management of dry mouth is mostly symptomatic and transiently ameliorative. Currently available medications are modestly effective but do little about the underlying process. Recent findings and exciting ongoing investigations promise more definitive relief of this uncomfortable feature of the syndrome.

FOR FURTHER READING

Becker H, Pavenstaedt H, Willeke P. Emerging treatment strategies and potential therapeutic targets in primary Sjögren's syndrome. *Inflamm Allergy Drug Targets.* 2010; 9(1): 10–9.

Brennan MT, Shariff G, Lockhart PB, Fox PC. Treatment of xerostomia: a systematic review of therapeutic trials. *Dent Clin North Am.* 2002; 46(4): 847–56.

Delaleu N, Jonsson MV, Appel S, Jonsson R. New concepts in the pathogenesis of Sjögren's syndrome. *Rheum Dis Clin North Am.* 2008; 34(4): 833–45.

Mavragani CP, Moutsopoulos HM. Conventional therapy of Sjögren's syndrome. *Clin Rev Allergy Immunol.* 2007; 32(3): 284–91.

Napeñas JJ, Brennan MT, Fox PC. Diagnosis and treatment of xerostomia (dry mouth). *Odontology.* 2009; 97(2): 76–83.

Ramos-Casals M, Tzioufas AG, Stone JH, et al. Treatment of primary Sjögren syndrome: a systematic review. *JAMA.* 2010; 304(4): 452–60.

Thelin WR, Brennan MT, Lockhart PB, et al. The oral mucosa as a therapeutic target for xerostomia. *Oral Dis.* 2008; 14(8): 683–9.

Tobón GJ, Pers JO, Youinou P, Saraux A. B cell-targeted therapies in Sjögren's syndrome. *Autoimmun Rev.* 2010; 9(4): 224–8.

Vitali C. Measurement of disease activity and damage in Sjögren's syndrome. *Rheum Dis Clin North Am.* 2008; 34(4): 963–71.

von Bültzingslöwen I, Sollecito TP, Fox PC, et al. Salivary dysfunction associated with systemic diseases: systematic review and clinical management recommendations. *Oral Surg Oral Med Oral Pathol Oral Radiol Endod.* 2007; 103 Suppl: S57. e1–15.

21

Management of Dry Eye

S. Lance Forstot, MD, FACS, and
Gary N. Foulks, MD, FACS

There is at present no cure for dry eye. Nevertheless, there has been significant improvement in the management of the disorder in the past 10 years.

The two major types of dry eye (aqueous-deficient and evaporative) have some management options in common, but also have options specific to the type of dry eye. Also, treatment is usually determined by the severity of the dryness and the severity of symptoms. It is important as a first management principle to have a complete eye examination to determine the type of dry eye that exists and to identify which of the factors producing dry eye are present. Once the mechanism and severity of dry eye have been determined, a stepwise approach to management can be recommended.

Minimizing the Aggravating Factors to Dry Eye

Since symptoms of dry eye are often aggravated by certain environmental stresses and physical or visual activities, it is often helpful for patients to anticipate and avoid or limit those situations. Dehumidified environments or those with strong air currents increase evaporation of the tear film. This is very common on long airplane trips, so patients should be prepared to supplement their tears on such excursions. Use of a room humidifier or furnace humidifier can help to improve the home environment.

Prolonged visual tasks also aggravate symptoms of dry eye because blinking is reduced during such activities as reading or using a computer. It is helpful in these situations to look away occasionally from the reading material to stimulate a blink or periodically to rest the eyes or even intentionally blink. Supplemental tears to stabilize the tear film or increase the volume of the tear film may be used during such periods of prolonged near work. Lowering computer terminal displays to below eye level can reduce the amount of the surface of the eye that is exposed to evaporation of tears.

The wearing of contact lenses can increase tear evaporation. Using contact lens wetting drops and limiting the duration of lens wear can reduce the drying effect of the contact lens and prolong wearing time. The use of punctal plugs to increase the volume of tears retained on the surface of the eye also may be needed to allow continued lens wear.

Management Strategies for Dry Eye

The treatment options for management of dry eye are listed in Table 21–1. In general, the sequence of treatments is determined by the severity of the dryness and the clinical response to each step of therapy.

TEAR SUPPLEMENTATION AND LUBRICANTS

Numerous topical formulations are available to supplement the tear film, and each category of drop has benefits and limitations. Table 21–2 lists some of the

TABLE 21–1
Treatment Options for Dry Eye

1. Supplementation or replacement of tears
2. Lubricants
   a. Solutions
   b. Gels
   c. Ointments
   d. Dissolvable inserts (Lacriserts)
3. Nutritional supplements: omega-3 essential fatty acids
4. Topical anti-inflammatory therapy
   a. Corticosteroids
   b. Cyclosporine
   c. Azithromycin (for evaporative dry eye)
5. Retention of tears
   a. Temporary punctal plugs
   b. Permanent punctal plugs
   c. Cautery closure of puncta
6. Stimulation of tear production
   a. Oral stimulants
   b. Topical stimulants (yet to be approved)
7. Control of filaments
8. Autologous serum therapy
9. Hormone therapy
10. Surgical options
    a. Partial closure of the eyelid

TABLE 21–2
Some of the Available OTC Tear Supplements and Lubricants

Major component(s)	Strength	Trade name	Preservative
Carboxymethylcellulose	0.5%	Refresh	purite
	1.0%	Celluvisc	none
	0.25%	Theratears	none
Glycerin	0.3%	Moisture Eyes	benzalkonium
Hydroxypropyl- methyl cellulose	0.2–0.3%	GenTeal	perborate
		GenTeal Gel	perborate
Hydroxypropyl-cellulose	5 mg/insert	Lacrisert	none
Hydroxypropyl-methylcellulose/Dextran 70		Bion Tears	none
Hydroxypropyl-methylcellulose/glycerin		Clear Eyes	sorbic acid/edta
Hydroxypropyl-methylcellulose/glycerin/Dextran 70		Tears Naturale	
		Tears Naturale free	none
			polyquad
Polyvinyl alcohol	1.4%	AKWA Tears	benzalkonium
Glycerin		Optive	purite
		Optive free	none
Glycerin/HP-Guar		Systane	polyquad
		Systane PF	none
Drakeol Oil emulsion		Soothe XP	PHMB
		Soothe	none
Ointment/lanolin		Lacrilube	none

available supplements. Most of these products are nonprescription, over-the-counter eye drops. The formulations containing preservatives should be used no more than four times per day; patients who need more frequent use should use unpreserved formulations. The other general features of these treatments are that the thicker the drop the greater the blur to vision, although the drop stays longer upon the surface of the eye.

Some of the enhanced artificial tears are designed not just to increase the volume of the tears but also to provide specific protection for the surface of the eye.

For example, Theratears is a solution that mimics the salt content of the tear film but with a lower concentration in an attempt to reduce the concentration (osmolarity) of the tear film. Since a more concentrated tear film results in both damage to the surface cells of the eye and stimulation of inflammation, the goal of Theratears is to prevent the damage and decrease the stimulus to inflammation. A different strategy is used by the drop Optive, which includes specific molecules in a solution to protect the surface cells against the highly concentrated tears of dry eye.

Lubricants are used to reduce the friction of the eyelid against the eyeball. These formulations also protect the ocular surface. Solutions containing special molecules to adsorb to the ocular surface include Systane (a guar base) and Oasis Tears Plus, or Blink (a hyaluronate base). The adsorbed layer both lubricates and protects the surface. Gels are more viscous than solutions and provide a longer duration on the surface of the eye but can blur the vision and are therefore usually recommended for use at night. Ointments are even thicker than gels and consequently last longer on the surface but produce even more blur in vision; they are also used before sleep.

Lipid-containing formulations, either as additives (Freshkote) or emulsion (Soothe, Systane Balance), are very helpful in preventing evaporation of the tear film and can be particularly helpful in treating the evaporative type of dry eye.

Particularly in patients who require frequent application of topical tear supplements or lubricants, another option is possible. Small inserts of dissolvable material that lubricates the surface of the eye can be placed behind the lower eyelid into the conjunctival cul-de-sac on a daily basis. Many patients find the convenience and effectiveness of these Lacriserts to be helpful and to reduce the need for frequent topical artificial tears.

NUTRITIONAL SUPPLEMENTS

Dietary supplementation with omega-3 essential fatty acids has been recommended for prevention and treatment of dry eye. The American diet has become deficient in omega-3 fatty acids, which are not produced by the body but which must be ingested in the diet. Since our diet is high in omega-6 essential fatty acids it is necessary to include omega-3 dietary supplements to balance the levels of fatty acid that protect against or reduce inflammation. Omega-3 fatty acids are present in deep water fish or flax seed, and therefore fish oil or flax seed oil dietary supplements are available. Preliminary studies suggest that 3,000 mg should be ingested per day. Patients taking anticoagulants such as warfarin (Coumadin) should consult their physician to avoid any interference with anticoagulation therapy. Side effects of fishy breath or a sensation of bloating can occur. The other option is to increase the amount of fish in the diet to more than four times per week.

TOPICAL ANTI-INFLAMMATORY THERAPY

Since inflammation of the lacrimal gland and the ocular surface has been found to cause and aggravate dry eye, treatments to reduce inflammation have been advocated. The most potent and fastest-acting anti-inflammatory drugs are the corticosteroids. These drugs are used intermittently for treatment of flare-ups of dry eye symptoms but are not used long term due to the side effects of glaucoma and cataract. They are helpful when beginning therapy with topical cyclosporine but are usually discontinued once the cyclosporine has begun to work.

Topical cyclosporine also reduces inflammation of the ocular surface and is at present the only prescription drop approved by the Food and Drug Administration (FDA) for decreased tear production due to inflammation. The drug is marketed under the brand name Restasis and is used twice daily. The onset of effect of the cyclosporine can take up to 2 months and the peak effect of the medication is not reached until 6 months of therapy, but the drug has been shown to be safe for long-term use. About 17% of patients using Restasis will notice stinging upon instillation and 3% may not tolerate such stinging. Artificial tear supplements are usually needed in conjunction with the Restasis therapy. New anti-inflammatory drugs are in clinical testing and the future will undoubtedly bring new drugs to the market for treating dry eye, but at the present time corticosteroids and cyclosporine are the only options.

When considering treatment options for dry eye, there is an additional approach for the evaporative dry eye. This form of dry eye is most often associated with eyelid margin disease (meibomian gland dysfunction) in which the lipid-secreting glands in the eyelid are plugged and have abnormal secretions that fail to provide adequate protection against evaporation of the tears. Such eyelid margin disease can be treated with topical azithromycin (AzaSite) or oral doxycycline, in addition to massage of the eyelid after application of a warm compress to the eyelid. The medications require at least a month of treatment but can improve symptoms of both eyelid inflammation and evaporative dry eye.

RETENTION OF TEARS

Once inflammation of the ocular surface is controlled, the volume of tears may still be below normal. Increasing the volume of tears is possible by occluding the ducts that drain tears from the surface of the eye. The lacrimal puncta can be closed by a number of methods. Dissolvable inserts can be placed that provide temporary closure of the ducts lasting 1 to 2 weeks. Permanent replaceable plugs can be inserted in the puncta that last until they are removed or fall out, which is usually months or years. Finally, closure of the puncta can be done with laser or cautery, but such closure is usually permanent and reversal requires surgery. Punctal plugging works well to increase the volume of tears and is often recommended in patients who have not had success with previous treatments.

STIMULATION OF TEAR PRODUCTION

A long-sought goal in management of dry eye has been drugs to stimulate tear secretion. There are no such drugs approved at present for stimulating tear secretion, but some options are available to help. Pilocarpine (Salagen) and cevimeline (Evoxac) are approved for stimulating saliva production and have been shown to increase tear production in some patients. Although not as potent in stimulating tears as they are for saliva, both drugs can be considered for dry eye patients. The downside is that both drugs are associated with some troubling side effects, including sweating and gastrointestinal upset, that limit their usefulness in dry eye disease.

Topical stimulants also are not yet approved, but some promising studies are under way to obtain approval. The topical options are not limited by as many side effects as the oral drugs.

TREATING FILAMENTARY KERATOPATHY AND MUCUS ADHERENCE

Since filamentary keratopathy is so painful to the patient, it is worthwhile to describe the management of both filaments and adherent mucus on the cornea. Single filaments can be removed by use of fine forceps after topical anesthesia of the eye. If numerous filaments are present or there is extensive mucus adherent to the cornea, a more reasonable approach is to use topical mucolytic drugs. Acetylcysteine 10% solution instilled three times per day for 2 or 3 weeks usually removes both filaments and adherent mucus.

AUTOLOGOUS SERUM THERAPY

There is some evidence that the application of topical serum (taken from a patient's vein and diluted with artificial tears) to the surface of the eye as a drop improves both symptoms and signs of dry eye. This treatment option, called autologous serum therapy, requires frequent (bimonthly) blood drawing, and the final product requires refrigeration during use. The risk of contamination of the serum drop with bacteria or fungus is present, and patients must use care in storing and applying the drop. Nonetheless, for patients who remain symptomatic with ocular surface damage despite other treatments, it is a reasonable option. Typically, the treatment is continued for several months and then other treatment is resumed once the surface has healed. It is thought that proteins and growth factors in the serum protect and stimulate the ocular surface.

HORMONE THERAPY

There is increasing evidence that loss of androgen stimulation and protection of the lacrimal glands contributes to dry eye. A logical attempt at treatment is to consider replacement of androgen hormone to the lacrimal gland and ocular surface. However, clinical trials to date have had limited success using androgen (testosterone) therapy, and no approved treatment is available. The systemic use of testosterone results in unacceptable side effects in women and little effectiveness in men. The topical use of androgen has had anecdotal positive effect, but the controlled clinical trials do not demonstrate effectiveness. Future research may provide a hormone replacement option.

SURGICAL THERAPY

A last option for therapy of severe dry eye where the surface is threatened by surface damage is to perform surgery to reduce the exposure of the ocular surface. This usually involves suturing the outside corners of the upper and lower eyelid together to reduce the opening of the eyelid. This procedure can increase the effect of the topical supplements and lubricants, but with some change in appearance.

Special Considerations

When surgery is necessary to treat other conditions such as cataract, it is important to have the dry eye under the best control possible. Since there is a possible delay in healing after surgery in the dry eye patient, patients should inform the surgeon of their dry eye therapy. It has been shown in several studies that the level of visual performance after cataract and refractive surgery is better when full treatment of dry eye is achieved before surgery. Also, refractive surgery such as LASIK can result in reduced sensation of the cornea that can aggravate dry eye, and it is wise to exclude or fully treat dry eye before any such refractive surgery.

Although protective eyewear, such as wraparound sunglasses, does not treat dry eye, it can reduce symptoms of irritation by reducing the evaporation of tears, and it provides a more controlled environment around the eyes. Several options for such protective eyewear are marketed, including Panoptik and MEG (microenvironment glasses).

Summing Up

Whether dry eye is due to aqueous production deficiency or excess evaporation, options for management exist. Manipulation of the environment or adjustment of the demands of prolonged visual tasks can reduce aggravation of dry eye symptoms. Stepwise treatment based upon the severity of dryness includes supplementation of tears, lubrication, and dietary supplementation with omega-3 fatty acids. If such measures are inadequate, anti-inflammatory therapy with topical cyclosporine and intermittent topical steroids as well as topical azithromycin or oral doxycycline for meibomian gland dysfunction can be employed. Punctal plugs can be used, and some patients may benefit from oral tear stimulants. If these options fail, the use of autologous serum therapy or eyelid surgery can be considered. New options for therapy are continuing in development and may join the list of options in the near future.

FOR FURTHER READING

Report of the International Dry Eye Workshop (DEWS) 2007. The Ocular Surface 2007; 5: 65–202.

American Academy of Ophthalmology Preferred Practice Pattern: Dry Eye.

Foulks GN: Treatment of dry eye disease by the non-ophthalmologist. *Rheum Dis Clin North Am.* 2008; 34: 987–1000.

22

Treatment of Other Sicca Symptoms

22A: DRY EARS, NOSE, AND SINUSES

Soo Kim Abboud, MD

Nasal Symptoms

Sjögren's patients often suffer from significant nasal dryness, which can lead to pain, crusting, epistaxis (bleeding), sinusitis (sinus infections), and even septal perforation (a hole in the septum, the piece of cartilage and bone that is found in the center of the nose and separates the right from the left nasal passageway). Conservative treatment is typically effective at improving the majority of nasal symptoms, and includes adequate humidification of the environment, saline irrigation, and the avoidance of medications such as decongestants and antihistamines that can further dry the nasal passages and promote pain, crusting, and bleeding. Nosebleeds occur due to significant dryness and usually originate from the front of the nose along the septum. Humidification, saline irrigation (with Simply Saline, Nasal Comfort, or Ocean Spray, among many other brands), and moisturization of the anterior septum with a nasal gel, Vaseline, or an over-the-counter antibiotic ointment such as Neosporin or Polysporin can significantly decrease the frequency and severity of nosebleeds. Regular use of secretagogues (Salagen, Evoxac) at moderate to high doses may also help. If the epistaxis persists despite these measures, silver nitrate cauterization of the offending blood vessels can be performed by an otolaryngologist in the office.

Patients with Sjögren's are at increased risk of suffering from allergic rhinitis (itching, sneezing, and nasal congestion due to allergies) and can benefit from a topical nasal steroid once or twice daily to decrease the inflammation. Nasal steroids can often improve the inflammation from rhinitis and decrease the severity and frequency of sinusitis, or sinus infections, which occur more commonly in this population due to the dryness, crusting, and swelling that can trap bacteria. Antibiotics can cure bouts of sinusitis; oral steroids may be needed in refractory cases when the swelling is severe or in chronic cases.

Auditory Symptoms

Patients with Sjögren's are at increased risk of hearing loss, both conductive (hearing loss occurs due to problems with the ear canal, eardrum, eustachian tube, or ear bones) and sensorineural (nerve deafness) types. Autoimmune hearing loss can occur; this is a type of sensorineural hearing loss that results from one's one antibodies attacking the auditory nervous system. Treatment is similar to other forms of autoimmune hearing loss and centers on oral steroids (e.g., prednisone 1 mg/kg for 3 weeks). Occasionally, other immunosuppressant drugs are used for steroid-sparing effects. Partial return of hearing can occur if treatment is prompt, although progressive deterioration is more common. Other causes of the hearing loss that are treatable must be evaluated prior to a patient being given the diagnosis of Sjögren's-related autoimmune hearing loss.

Tinnitus, or ringing in the ears, also occurs more frequently in patients with Sjögren's. In patients with sensorineural hearing loss, tinnitus also frequently occurs. However, even Sjögren's patients with normal hearing complain of tinnitus. The reason for this is unknown. Tinnitus occurs more often in patients with anxiety and depression; on many occasions, treating the anxiety and depression can improve the patient's subjective tinnitus. While most patients are able to live with the tinnitus, some patients will suffer so greatly that more aggressive treatment such as tinnitus maskers or biofeedback may be necessary.

Otalgia, or ear pain, can occur in as many as 25% of Sjögren's patients. The origin of the ear pain is also largely unknown, although many suspect that the dryness in the upper airway can lead to eustachian tube dysfunction. The role of the eustachian tube is to equalize pressure within the middle ear; when the eustachian tube is diseased, the middle ear develops negative pressure, which can lead to pain, hearing loss, fluid accumulation, and even infection. The treatment of eustachian tube dysfunction depends on the severity of the disease; avoiding decongestants and using a nasal steroid and nasal saline to improve function is usually all that is necessary. In severe cases of eustachian tube dysfunction patients may suffer from recurrent fluid buildup in the middle ear and even infections. Patients with this level of disease may benefit from antibiotics or even a myringotomy tube (a tube is placed in the eardrum to drain the middle ear and bypass a defective or diseased eustachian tube).

Ear pain, redness, and swelling may also occur due to relapsing polychondritis. This condition causes autoimmune inflammation of ear cartilage as well as other cartilaginous structures in the head and neck and may occur as an isolated condition or in association with other autoimmune diseases like

Sjögren's. It is usually treated with high-dose oral steroids and other immuno-suppressant drugs.

The Larynx

Patients with Sjögren's are at higher risk of suffering from laryngeal (voice box) symptoms due to salivary gland dysfunction and upper airway dryness. This can lead to hoarseness or laryngitis, dysphagia (difficulty swallowing), globus sensation (lump in the throat sensation), dyspnea (difficulty breathing), or coughing. Laryngeal dryness can be improved with humidification and adequate hydration. Secretagogues, as mentioned above, may also provide relief. When laryngeal dryness leads to thick mucus and difficulty clearing this, a mucus thinner such as long-acting guaifenesin 600 mg twice daily can be employed with some benefit.

While the exact causal relationship is unknown, many patients with Sjögren's suffer from gastroesophageal reflux disease (GERD). Patients with extra-esophageal manifestations of GERD commonly suffer from hoarseness, dysphagia, globus sensation, constant clearing of the throat with or without thick phlegm, cough, or recurrent sore throat. Many patients with these symptoms do not suffer from heartburn or indigestion and may be misdiagnosed with other conditions. Patient symptoms often improve with medication that decreases the amount of acid produced in the stomach. These include over-the-counter H2 blockers like Tagamet and Zantac or proton pump inhibitors such as Prilosec, Prevacid, Aciphex, Protonix, Nexium, and Zegerid. These medications are taken for a minimum of 2 months and may need to be taken long term. Patients should take them at least 30 to 60 minutes before mealtime once or twice daily depending on the severity of symptoms. Dietary and lifestyle modifications are equally important for the successful treatment of GERD and extra-esophageal reflux. A few recent studies have suggested that there is an increased risk of osteoporosis and hip fractures in patients taking proton pump inhibitors long term. Therefore, regular monitoring of bone mineral density by DEXA scanning is also recommended.

Summing Up

The underlying cause of nasal, otologic, and oral symptoms of Sjögren's should first be ascertained. A general principle is to promote humidification measures, avoid drying agents (e.g., antihistamines), and use irrigation as needed (nasal saline). Associated inflammatory conditions such as chondritis or vestibulitis respond to corticosteroids or other immunosuppressives. Ear pain can be relieved with a variety of approaches that decrease eustachian tube dysfunction. The management of laryngeal involvement consists of antireflux measures such as proton pump inhibitors and mucolytic agents.

FOR FURTHER READING

Patient information can be found on the following American Academy of Otolaryngology websites: http://www.entnet.org/HealthInformation/WhatIsGERD.cfm http://www.entnet.org/HealthInformation/autoimmuneInnerEar.cfm

22B: DRY SKIN

Theresa L. Ray, MD, and John R. Fenyk, Jr., MD

Skin manifestations are seen in many patients with Sjögren's syndrome and include a wide variety of diseases ranging from cutaneous vasculitis to annular erythema (red rings). However, the most common skin complaint is xerosis (dryness), which occurs in up to 50% of patients. While the exact mechanisms for dryness in Sjögren's are unknown, they may result from an attack on the structures that moisturize and lubricate the skin, similar to that observed in the salivary glands. When a skin biopsy is performed, lymphocytic infiltrates are sometimes seen around the various structures in the dermis (lower layer skin), including hair follicles, oil glands, as well as eccrine (sweat) glands. Once destroyed, these oil and sweat glands cannot be restored.

The major features of dry skin (xeroderma) are scaling, redness, itching, and cracking of the skin. Treatment of xeroderma in patients with Sjögren's does not differ significantly from treatment of other causes of dry skin. Suggestions for dealing with this problem include the following:

1. Take short, lukewarm baths or showers. Lukewarm water does not remove skin oils as completely as hot water.
2. Use gentle bath bars (e.g., Dove, Basis, Cetaphil) or the low/ no-residue glycerin bars (e.g., Neutrogena), not harsh deodorant soaps. Often, "cleansers" are better able to control the acid–base balance of the skin than true "soaps." Liquid cleansers (Cetaphil, Purpose, Olay) sometimes contain a higher content of moisturizers than the bath bars; however, liquids may also contain preservatives that can act as potential allergens or irritants. Therefore, any product that irritates the skin should be discontinued.
3. After bathing, pat dry and use one or more of the moisturizing techniques mentioned below.

4. Moisturize frequently. In reality, there are relatively few ways of maintaining or adding to the skin's moisture content:
   a. Trap moisture in the skin, immediately after bathing or showering. While the skin is still damp or moist, apply a thin layer of petrolatum (Vaseline), bath oil (RoBathol, Neutrogena body oil), or even some cooking oils such as safflower oil, canola oil, or Crisco. In general, the thicker and greasier a moisturizer is, the better it is at trapping moisture in the skin.
   b. "Drag" moisture into the skin. This is done with products that contain chemicals such as urea, glycerin, lactic, or similar "metabolic" or alpha-hydroxy acids (AmLactin Cream, Carmol).
   c. Repair the skin's protective barrier function and thereby retain or trap the skin's natural moisture. The products in this group are relatively new and are based on naturally occurring chemicals called ceramides (CeraVe, Aveeno Eczema Care).
5. Avoid fabric softeners, whether in the washer or in the dryer. They may irritate or dry the skin. Use laundry detergents that are free from dyes, fragrances, and preservatives. Many brands have a "Free and Clear" option for laundry detergents that meet these criteria.
6. Drink plenty of water; remain well hydrated.
7. Use a humidifier, especially if the house has forced air heat, which is especially drying.
8. Swimming is permissible but may also irritate or dry the skin. Patients should shower after swimming and then immediately use a moisturizer.

Summing Up

Sjögren's syndrome causes a wide variety of skin problems, especially dryness. Care must be taken to avoid products or habits that dry or irritate the skin and to use an adequate amount of moisturizers. This tends to be a chronic problem but can be successfully managed, especially with professional help.

FOR FURTHER READING

DeWinter S, Van Buchern M, Vermeet MH. Annular erythema of Sjögren's syndrome. *Lancet.* 2006; 367: 1604.

Fox RI. Sjögren's syndrome. *Lancet.* 2005; 366: 321–31.

Fox RI, Liu AY. Sjögren's syndrome in dermatology. *Clin Dermatol.* 2006; 24: 393–413.

Soy M, Piskin S. Cutaneous findings in patients with primary Sjögren's syndrome. *Clin Rheumatol.* 2007; 26: 1350–52.

22C: VAGINAL DRYNESS

Elisa Rodriguez Trowbridge, MD

Prevalence of Vaginal Dryness

Vaginal dryness is a common problem among women, especially after menopause, and can occur with even greater frequency and severity in patients with
Sjögren's syndrome. One study described a group of women with Sjögren's
who had painful intercourse associated with vaginal dryness as the presenting
manifestation of the disease. Interestingly, in this particular group, the gynecological symptoms preceded the onset of dry eyes and dry mouth by many
years. Other studies of gynecological manifestations reported that Sjögren's
patients more frequently complained of vaginal dryness (53% to 55%) compared to healthy subjects (29% to 33%) and that this symptom was two to three
times more common among postmenopausal women in both groups. Thus,
the complaint of vaginal dryness in many Sjögren's patients is likely due to
multiple factors, including an exacerbation of vaginal atrophy or atrophic vaginitis. Atrophic vaginitis refers to a condition that usually occurs after menopause and is characterized by dryness and inflammation of the vagina with
thinning of the epithelium (surface lining) due to estrogen deficiency. Estrogen
provides multiple benefits that are essential to vaginal health (Table 22–1).

During menopause, there is a dramatic reduction in estrogen production,
with a 95% decrease in estrogen concentration. Less commonly, estrogen deficiency can also occur in younger women with premature ovarian failure or can
result from other causes. Factors other than low estrogen levels can also contribute to the level of vaginal atrophy, including tobacco use, vaginal nullipar-
ity (no vaginal births), and cessation of coital activity.

Diagnosis, Symptoms, and Signs

The diagnosis of atrophic vaginitis is clinical and based on characteristic symptoms and physical findings. Women complaining of vaginal dryness may also

TABLE 22–1
Vaginal Effects of Estrogen

Maintains vaginal thickness and elasticity
Keeps vaginal lining moist
Preserves vaginal blood flow
Promotes growth of helpful bacteria
Maintains acidic vaginal environment
Protects against vaginal and urinary tract infections

experience symptoms of vaginal burning, pain with intercourse, vaginal itching, a white or yellowish discharge, and vaginal spotting or bleeding. In addition, urinary tract symptoms (painful urination, urinary frequency, urgency, or leakage) may also be reported.

Typical physical examination findings of vaginal atrophy include thinning pubic hair, narrowing of the vaginal introitus (opening), petechiae (small hemorrhages) of vaginal tissues, loss of rugae (vaginal folds), fusion of the labia minora, and decreased vaginal moisture. The examination should be performed with caution since some women with vaginal atrophy can have a small vaginal opening. Before attempting a speculum examination, a digital examination with one lubricated finger should be performed to assess the vaginal width and length. A small Pederson speculum is generally more comfortable for patients.

Laboratory tests are not necessary and generally not diagnostic of atrophic vaginitis. They are mainly used to exclude other conditions that cause similar symptoms, including (1) vaginal infections (candidiasis, bacterial vaginosis, trichomoniasis); (2) localized reactions to environmental agents (soaps, perfumes, detergents, sanitary napkins, lubricants); (3) vaginal lichen planus or lichen sclerosis; or (4) gynecological cancers. A wet mount should be performed whenever a vaginal discharge is present to determine the cause.

Treatment of Vaginal Dryness

Treatment of vaginal dryness differs according to the severity of the patient's symptoms. The impact of symptoms on quality of life and patient goals should also be assessed. Women with mild symptoms of vaginal dryness can first be treated with daily vaginal moisturizers. Luvena is a pro-biotic moisturizer that has recently come on the market from the creators of Biotene products for dry mouth. Replens, a long-acting vaginal moisturizer, is a bioadhesive that binds to the vaginal epithelium, releasing purified water and thus producing a moist layer over the vagina. Replens has been found to be as effective in improving symptoms of vaginal dryness as vaginal estrogen. In addition, women may use water-soluble lubricants when engaging in sexual activity (e.g., K-Y Personal Lubricants and Astroglide).

For women with moderate to severe symptoms related to estrogen deficiency, the most effective treatment is vaginal estrogen. Moisturizers and lubricants can be helpful in improving symptoms of vaginal dryness but typically do not reverse the atrophic vaginal changes. Although use of systemic (i.e., oral) estrogen can help relieve symptoms of vaginal dryness, the use of low-dose local estrogens is preferred because of decreased systemic absorption and less estrogen exposure to other organs.

Localized use of estrogen can be administered in various forms, including (1) vaginal creams (e.g., Premarin cream, Estrace cream); (2) vaginal rings (e.g., Estring, Femring); or (3) vaginal suppositories (e.g., Vagifem). A systematic review of 16 randomized trials evaluating the efficacy of local estrogen therapy in treating vaginal atrophy found that creams and pessaries were equally effective. However, vaginal creams are generally the most popular first-line therapy. Patients should be seen for regular follow-up examinations to monitor treatment efficacy and side effects and to perform dosage adjustments as needed.

For women who wish to avoid hormones or for whom hormonal treatments are contraindicated (e.g., those with estrogen-receptor–positive breast cancer), moisturizers and other therapies are preferred. Replens has been shown to improve symptoms of vaginal atrophy and decrease pain with intercourse.

Summing Up

It is important to evaluate and treat symptoms of vaginal discomfort and dryness in women with Sjögren's. Estrogen deficiency is a frequent concomitant problem that also needs to be addressed. Therapeutic decisions are based on the severity of symptoms as well as other medical problems. Treatment of vaginal dryness and associated symptoms is not only effective but also safe and well tolerated by almost every patient.

FOR FURTHER READING

Bygdeman M, Swahn ML. Replens versus dienoestrol cream in the symptomatic treatment of vaginal atrophy in postmenopausal women. *Maturitas.* 1996; 23: 259–63.

Haga HJ, Gjesdal CG, Irgens LM, Ostensen M. Reproduction and gynaecological manifestations in women with primary Sjögren's syndrome: a case-control study. *Scand J Rheumatol.* 2005; 34(1): 45–8.

Marchesoni D, Mozzanega B, De Sandre P, et al. Gynaecological aspects of primary Sjögren's syndrome. *Eur J Obstet Gynecol Reprod Biol.* 1995; 63(1): 49–53.

Mulherin DM, Sheeran TP, Kumararatne DS, et al. Sjögren's syndrome in women presenting with chronic dyspareunia. *Br J Obstet Gynaecol.* 1997; 104(9): 1019–23.

Suckling J, Lethaby A, Kennedy R. Local oestrogen for vaginal atrophy in postmenopausal women. *Cochrane Database Syst Rev* 2003; CD001500.

Van der Laak JA, de Bie LM, de Leeuw H, et al. The effect of Replens on vaginal cytology in the treatment of postmenopausal atrophy: cytomorphology, versus computerized cytometry. *J Clin Pathol.* 2002; 55: 446.

23

Diagnosis and Management of Fatigue

Richa Mishra, MD, and
Frederick B. Vivino, MD, MS, FACR

What is Fatigue and How Do We Define It?

Fatigue is a common and disabling symptom for patients with Sjögren's syndrome and is best defined as a low-energy state characterized by physical or mental weariness. This typically results in an inability to sustain normal activities or, in a worst-case scenario, any activity whatsoever. In some cases the fatigue is severe enough to lead to misdiagnosis of Sjögren's as chronic fatigue syndrome; the latter diagnosis, however, is always considered a diagnosis of exclusion. Fatigue may take a variety of forms and have a variety of causes. Although constantly present, fatigue is also a dynamic state with waxing and waning intensity that responds to various physiological and situational influences, including emotional state, recent activities, disease activity, weather patterns, medication use, sleep patterns, and diurnal variation.

How Often Does Fatigue Occur in Sjögren's and What Is its Impact?

Fatigue is found in the majority of patients with Sjögren's, and the prevalence varies according to the method of assessment used in different studies. One survey of Sjögren's Syndrome Foundation members completed in the late 1990s listed fatigue as the third most troubling symptom (prevalence 77%), after dry eyes (90%) and dry mouth (88%). Since then at least four different studies have documented significantly diminished quality of life among people with Sjögren's compared to normal individuals. These results parallel the diminished quality of life found in other patient groups, including people with rheumatoid arthritis (RA) and fibromyalgia. In 2009 Segal and colleagues reported that fatigue and pain are two of the most important factors that affect quality of life (i.e., physical and emotional well-being) in Sjögren's. Additionally, when compared to healthy people of the same age and background, Sjögren's patients have lower rates of employment and higher rates of disability.

What Do You Feel, and What Is Causing Your Fatigue?

The majority of patients with connective tissue disorders, including lupus, RA, and Sjögren's, suffer from fatigue. Fatigue has many forms and descriptions. Basic fatigue is always present but worsens during periods of peak disease activity (disease flares). It is most common in individuals with involvement of the internal organs and sometimes is associated with flu-like symptoms. The exact cause is unknown but may be related to the release of cytokines (chemical mediators of inflammation) in the blood—a sign of systemic inflammation. Another possible cause of fatigue is neuroendocrine dysfunction, a type of hormonal imbalance.

Many Sjögren's patients are notoriously poor sleepers and wake up frequently at night or complain of "nonrestorative" sleep. This causes a sensation of fatigue immediately upon awakening (i.e., waking up tired) and can occur for multiple reasons, including restless leg syndrome, periodic limb movement disorder of sleep, sleep apnea, medication side effects, or discomfort from dry eyes and mouth. This kind of fatigue is sometimes associated with impaired concentration and memory, termed "brain fog."

Some of the most important causes of fatigue in Sjögren's are listed in Table 23–1.

Immobilizing or "rebound" fatigue sometimes occurs during periods of disease quiescence due to a sudden increase in activity levels (i.e., overdoing it the preceding day) beyond what the body can tolerate. Sudden fatigue or the "crumple and fold" phenomenon that is not related to a change in activity levels raises the possibility of infection, especially when a fever is present. Weather-related fatigue that feels like a sweeping wave and is associated with muscle aches suggests fibromyalgia.

Fibromyalgia is commonly associated with Sjögren's (prevalence up to 47%) and is characterized by diffuse body pain, chronic fatigue, nonrestorative sleep, morning stiffness, a subjective feeling of swelling, and modulation of the symptoms by the weather. It is often associated with other disorders, including depression, irritable bowel syndrome, temporomandibular joint dysfunction, migraine headaches, pelvic urethral (spastic bladder) syndrome,

TABLE 23–1
Some Causes of Fatigue in Sjögren's Syndrome

Systemic inflammation	Hypothyroidism
Disturbed sleep	Muscle inflammation
Anxiety and depression	Vitamin D deficiency
Fibromyalgia	Severe anemia
Medication side effects	Infection
Vitamin B_{12} deficiency	Celiac disease

and costochondritis (inflammation of a rib and adjoining cartilage, causing chest pain).

Fatigue with the "molten lead phenomenon," like someone has poured molten lead into the limbs during sleep or like walking with heavy weight, suggests inflammatory arthritis (especially with morning stiffness for more than 1 hour). A similar phenomenon can also occur due to proximal muscle weakness; the latter is suspected when a patient has difficulty lifting the limbs (e.g., getting out of a chair or raising the arms to comb one's hair). It can be caused by myositis (muscle inflammation), steroid myopathy, hypothyroidism, or vitamin D deficiency. Vitamin D deficiency is common in the general population, especially among autoimmune disease patients. It has been implicated as a cause of not only fatigue and weakness but also generalized muscle and bone pain. Fatigue related to other physical causes such as thyroid problems or anemia makes people feel as if they are climbing a steep hill while walking on level ground.

A "tired-wired" feeling can result from use of certain medications like prednisone or too much caffeine. With this type of fatigue the body feels tired but the mind wants to keep going and can't let the body rest. Prednisone typically causes insomnia and is therefore best taken in the morning. Some medications, such as painkillers (for example, tramadol [Ultram], oxycodone [OxyContin], or gabapentin [Neurontin]), may cause drowsiness and therefore are best taken at night.

People who suffer from chronic illnesses frequently develop psychosocial problems. Prevalence rates for depression and anxiety as high as 48% have been reported in individuals with Sjögren's. In some cases the energy spent fighting these illnesses causes severe emotional fatigue that at times can seem overwhelming. Anxiety and depression also may interfere with restful sleep and further exacerbate the fatigue; these disorders also may worsen chronic pain, headaches, and other symptoms.

How Do We Approach this Problem?

Fatigue can be alleviated in most patients after finding the proper cause. However, since so many different types of fatigue occur in Sjögren's and more than one cause may coexist in the same patient, finding the answer often poses a difficult challenge. The approach to this complex problem always begins with a thorough history and physical examination to identify clues that help characterize the type of fatigue and distinguish one cause from another. Medication lists should be reviewed. Patients should be questioned about sleep disturbances and screened for depression (Table 23–2). The examination should include palpation of the joints for swelling and tenderness as well as palpation of muscle tender points to screen for fibromyalgia. The skin, thyroid,

TABLE 23–2
Screening for Depression

A simple way to screen for depression is to ask the patient, "During the past month, have you often been bothered by the following?"

*Loss of interest or pleasure in doing things (anhedonia)

*Feeling down, depressed, or hopeless (depressed mood)

If one answer is "yes," probe for the core symptoms of depression (**SALSA**) by asking, "Have you experienced any of the following feelings nearly every day for the past 2 weeks?"

*Sleep disturbance

*Anhedonia

*Low Self-esteem

*Appetite decrease

The presence of two or more core symptoms correlates with a diagnosis of major depression.

lymph nodes, lungs and abdomen are also examined. Muscle strength and reflexes are tested to look for objective evidence of weakness.

Various blood tests are ordered to screen for systemic inflammation. Abnormalities may include elevation of blood test markers for inflammation (e.g., erythrocyte sedimentation rate or C-reactive protein) and/or the presence of autoantibodies (rheumatoid factor [RF], ANA, anti-SSA, anti-SSB) or high levels of inflammatory proteins (cryoglobulins, serum beta-2 microglobulin, IgG, IgM, IgA). Other useful studies include thyroid functions tests (free T4, TSH), muscle enzymes (CPK, aldolase), vitamin D level (25-hydroxyvitamin D), and complete blood cell counts.

Patients who frequently awaken at night for unknown reasons or who arise in the morning feeling tired should be referred for polysomnography (sleep study). An EMG/NCV (electromyography/nerve conduction velocity) study is sometimes performed by a neurologist or physiatrist to determine whether weakness is due to a nerve or muscle problem.

What Treatments Are Most Helpful?

Obviously, the successful treatment of fatigue depends heavily on correct identification of the causes. Additional rest always helps but, unfortunately, provides only temporary relief.

A variety of immunosuppressive drugs can decrease systemic inflammation, alleviate fatigue associated with active disease, and decrease the frequency of disease flares. These may include medications such as hydroxychloroquine (Plaquenil), corticosteroids (prednisone, methylprednisolone [Medrol]), and methotrexate. A study published in 2008 suggested that treatment with intravenous rituximab (Rituxan) may alleviate fatigue as well. Likewise, muscle inflammation is treated with immunosuppressives (steroids, methotrexate,

TABLE 23–3
Tips To Achieve Restful Sleep

1. Keep a regular sleep schedule for going to bed and getting up.
2. Avoid taking daytime naps.
3. Try to get at least 8-1/2 hours of sleep per night, or longer if you wake up a lot.
4. Do not use caffeine within 6 hours of bedtime.
5. Try to exercise regularly for at least 20 minutes a day, but don't exercise right before bed.
6. Create a dark, cool, quiet, and secure environment for sleep.
7. Do not go to bed hungry.
8. Do not work or watch TV in the bedroom.
9. Try a warm bath before bedtime to relax aching muscles and relieve stress.

azathioprine [Imuran]) followed by physical therapy. The choice of medication depends on physician experience, side effects, and the presence of other disease-related and/or medical problems.

Patients who are sleep-deprived may benefit from counseling on "sleep hygiene" (Table 23-3).

In Sjögren's, nocturnal dryness of the eyes and mouth may also disturb sleep. A room air humidifier can be helpful. Patients are encouraged to use ocular lubricants (e.g., Refresh PM) or gels (e.g., GenTeal gel) instead of artificial tears before bed for longer-lasting relief. Bedtime doses of oral secretagogues (e.g., pilocarpine [Salagen] or cevimeline [Evoxac]) are also very useful. The mouth and inner cheeks can also be coated with over-the-counter moisturizing gels (Oral Balance, Orajel) or vitamin E oil to alleviate nighttime symptoms.

Treatment of fibromyalgia is also focused on the development of good sleep habits, treatment of dryness, and use of medications to relieve muscle pain and promote restful sleep. The current FDA-approved treatments, pregabalin (Lyrica), duloxetine (Cymbalta), and milnacipran (Savella), are all helpful but can be drying and are best used at low doses. Other choices that are sometimes better tolerated include trazodone (Desyrel), venlafaxine (Effexor), tizanidine (Zanaflex), and zaleplon (Sonata). After improvement of pain, the next step is to start a regular exercise program that includes stretching and aerobics. If the above treatment does not work, then a sleep study is strongly recommended to look for treatable causes of nonrestorative sleep.

Vitamin D deficiency is treated with over-the-counter supplements or prescription vitamin D. Replacement doses vary according to the degree of deficiency. A follow-up blood test in 3 months is recommended to confirm improvement. Vitamin B_{12} deficiency is treated by replenishing vitamin B_{12} by the sublingual, or intramuscular injection route. Levels of vitamin B_{12} should be checked in the blood on a regular basis. Treatment of celiac disease is discussed in another chapter.

Depression is common in people with chronic illnesses and should be treated under medical supervision. In Sjögren's, management of depression should also focus on better treatment of the underlying disease, counseling, and the development of a support system to help deal with physical or mental stress. Regular exercise also helps fight depression and fatigue. In severe cases medications are used, with special care to choose an agent (e.g., venlafaxine) that does not make dryness worse. Over-the-counter St. John's wort should be avoided because of its drying side effects.

The treatment of hypothyroidism requires thyroid hormone replacement with medications (levothyroxine [Synthroid], thyroid tablets [Amour Thyroid]). Follow-up blood tests are frequently needed (e.g., every 6 months) to ensure optimal dosing.

When all else fails, patients can try the "Fatigue Fighters" listed in Table 23–4, or a trial of modafinil (Provigil) can be considered. This medication is normally used to treat narcolepsy; however, a recent study suggests that it helps fatigue in multiple sclerosis patients as well. Therefore, it may be useful in Sjögren's.

Summing Up

Fatigue adds to the burden of illness in Sjögren's and has a significant impact on patients' quality of life and disability. It has many faces and can result from

TABLE 23–4
Fatigue Fighters

1. Know your limits and pace yourself.
2. Plan to do no more than one activity on your bad days. Do more on your good days, but don't overdo it!
3. Listen to your body and take a 20-minute time-out every few hours to help you get through the day.
4. Educate your friends and family about what you are going through and how the fatigue in Sjögren's syndrome can come and go.
5. Develop a support system to help you with chores. Ask family and friends to be prepared to do one or two tasks for you on your bad days. Give them specific instructions in advance and be reasonable in your expectations.
6. Get your body moving every day. Start with 5 minutes of aerobic exercise (e.g., walking, biking, elliptical, treadmill) and increase by an additional 2 to 3 minutes each month up to a maximum of 25 minutes daily. If you have a heart or lung condition, consult your doctor first.
7. Identify the major stressors in your life, and work with a mental health professional or your support system to minimize their impact.
8. If you are still employed, ask your employer for accommodations because of your medical condition.
9. Try to work from home, if possible, to gain more flexibility with your work routine.
10. Resources (search "chronic fatigue") that provide more information on work accommodations and/or career options include the Disability and Business Technical Assistance Center (www.dbtac.vcu.edu) and the Job Accommodation Network (askjan.org).

a variety of mechanisms. Finding the etiology can be a complex challenge for even the best clinician since more than one cause can coexist in the same individual. Every patient with moderate to severe fatigue deserves a thorough evaluation. A wide variety of disease-specific and general treatments may help. An improved understanding of the neurobiology of pain and fatigue in future years will no doubt open the door to new treatments as well.

FOR FURTHER READING

Al-Said Y, Al-Rached H, Al-Qahtani H, Jan M. Severe proximal myopathy with remarkable recovery after vitamin D treatment. *Can J Neurol Sci.* 2009; 36: 336–39.

Brody D, Hahn S, Spitzer R, et al. Identifying patients with depression in the primary care setting: a more efficient method. *Arch Intern Med.* 1998; 158: 2469–75.

Dass S, Bowman, S, Vital E, et al. Reduction of fatigue in Sjögren's syndrome with rituximab: results of a randomized, double-blind placebo-controlled pilot study. *Ann Rheum Dis.* 2008; 67: 1541–4.

Gudbjornsson B, Broman JE, Helta J, Hällgren R. Sleep disturbances in patients with primary Sjögren's syndrome. *Br J Rheumatol.* 1993; 32: 1072–6.

Holick MF. Vitamin D deficiency. *N Engl J Med.* 2007; 357: 266–81.

Plotnikoff GA, Quigley JM. Prevalence of severe hypovitaminosis D in patients with persistent, nonspecific musculoskeletal pain. *Mayo Clin Proc.* 2003; 78: 1463–70.

Segal B, Bowman S, Fox P, et al. Primary Sjögren's syndrome; health experiences and predictors of health quality among patients in the United States. *Health and Quality of Life Outcomes.* 2009; 7: 46.

Strombeck B, Ekdahl C, Manthorpe R, et al. Health-related quality of life in primary Sjögren's syndrome, rheumatoid arthritis and fibromyalgia compared to normal population data using the SF-36. *Scand J Rheumatol.* 2000, 29: 20–8.

Valtysdottir ST, Gudbjornsson B, Hallgren R, Hetta J: Psychological well-being in patients with primary Sjögren's syndrome. *Clin Exp Rheumatol.* 2000; 18(5): 597–600.

24

Management of Chronic Musculoskeletal Pain
Lan Chen, MD, PhD

Chronic musculoskeletal pain is a frequent complaint among Sjögren's syndrome (SS) patients. The causes for pain include neuropathic, arthritic, para-articular (e.g., tendinitis, bursitis), and/or diffuse muscle pain such as fibromyalgia, which is one of the most common comorbidities in Sjögren's.

Evaluating Chronic Pain

The first step for management of chronic pain in Sjögren's patients is to identify the cause. As with any medical workup, it begins with a thorough history and physical examination. Several questions can focus the evaluation: How did the pain begin? Where is it located? Is it localized or diffuse, inside or outside the joint? If nerve pain is suspected, does it occur in a dermatomal distribution (area of skin supplied by branches of a single spinal nerve) or a non-dermatomal distribution?

Second, physicians must keep in mind that the response to pain varies greatly from one patient to another one. A patient's culture, education, and psychological status can influence his or her pain expression. It is important to let the patient describe the pain using his or her own words. Uncovering emotional feelings in patients can be a helpful part of therapy.

Third, patients should be asked what improves the pain. Factors that improve patients' pain may prove helpful in directing the treatment. Determine what other types of therapy the patient has tried and what benefit, if any, he or she had. Inquire specifically about injections, surgery, medications (including past corticosteroid use), physical therapy, chiropractic, biobehavioral, and other complementary methods.

Fourth, inquire about how the symptoms have affected the patient's life at home, with friends, and at work. Is the pain preventing the patient from caring for a child or her loved one, maintaining her job, or performing basic activities of daily living? Patients with pain that is severe or longstanding are vulnerable to physical or psychological dysfunction and job-related issues, such as disability, which all have an impact on pain management.

Last, but not least, the presence of coexisting psychological disorders, such as depression, anxiety, or mood disorders, may add further complexity to the treatment of chronic pain, particularly when associated with drug or alcohol addiction. Additional therapy for these coexisting psychological disorders is always necessary for more effective pain management. However, these issues should not lead the clinician away from seeking a primary chronic pain diagnosis and treatment.

Available Pharmacological and Non-Pharmacological Therapies for Chronic Pain

NONSTEROIDAL ANTI-INFLAMMATORY DRUGS

The analgesic and anti-inflammatory effects of nonsteroidal anti-inflammatory drugs (NSAIDs) (e.g., Motrin, ibuprofen) play a central role in the management of many conditions. It is now known that NSAIDs also act centrally, at least in certain pain states. NSAIDs are primarily indicated for mild to moderate pain, particularly for arthritis, tendinitis, or bursitis. There are many NSAIDs from which to choose. Although the efficacy of various NSAIDs is similar, an individual's response to therapy can be highly variable. Thus, a patient who does not tolerate or respond to a particular NSAID may do well on another. The reluctance of many patients and physicians to use NSAIDs is in part due to many side effects associated with these drugs. Most NSAIDs interfere with platelet aggregation and may cause bleeding; NSAIDs produce adverse gastrointestinal side effects, including dyspepsia and gastric ulceration. There are also a variety of kidney side effects associated with NSAID use, including salt and water retention and reversible renal insufficiency due to renal vasoconstriction, acute interstitial nephritis, or acute tubular necrosis. Therefore, NSAIDs should be prescribed with caution in patients with hypertension, preexisting renal insufficiency, or heart failure. Other side effects of NSAIDs include hepatic toxicity, confusion, an inability to concentrate, and allergic reactions. Under medical supervision NSAIDs can, however, be prescribed safely and effectively for management of short-term pain or for chronic therapy in selected patients, especially when used on an as-needed basis.

DISEASE-MODIFYING THERAPIES

A small subset of patients with Sjögren's will develop a rheumatoid-like arthritis with painful swelling of large and small joints. More patients will develop inflammatory joint pain (polyarthralgia) in the absence of obvious swelling. A wide variety of immunomodulating drugs and disease-modifying therapies such as hydroxychloroquine (Plaquenil) are available for treatment, following an approach similar to that used to treat true rheumatoid arthritis. Treatment decisions are based on the severity of arthritis, the patient's other health problems, and the patient's comfort level for certain side effects (e.g., infections, low blood counts).

TRICYCLIC ANTIDEPRESSANTS

Amitriptyline (Elavil) has been the most widely studied tricyclic antidepressant (TCA) in chronic pain, although a number of others, including doxepin (Sinequan, Adapin), imipramine (Tofranil), nortriptyline (Pamelor), and desipramine (Norpramin), also have been used with success. TCAs are believed to have independent analgesic effects as well as an ability to relieve the depressive symptoms associated with chronic pain. The mechanism of their analgesic action has been theorized to relate to the analgesic properties associated with their properties as serotonin and norepinephrine reuptake inhibitors. There is also some evidence that TCAs potentiate the endogenous opioid system. TCAs prescribed for chronic pain have typically been given to fibromyalgia patients at doses lower than those used in depression. TCAs can cause wide-ranging adverse effects. Aside from anticholinergic (drying) effects, most of the more troubling or serious side effects involve the gastrointestinal, cardiovascular, and neurological systems. Physicians must explain to the patient why TCAs are used, how to administer them, and what benefits and side effects might be expected. It is also important for Sjögren's patients to know of possible unpleasant side effects, such as dry mouth.

ANTICONVULSANTS

A number of anticonvulsants are effective for chronic pain therapy, particularly for neuropathic pain. Phenytoin (Dilantin), carbamazepine (Tegretol), oxcarbazepine (Trileptal), valproic acid (Depakene), and clonazepam (Klonopin), as well as the newer agents gabapentin (Neurontin) and pregabalin (Lyrica), have been used, frequently with reasonable results. Mechanisms of action for the anticonvulsants are different and not fully understood. Carbamazepine, which is pharmacologically related to the TCAs, prevents repeated discharges in neurons, an action that is consistent with its ability to relieve lancinating pain.

Pregabalin is similar in structure to gabapentin. Many physicians will begin with gabapentin since it is inexpensive and well tolerated, even at high doses. Plasma levels do not need to be followed as they do with phenytoin and carbamazepine. Pregabalin can be given less frequently (twice daily) than gabapentin (usually three times daily) and may cause euphoria. It is a Schedule V controlled substance.

OPIOIDS

The role of opioid (narcotic) therapy in the more severe forms of acute pain and in malignant pain is well established, but opioid administration in chronic nonmalignant pain remains controversial. For patients with chronic non-malignant pain like most Sjögren's patients, the decision to begin long-term opioid therapy must be weighed carefully against the potential for side effects. Opioids are employed usually after other therapies have failed. A psychological evaluation should take place initially, with an emphasis on uncovering comorbidity that may be interfering with current treatment strategies. It is essential that patients continue to receive emotional support. Opioid candidates should be evaluated and overseen by a pain management specialist experienced in prescribing these agents. Most such specialists have patients sign a "pain contract," which is in fact a detailed informed consent. Nearly 100,000 people die annually from complications of opioid abuse/overdose in the United States, so use must be closely monitored by a specialist.

Patients may receive substantial relief of pain from opioid therapy. In short-term use, opioids are effective in relieving chronic neuropathic pain and can be prescribed safely without the development of tolerance or addiction. These problems, however, are likely to occur with chronic use. Patients should be closely monitored, especially after initiation of opioid therapy, since the risk for an adverse event is greatest shortly after initiation. Additionally, patients receiving higher doses are at increased risk for overdose. The most profound analgesic effects of opioids are mediated by the mu receptors, which are found in large numbers in the central nervous system, such as midbrain periaqueductal gray matter and the substantia gelatinosa in the dorsal horn of the spinal cord. This explains why opioids induce intense analgesia and euphoria, as well as other effects, such as bradycardia, sedation, physical dependence, and respiratory depression. Opioids may also have anticholinergic effects. Patients should be continuously educated about side effects.

TRAMADOL

To some degree, Tramadol (Ultram) is a novel analgesic that has some activity at mu receptors. It also inhibits the reuptake of serotonin and norepinephrine and may provide analgesia through this mechanism. Its side effect profile is similar to that of other weak opioids, although the incidence of gastric upset seems to be higher. Seizures are an additional risk, particularly in patients on antidepressants, neuroleptics, or other drugs that decrease the seizure threshold. A systematic review found that tramadol was effective for relief of neuropathic pain. Another review concluded that tramadol improved functional outcomes and pain in patients with fibromyalgia. That same systematic review, however, did not find tramadol more effective than NSAIDs or nortriptyline for relief of other chronic pain.

TOPICAL PHARMACOLOGICAL THERAPIES

An attractive approach to pain control is to apply drugs locally to the peripheral site of pain. Topical applications include creams, lotions, gels, oils, aerosols, or patches to involved sites. These topical remedies concentrate a large amount of the medication at the site of the pain with lower or negligible systemic drug levels, thus producing fewer or no adverse drug effects. Other advantages of topical application are lack of drug interactions and the ease of use. Topical applications of NSAIDs (e.g., 1% diclofenac gel) are available for prescription use and help localized arthritic pain. Local anesthetic patches (e.g., 5% Lidoderm patch) or gels are also effective treatments for many painful conditions.

Capsaicin is a natural constituent in pungent red chili peppers. It can selectively activate, desensitize, or exert a neurotoxic effect on sensory neurons depending on the concentration and the delivery mode. Topical capsaicin cream is an over-the-counter preparation that is available in two strengths (0.025% and 0.075%) and is FDA approved for treatment of osteoarthritis and rheumatoid arthritis. Interestingly, this extract from red chili peppers has long been used in traditional topical Chinese medication mixes for joint pain.

NONPHARMACOLOGICAL THERAPIES

Nonpharmacological therapies encompass a wide array of treatments which may be grouped into the physical interventions, including physical therapy,

TABLE 24–1
Medications used in Sjögren's Patients for Chronic Musculoskeletal Pain

A. Inflammatory pain
  Nonsteroidal anti-inflammatory drugs or aspirin
  Disease-modifying agents
  Hydroxychloroquine (Plaquenil)
  Immune suppressives, including methotrexate, azathioprine (Imuran)
  Biologics, including rituximab (Rituxan)
B. Noninflammatory pain (e.g., deformities, fibromyalgia, mechanical, neuropathic pain)
  Tricyclic antidepressants
  Anticonvulsants
  Tramadol (Ultram)
  Narcotic analgesics, including opioids

acupuncture, chiropractic manipulation, and massage, and psychoeducational interventions, such as cognitive-behavioral therapy, family therapy, patient education, and psychotherapy.

Summing Up

Chronic pain is a summation of physical and psychological derangements, so successful management requires addressing all of its various aspects. A number of interventions can help. Therapeutic selections are based on the etiology of pain and the patient's other medical problems. Proper patient education is crucial in order to achieve optimal results. For most individuals, as studies suggest, a combination of therapies is more effective than any single approach for maintaining long-term gains.

FOR FURTHER READING

Allegrante JP. The role of adjunctive therapy in the management of nonmalignant pain. *Am J Med.* 1996; 101: 33S.

Ballantyne JC, Mao J. Opioid therapy for chronic pain. *N Engl J Med.* 2003; 349: 1943.

Chen LX. Fibromyalgia: a commonly co-existing condition in Sjögren's patients. *Sjögren's Quarterly.* 2009; 4(1): 1.

Chen LX, Goldman J, Pullman-Mooar S. Chapter 30: Local therapy for chronic pain. In Wallace D, Clauw D, eds. *Fibromyalgia and Other Non-Neuropathic Pain Syndromes.* Lippincott Williams & Wilkins, 2005.

Dobscha SK, Corson K, Perrin NA, et al. Collaborative care for chronic pain in primary care: a cluster randomized trial. *JAMA.* 2009; 301: 1242.

Duhmke RM, Cornblath DD, Hollingshead JR. Tramadol for neuropathic pain. *Cochrane Database Syst Rev.* 2004; CD003726.

Eisendrath SJ. Psychiatric aspects of chronic pain. *Neurology.* 1995; 45: S26.

Fields HL. Pain. New York: McGraw-Hill Information Services Company, Health Profession Division, 1987.

Holzer P. Capsaicin: cellular targets, mechanisms of action, and selectivity for thin sensory neurons. *Pharmacol Rev.* 1991; 43(2): 143–201.

Jaeschke R, Adachi J, Guyatt G, et al. Clinical usefulness of amitriptyline in fibromyalgia: The results of 23 N-of-1 randomized controlled trials. *J Rheumatol.* 1991; 18: 447.

Joranson DE, Ryan KM, Gilson AM, Dahl JL. Trends in medical use and abuse of opioid analgesics. *JAMA.* 2000; 283: 1710.

McCormack K. Non-steroidal anti-inflammatory drugs and spinal nociceptive processing. *Pain.* 1994; 59: 9.

Pilowsky I, Hallett EC, Bassett DL, et al. A controlled study of amitriptyline in the treatment of chronic pain. *Pain.* 1982; 14: 169.

Swerdlow M. Review: Anticonvulsant drugs and chronic pain. *Clin Neuropharmacol.* 1984; 7: 51.

25

Management of Serious Internal Organ Manifestations

Daniel Small, MD, M.M.Sc., F.A.C.P., F.A.C.R.

The treatment of serious internal organ system involvement in Sjögren's syndrome requires the active participation of a rheumatologist coordinating the care of the patient in concert with specialist physicians. In the experience of this author, specialist physicians often treat patients with serious organ system involvement in a piecemeal manner, treating or not treating serious internal organ system disease without knowledge of the etiological role that Sjögren's may be playing in the disease process. To complicate this treatment process, there are relatively few FDA-approved indications for therapy of serious organ system involvement. When a physician may choose to treat a disease process, the patient's insurer may not approve such a therapy due to the lack of an FDA indication for the particular medication that the physician has chosen to use. The patient with serious organ system involvement must find physicians who are knowledgeable about the systemic manifestations of Sjögren's and who are willing to follow the patient closely and be advocates for the patient. The physician may have to steer the patient through a morass of blockades to diagnosis and therapy that third-party insurers may throw up in their zeal for cost containment.

Treating serious internal organ system involvement in Sjögren's requires careful monitoring of both the organ damage and the potential side effects of the medication chosen. Because the course of a particular organ system involvement may be highly variable, reasonable goals for therapy should be arrived at once a decision to treat has been made. While reversal of major organ system damage is always an ideal goal, many times it cannot be reasonably met, and stabilization and prevention of further deterioration may be the best result that can be expected. Due to the tremendous capacity for damage and repair of which major organs are capable, many patients may not present with organ-specific symptoms until significant damage has already taken place. For example, a person with a sedentary lifestyle, living at sea level, with pulmonary hypertension may not experience shortness of breath until he or she has fairly advanced disease. Early recognition, monitoring, and treatment are keys to successful outcomes for patients with serious internal organ system involvement with Sjögren's.

Treatment of Pulmonary Involvement

Bronchopulmonary disease may be variable, with involvement of some or all anatomical components of the lung. Involvement of other intrathoracic structures (pleura, respiratory muscles, heart, rib cage) can also occur. The most common manifestations include interstitial lung disease and pulmonary hypertension. Patients may present with cough and progressive shortness of breath. Critical to the diagnosis and long-term follow-up of lung involvement is early recognition and referral to the pulmonologist for serial observation and testing. The diagnosis of interstitial lung disease is aided by abnormalities on high-resolution CT scanning of the chest and diminished carbon monoxide-diffusing capacity on pulmonary function studies, along with restrictive lung disease. These measurements can be performed serially for staging progress of therapy. There are other infectious etiologies as well as environmental and occupational etiological factors that can mimic interstitial lung disease associated with connective tissue disease; thus, appropriate cultures and biopsies may be necessary for a definitive diagnosis of interstitial lung disease associated with Sjögren's.

Once the diagnosis is established, a short course of moderate-dose steroids will help the pulmonologist and rheumatologist determine the degree of reversibility of the pulmonary involvement. Symptomatic improvement, along with improvement in the pulmonary function studies and CT scan of the chest, suggests a favorable prognosis and provides the basis for going ahead with long-term therapy with immunosuppressive drugs. Whereas the pulmonologist may initiate steroid therapy, the rheumatologist usually will initiate and manage long-term immunosuppressive therapy. There are currently no FDA-approved indications that include interstitial lung disease, but there is a wealth of literature showing successful outcomes with the use of several immunosuppressive agents in interstitial lung disease. Azathioprine (Imuran, Azasan), cyclophosphamide (Cytoxan), mycophenolate mofetil (CellCept), cyclosporine (Sandimmune), and chlorambucil (Leukeran) have all been shown to improve clinical outcomes in patients with interstitial lung disease.

Immunosuppressive therapy requires close physician management for surveillance for side effects, infections, and the possible long-term complication of development of malignancies. If corticosteroids are required for long-term management, surveillance for the development of diabetes, hypertension, and osteoporosis is important. Prophylactic bisphosphonate or teriparatide therapy is commonly used with long-term corticosteroid therapy.

Close monitoring of patients undergoing long-term treatment with immuno-suppressive therapy for chronic lung disease is important, as during follow-up, progressive respiratory diseases may occur due to the underlying disease, treatment, infections, pulmonary embolism, or neoplasms.

Serial echocardiograms are helpful in detecting the development of pulmonary hypertension in patients with interstitial lung disease and also in patients with Sjögren's with unexplained shortness of breath. A number of therapies are now available for treating pulmonary hypertension (PAH) that can improve the long-term prognosis for patients with this condition. Standard PAH therapy (endothelin receptor antagonists, phosphodiesterase type 5 inhibitors, or prostanoids) is effective in some patients, but there are short-term and long-term failures. In patients with interstitial lung disease with PAH and those with PAH with signs of active systemic disease (elevated inflammatory markers), immunosuppressant therapy has been helpful. Unfortunately the best treatment strategy for PAH remains to be defined.

Some patients have mild lung involvement with very irritating symptoms. Patients with bronchial involvement may complain of cough and hoarseness but may not have serious progressive lung disease. Cough suppressants and steroid inhalers may provide symptomatic improvement without significant systemic side effects. If there are significant signs of systemic activity (elevated inflammatory markers), aggressive therapy of their Sjögren's with disease-modifying agents may result in improvement of some of their respiratory symptoms.

Therapy of Renal Disease

Interstitial nephritis with mild proteinuria and tubular dysfunction is the most common renal manifestation of Sjögren's, but glomerular involvement due to immune complex deposition may also rarely occur. A potassium-losing nephropathy is another manifestation of Sjögren's, usually caused by a tubular defect. Potassium replacement is necessary for these patients.

The interstitial nephritis that is seen in Sjögren's can often result from the use of nonsteroidal anti-inflammatories (NSAIDs) for treatment of joint or muscle pain occurring in active Sjögren's. This kind of nephritis is quite responsive to steroids and usually is short-lived and will resolve with cessation of the use of NSAIDs for that patient. Some patients may develop interstitial nephritis as a result of lymphocytic infiltration into the kidney tissue without concomitant NSAID use. Corticosteroid and immunosuppressant therapy may be necessary to lessen proteinuria and improve long-term renal function in such patients. Renal biopsy may be necessary to differentiate patients with interstitial nephritis, glomerulonephritis, or both. Serial urine protein measurements, repeated urinalyses, and creatinine clearance measurements will help the nephrologist determine whether treatment has been successful.

Glomerulonephritis is rare in patients with Sjögren's. Usually corticosteroids along with immunosuppressive therapy are necessary for successful treatment. Renal biopsy and serial 24-hour urine measurements of protein, along with urinalysis looking for active urinary sediment that denotes kidney inflammation, are important for monitoring patients with glomerulonephritis. Azathioprine (Imuran, Azasan), cyclophosphamide (Cytoxan), and mycophenolate mofetil (CellCept) have all been helpful in treating glomerulonephritis. Recent studies in patients with lupus nephritis suggest that mycophenolate mofetil therapy achieves similar outcome as cyclophosphamide, with fewer side effects.

Therapy of Neurological Disease

The neurological manifestations of Sjögren's include both central (CNS) and peripheral nervous system involvement. The wide spectrum of CNS involvement includes focal (sensory and motor deficits, brain stem, cerebellar lesions, seizure disorder, migraine headaches) or nonfocal (encephalomyelitis, aseptic meningitis, neuropsychiatric disease), spinal cord (myelopathy, transverse myelitis, motor neuron disease) findings of multiple sclerosis (MS)-like illness and optic neuritis. Evolving imaging techniques such as single photon emission computed tomography (SPECT), magnetic resonance spectroscopy, or magnetization transfer imaging are being used as research tools for understanding the nature of CNS involvement in Sjögren's. Most medical centers use MRI, brain mapping, and analysis of cerebrospinal fluid to determine disease activity in patients with neurological symptoms.

By far the most common involvement is peripheral neuropathy. The treatment of peripheral neuropathy entails treatment of the symptoms and aggressive management of the underlying Sjögren's. This author has found that aggressive management of the systemic signs of inflammation of Sjögren's leads to less progression of peripheral neuropathy. Most patients with peripheral neuropathy develop a sensory neuropathy and, less commonly, motor nerve involvement. They may experience dysesthesias—burning, sharp pain, and numbness and altered temperature sensation. The medications that are used for peripheral neuropathy symptoms will often help symptoms of pain, but do little to alter the symptoms of numbness and altered temperature sensation.

Cranial neuropathy is another treatable neurological manifestation. This author has seen many different manifestations, from facial paralysis, fifth cranial nerve abnormalities, and oculomotor palsies to disorders of hearing and balance. Fortunately most patients experience only temporary symptoms, but sometimes permanent disability can result. A short-term course of moderate corticosteroids may speed the time course for recovery in some patients. MRI of the brain with contrast should be performed if possible, specifically looking for malignancy and more widespread CNS disease such as vasculitis, meningitis, or localized lesions that may need a different therapy. Remaining dysesthesias may respond to antiseizure medications such as gabapentin (Neurontin), carbamazepine (Tegretol), phenytoin (Dilantin), and valproic acid (Depakene, Depakote) or the newer neurological medications pregabalin (Lyrica) or duloxetine (Cymbalta).

The CNS manifestations of Sjögren's are controversial. Rapidly progressive neurological signs and symptoms with widespread CNS disease seen on MRI of the brain, though rare, are an indication for aggressive management with steroids and immunosuppressive therapy. On the other end of the spectrum is the patient who describes "brain fog" with minimal findings on MRI of the brain. To determine who and how to treat, the recruitment of a knowledgeable neurologist is critical not only for initial diagnosis but also for long-term follow-up. Serial brain MRIs may be necessary to assess the rapidity of neurological change. Neuropsychiatric studies and brain mapping may show subtle changes over time that may be critical to making a decision to treat aggressively. Lumbar puncture and analysis of cerebrospinal fluid may be necessary to look for active CNS inflammation.

Patients with active CNS disease may be helped by the use of high-dose systemic corticosteroids followed by the use of immunosuppressive therapy. Clinical endpoints may be difficult to come by, and the mere prevention of further deterioration may be considered a successful result in some patients with severe CNS involvement. To date there have been no prospective randomized trials of treatment of patients with CNS disease; all reports are anecdotal or descriptions of nonrandomized patient series that contain heterogeneous groups of patients with CNS disease. Patients who are currently on immunosuppressive therapy for other systemic or serious organ system involvement who develop signs of CNS disease should be carefully screened for possible CNS infection. Manifestations of chronic CNS infection can mimic the signs and symptoms of CNS Sjögren's.

Patients who present with a MS-like process present a special diagnostic and therapeutic dilemma. Are they patients with Sjögren's who have developed CNS disease that looks just like MS, or are they patients with MS who also have Sjögren's? Because patients with MS can have a highly variable course, appropriate endpoints for management may be very difficult to determine, and lack of progression may be as good an outcome as any. This author has several patients who have been diagnosed as having MS with Sjögren's at one major medical center and Sjögren's with CNS disease that is MS-like by another center. These patients often have very slowly progressive disease, and it has been difficult to assess benefit from either aggressive therapy of their CNS Sjögren's or aggressive therapy of their MS.

Therapy of Serious Gastrointestinal Disease

The manifestations of serious gastrointestinal (GI) disease include motility disorders and pancreatic and hepatic disease. This author has seen everything from hypermotility to amotility of the GI tract in patients with Sjögren's. Hypomotility and amotility disorders may respond to the use of metoclopromide (Reglan), domperidone (Motilium), erythromycin, and other pro-motility agents. Gastroesophageal reflux often accompanies motility disturbances, and proton pump inhibitors have been helpful in decreasing symptoms associated with hyperacidity, reflux esophagitis, and gastritis. Chronic pancreatitis is infrequently seen as a complication of alterations of motility of the pancreatic and biliary outflow tracts. Analgesics, avoidance of alcohol, rest of the GI tract, and careful exploration of the biliary and pancreatic ducts looking for other causes of obstruction are the mainstays of therapy for pancreatic disease.

The hepatic disorders include primary biliary cirrhosis, sclerosing cholangitis, and granulomatous hepatitis. Cryptogenic cirrhosis may occur as a result of long-term chronic inflammation of the liver. Symptomatic therapy with ursodiol (Actigall, Urso) can reduce the elevated bilirubin levels seen in primary biliary cirrhosis and sclerosing cholangitis. This author has found that patients treated with hydroxychloroquine (Plaquenil) often have a more benign course with primary biliary cirrhosis. The incidence of other liver pathology (unexplained cirrhosis, steatohepatitis) appears to be less frequent in patients treated with hydroxychloroquine as well. Patients with sclerosing cholangitis and granulomatous hepatitis may respond to oral methotrexate therapy.

There is a strong association of patients with chronic hepatitis C having manifestations similar to those of patients with Sjögren's. This author has found that those patients, when treated with interferon and ribavirin to lower their circulating levels of hepatitis C virus, improve clinically from their hepatitis and from the systemic manifestations that are similar to those of patients with Sjögren's.

Therapy of Hematological Disease

The manifestations of hematological disease in Sjögren's include the anemia of chronic disease, development of thrombocytopenia, leukopenia, coagulopathies, and lymphadenopathy. Patients are often asymptomatic, and the abnormalities are found on routine laboratory testing. The majority of these patients have signs of active systemic disease. Treating their connective tissue disease and following their inflammatory markers usually result in improvement of their hematological manifestations. Specific treatment with corticosteroids, blood, or specific cell transfusions may be necessary for acute life-threatening manifestations. Methotrexate, azathioprine (Imuran, Azasan), and corticosteroids have been beneficial for treatment of lymphadenopathy. Lymphadenopathy may be the forerunner of lymphoma. This author has found on occasion that long-term treatment of Sjögren's with methotrexate has led to the development of lymphadenopathy, which has responded to the use of corticosteroids and the cessation of methotrexate therapy. The progression of lymphadenopathy to lymphoma and its treatment is covered elsewhere in this text.

Other Major Organ System Involvement

Sometimes patients present with severe skin involvement. The SSA/Ro antibody associated with Sjögren's is also associated with subacute cutaneous lupus. Thus, widespread skin rash, often in sun-exposed areas, can occur. Skin rashes often respond to topical and systemic steroids but may recur. Chronic skin rash usually responds to more aggressive therapies for the underlying Sjögren's. Hydroxychloroquine (Plaquenil) is often beneficial for skin involvement, but for patients who are intolerant to hydroxychloroquine, or when it may be less effective than desired, dapsone, methotrexate, and azathioprine (Imuran, Azasan) may be beneficial.

Vasculitis can occur in patients with Sjögren's. The manifestations may range from a mild process, such as the hypergammaglobulinemic purpura that presents with relatively asymptomatic pinpoint purpura on the lower extremities and leads to hyperpigmentation, to a severe systemic vasculitis with multiple organ system involvement. Careful investigation with biopsies of the lesions, evaluation of the degree of organ system involvement, search for infectious etiologies such as endocarditis or hepatitis, cryoglobulins, or other associated problems will lead to proper therapy. If no other specific etiology is found, corticosteroids followed by immunosuppressive agents or even immunosuppressive agents and plasmapheresis may be necessary in such patients. The specific treatment depends on the type of vasculitis found, the organ systems involved, and the general health of the patient.

Cardiac involvement with pericarditis, rhythm disturbances, and coronary vasculitis is not common but has been seen in a few patients. Pericarditis usually responds to corticosteroids but may herald other systemic problems. Aggressive management of the other systemic manifestations of Sjögren's will usually lead to improvement in these manifestations as well.

A unique problem can occur after pregnancy. Since the SSA/Ro antibody can pass through the placenta and enter the fetal circulation, babies born of women with SSA/Ro positivity can develop manifestations of neonatal lupus and have congenital heart block. It is important for women with Sjögren's who have SSA/Ro positivity to inform their obstetricians of this so that their babies can be monitored closely after birth. Babies who develop neonatal lupus and/ or congenital heart block usually do well with supportive therapy. The SSA/Ro antibody will gradually be metabolized, and the baby's symptoms will slowly improve over 1 to 2 weeks.

Summing Up

The major approaches to managing organ involvement in Sjögren's include several factors. First, local symptomatic treatment that targets a specific area of involvement is used. This might include proton pump inhibitors for GI involvement, mucolytics and humidification measures for pulmonary disease, or diuretics for renal manifestations. Next, agents can be prescribed for generalized dryness, such as pilocarpine derivatives. Sjögren's is also an inflammatory process, and disease-modifying agents can be useful. These include hydroxychloroquine for milder manifestations, corticosteroids for organ inflammation (e.g., interstitial lung disease), immune suppressive measures (e.g., azathioprine) as steroid-sparing agents, and biologics (e.g., rituximab) for serious organ involvement. Disease-modifying drugs usually work systemically and can have beneficial effects on more than one area of involvement at a time.

FOR FURTHER READING

Launay D, Hachulla E, Hatron PY, et al. Pulmonary arterial hypertension: a rare complication of primary Sjögren syndrome: report of 9 new cases and review of the literature. *Medicine (Baltimore)*. 2007; 86(5): 299–315.

Mavragani CP, Moutsopoulos HM. The geoepidemiology of Sjögren's syndrome. *Autoimmun Rev*. 2009, Nov. 10.

Pertovaara M, Korpela M, Pasternack A. Factors predictive of renal involvement in patients with primary Sjögren's syndrome. *Clin Nephrol*. 2001; 56(1): 10–8.

Rogers SJ, Williams CS, Román GC. Myelopathy in Sjögren's syndrome: role of nonsteroidal immunosuppressants. *Drugs*. 2004; 64(2): 123–32.

Schneider A, Merikhi A, Frank BB. Autoimmune disorders: gastrointestinal manifestations and endoscopic findings. *Gastrointest Endosc Clin North Am*. 2006; 16(1): 133–51.

26

Evaluation and Management of the Neurological Manifestations of Sjögren's Syndrome

Steven Mandel, MD, Carla LoPinto-Khoury, MD,
Ramon Manon-Espaillat, MD, MA, William Neil, MD,
Scott Pello, MD, David Roshal, DO, and
Meredith Snapp, MD

Involvement of the nervous system is a common extra-glandular manifestation of Sjögren's syndrome. On review of epidemiological studies, between 20% and 70% of patients with primary Sjögren's develop associated neurological symptoms. Variations among study design account for a wide range in reported prevalence. Peripheral nervous system (PNS) involvement (i.e., affecting nerves in the arms and legs) is more common than central nervous system (CNS) (i.e., affecting brain and spinal cord) manifestations. For example, an investigation of 87 Italian patients with primary Sjögren's who were clinically tested for neurological abnormalities found that 7% had CNS dysfunction while almost 14% showed PNS dysfunction.

The number of Sjögren's patients with active neurological complaints may sometimes underestimate the actual number with neurological complications. This was suggested by another study of 62 patients with Sjögren's who were evaluated for peripheral neuropathy. Thirty-seven patients were diagnosed with PNS involvement based on clinical examination; however, after objective testing with nerve conduction studies, an additional 28% were found to have abnormalities suggestive of this complication. Therefore, asymptomatic, subclinical neuropathies may also exist.

The onset of neurological symptoms often precedes the classic sicca symptoms of Sjögren's. Delande and colleagues conducted a large epidemiological study of 82 patients with neurological manifestations of Sjögren's. They reported that 81% of patients had neurological symptoms that preceded the diagnosis of Sjögren's, and 47% of patients noticed neurological complaints before sicca symptoms. Physicians should therefore maintain a high index of suspicion for underlying Sjögren's in patients who present with primary neurological complaints, even when dryness is absent.

Although a wide variety of neurological symptoms are reported in patients with Sjögren's, the causal relationship to Sjögren's is not always clear. The possibility of two separate diseases occurring within the same individual cannot be excluded. One study compared the neurological involvement in systemic lupus erythematosus, scleroderma, and Sjögren's and found a similar incidence of neurological disease in all three groups. In 25% to 34% of cases, secondary factors were identified that may have contributed to the neurological manifestations and were not related to the underlying connective tissue disease. Therefore, one cannot assume that neurological complaints are the direct result of Sjögren's unless a thorough neurological evaluation is performed to exclude other common causes of similar symptoms.

Peripheral Nerve Manifestations in Primary Sjögren's Syndrome

The prevalence of peripheral neuropathy in Sjögren's syndrome varies between 10% and 60% in different studies, and many types of neuropathy occur. These neuropathies may involve nerves that control sensation (sensory neuropathy), muscle power (motor neuropathy), or essential body functions like heart rate, blood pressure, or intestinal function (autonomic neuropathy). In some cases patterns are mixed. Distal sensorimotor polyneuropathy and distal sensory polyneuropathy are the most common types (Table 26–1).

SENSORY NEUROPATHIES

Small-fiber sensory neuropathy and sensory ataxic neuropathy are well-known peripheral nervous system manifestations of Sjögren's. Initial symptoms include distal paresthesias (abnormal sensations) such as burning or tingling

TABLE 26–1
Categories of Peripheral Neuropathy in Sjögren's Syndrome

Distal sensory polyneuropathy

Distal sensorimotor polyneuropathy

Sensory ataxic neuronopathy (dorsal root ganglionitis)

Mononeuritis multiplex

Demyelinating neuropathy

Polyradiculopathy

Cranial neuropathy

Autonomic neuropathy

of both feet that gradually spread more proximally to involve the hands and other parts of the legs. The timing and pattern of progression vary in different patients. In advanced cases, patients may lose proprioception (sense of position), resulting in poor coordination and difficulty walking due to an inability to sense the ground. Pseudoathetosis in the hands may occur when the upper extremities are involved.

On neurological examination of the extremities, patients are typically found to have decreased sensation to pain (pinprick) in a stocking-and-glove distribution, and, in more advanced cases, loss of position/vibration sensation, loss of reflexes, decreased coordination, and a positive Romberg sign. Dorsal root ganglionitis, which is histologically described as lymphocytic infiltration with resulting neuronal degeneration and neuron loss, is the pathological process that is believed to be the cause of sensory ataxic neuronopathy.

LARGE-FIBER NEUROPATHIES

Neuropathies involving large-diameter nerve fibers have also been described in Sjögren's and frequently exhibit evidence of symmetrical motor nerve involvement. They often cause limb weakness in addition to the symptoms described above. These neuropathies most commonly cause damage to axons (slender portion of the nerve cell that conducts electrical impulses) or the myelin sheath (insulation layer) around the nerves (see below) (Fig. 26–1). Examples include sensorimotor, motor, and sensory axonal neuropathy, demyelinating polyneuropathy, and demyelinating polyradiculopathy.

In a retrospective study, Mellgren and colleagues reported that a symmetrical sensorimotor axonal polyneuropathy occurred most frequently (68%) among this group, followed by a symmetrical sensory axonal neuropathy (32%). In some cases motor symptoms predominate and sensation remains

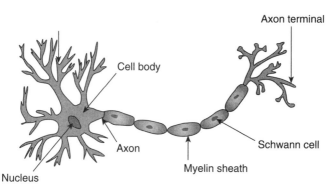

FIGURE 26–1 **Anatomy of a Nerve Cell.**

relatively intact. An EMG nerve conduction (described below) study is typically performed to better characterize the type of nerve involvement.

MONONEURITIS MULTIPLEX

In some cases, patients may develop sensory symptoms in a limb associated with motor weakness (wrist drop or foot drop) that occurs in an asymmetrical pattern (i.e., some nerves or portions of nerves are more severely affected than others). Differences may be seen between the extremities. An EMG nerve conduction study best demonstrates the asymmetrical pattern, and biopsy of the involved nerve will frequently reveal vasculitis.

AUTONOMIC NEUROPATHY

Different patterns of autonomic nerve fiber involvement have been documented in Sjögren's. The autonomic nervous system regulates essential body functions including heart rate, blood pressure, bowel motility, and bladder function. Reported manifestations in Sjögren's patients are usually described as mild and are summarized in Table 26–2.

The pathogenesis of the autonomic neuropathy in Sjögren's has been speculated to be caused by both ganglioneuronopathy and vasculitic lesions in peripheral nerves affecting autonomic fibers. Klein and colleagues reported that among 18 patients with autoimmune autonomic neuropathies, 4 had a high ganglionic acetylcholine receptor antibody titer (blocking antibodies), sicca symptoms, abnormal pupils, and other autonomic abnormalities as part of severe autonomic dysfunction. Controversy still remains regarding the prevalence of autonomic dysfunction in primary Sjögren's. Niemela and colleagues performed a battery of autonomic tests (Valsalva maneuver, deep-breathing test, active orthostatic test, measurements of baroreflex sensitivity with phenylephrine, 24-hour heart rate variability) on 30 patients with primary Sjögren's and 30 healthy age- and sex-matched controls. They found no significant differences between the Sjögren's patients and the healthy controls in any

TABLE 26–2
Manifestations of Autonomic Neuropathy

Adie's tonic pupils

Fixed tachycardia

Anhidrosis

Bowel dysfunction

Gastroparesis

Bladder dysfunction

Orthostatic hypotension

of the above tests. Therefore, the prevalence and type of autonomic neuropathy seen in Sjögren's may vary according to how the nerves are tested.

Central Nervous System Disease

CNS involvement in Sjögren's was first recognized in the early 1980s by Alexander and colleagues and is now known to cause a wide variety of neurological problems. Some of these problems are listed in Table 26-3.

The clinical course can be self-limited, relapsing, or progressive. The neurological deficits can be focal (e.g., hemiparesis) or diffuse (e.g., cognitive dysfunction). These abnormalities are thought to result from lymphocytic infiltration (inflammation) of the brain and spinal cord and damage to the myelin layer surrounding nerve cells. In rare instances, true vasculitis (inflammation of the blood vessels) of the brain is found. Neurological signs and symptoms and results of imaging studies, spinal tap, and so forth greatly overlap those of other disorders such as multiple sclerosis or CNS lupus. Therefore, great care must be taken to exclude these disorders before the diagnosis of CNS Sjögren's is firmly established.

Cranial Neuropathies

The 12 paired cranial nerves that arise from the brain or brain stem control various special senses (sight, hearing, smell, etc.) and are sometimes affected by Sjögren's. Some cranial neuropathies are classified as CNS disorders, while others belong to the PNS.

TABLE 26–3
Spectrum of Central Nervous System Disorders in Sjögren's Syndrome

Hemiparesis (one-sided weakness) or monoparesis
Hemisensory or monosensory loss
Aphasia
Seizures
Strokes, transient ischemic attacks
Movement disorders, tremors
Encephalopathy
Aseptic meningitis
Dementia
Cognitive dysfunction
Neuropsychiatric disorders
Optic neuritis
Transverse myelitis

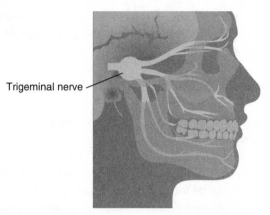

Trigeminal nerve

FIGURE 26–2 **Cranial Neuropathies.**

Trigeminal sensory neuropathy (trigeminal neuralgia) is classically seen in Sjögren's and may also occur in other connective tissue diseases (Fig. 26–2). Patients typically present with numbness, paresthesias (abnormal sensations), and lancinating pain on one or both sides of the face. Symptoms may be aggravated or precipitated by facial movements, including eating and speaking, touching the skin, or exposure of the face to cold air. Examination may reveal diminished sensation to pinprick in a trigeminal nerve distribution.

The symptoms sometimes start on one side and then become bilateral. The etiology is unknown; however, since trigeminal sensory neuropathy is sometimes the presenting symptom of a sensory ataxic neuronopathy (described above), it has been suggested that its pathogenesis may be the same.

Optic neuritis, which is characterized by inflammation of the optic nerve resulting in pain and visual impairment, is well documented in Sjögren's and may lead to permanent blindness if not promptly diagnosed and treated.

One retrospective study published in 2004 looked at 82 patients with primary Sjögren's and neurological manifestations and found a surprisingly high rate of cochlear nerve (eighth nerve) impairment that caused hearing loss.

Other symptoms caused by cranial neuropathies include facial muscle weakness (Bell's palsy) caused by facial nerve (seventh nerve) paresis or paralysis and loss of olfaction (smell), presumably secondary to cranial nerve I involvement. Some patients may present with multiple cranial neuropathies occurring simultaneously. The remaining cranial nerves can also be affected.

Muscle Involvement in Primary Sjögren's

In primary Sjögren's syndrome, according to some studies, up to one third of patients complain of muscular pain and/or weakness. In many cases this is due to fibromyalgia, a chronic pain syndrome. In about 3% of patients, however, inflammatory disease of the muscles (myositis) occurs in Sjögren's and represents a much more serious problem. Muscular signs and symptoms are similar to those seen in diseases like polymyositis and dermatomyositis. Patients typically present with prominent proximal muscle weakness as well as elevated serum muscle enzymes and abnormal EMG and muscle biopsy. The EMG shows characteristic small motor unit potentials with short duration and early recruitment pattern. A muscle biopsy will show inflammation.

Sjögren's can also coexist with another type of muscle disease called inclusion body myositis. In this disease patients may present with both distal muscle weakness, especially the foot extensors and finger flexors, and proximal muscle weakness. There is sometimes an associated neuropathy. The muscle weakness and atrophy can be asymmetrical, with selective involvement of the quadriceps, iliopsoas, triceps, and biceps. The diagnosis is confirmed by performing a muscle biopsy for special stains and electron microscopy.

Evaluation of the Patient with Suspected Neurological Sjögren's

The diagnosis of neurological Sjögren's always begins with the clinical history and examination. It is important to have a firm diagnosis of Sjögren's according to current diagnostic criteria and to exclude other disorders that cause similar symptoms.

Careful questioning about neurological symptoms should include the presence or absence of pain in the face or extremities, numbness or tingling in the extremities, the exact distributions of the areas affected, gait instability, and fatigue or weakness of the proximal large muscles (i.e., do you have difficulty raising your arms, do you have difficulty standing from a sitting position) or distal muscles (i.e., difficulty with fine motor tasks such as writing or foot drop). A history of autonomic dysfunction may be elicited by inquiring about bladder or bowel incontinence or orthostasis (e.g., dizziness when arising from a chair). Spinal cord symptoms can mimic features of peripheral involvement, including weakness, sensory change (e.g., numbness below the waist), gait problems, or bladder and bowel symptoms. A history of painful visual loss may indicate optic neuritis. Hearing loss or vertigo would imply eighth cranial nerve lesions. Brain involvement might manifest as cognitive changes or seizures.

A full examination by a neurologist must be performed with particular attention to the cranial nerves, funduscopy, motor testing, reflexes, and a complete sensory examination. Cranial nerve findings may include abnormal pupillary constriction and sensory change in the trigeminal nerve distribution. Motor examination may reveal distal muscle atrophy and weakness in the case of a peripheral neuropathy, or spasticity of the limbs if involving the spinal cord. Reflexes, especially at the ankle, may be absent in a peripheral neuropathy or brisk with spinal cord involvement. Sensory testing likely will reveal decreased perception of vibration at the fingers and toes, decreased sense of joint position in space, and diminished pinprick and temperature sensation. A Romberg test (testing of balance with the eyes closed) may tell whether or not proximal position sense is impaired. The gait examination may be markedly impaired with a sensory ataxia.

Suspicion of a peripheral neuropathy based on clinical symptoms and the examination should warrant neurophysiological testing. This includes a nerve conduction study and needle electromyography (EMG) performed by a qualified neurophysiologist to distinguish patterns of sensory, motor, and mixed neuropathies. As a distal symmetrical sensory neuropathy is common in Sjögren's, abnormal sural nerve action potentials and denervation are frequently found, although the findings can be variable. Nerve conduction studies and EMG can also help to diagnose nerve root dysfunction (radiculopathies) and muscle disorders (myopathies). Sympathetic skin response may be absent when tested and indicative of autonomic nerve dysfunction. Other neurophysiological testing includes Somatosensory evoked responses and visual evoked response if CNS disorders are suspected.

Laboratory tests, including anti-SSA/SSB, are important to confirm the diagnosis of Sjögren's and to exclude other causes of neurological disease. Anti-SSA and anti-SSB antibodies have been respectively found in 41% to 48% and 13% of suspected cases of neurological Sjögren's. The prevalence of these autoantibodies in PNS and CNS diseases is roughly the same. In the absence of anti-SSA and SSB, the diagnosis of Sjögren's must be confirmed by a lip biopsy. If myopathy is suspected, muscle enzymes (creatinine kinase, aldolase) should be assessed.

Blood tests for common metabolic causes of peripheral neuropathy should be performed, including diabetes mellitus with hemoglobin A1C, thyroid antibodies, and vitamin levels, especially B_{12}. Serological testing for infectious conditions, including hepatitis C, which is frequently associated with SS or an SS-like illness, may reveal the need for additional treatment with interferon therapy, especially when liver function tests are abnormal. HIV-infected patients can develop a Sjögren's-like syndrome from CD8 lymphocyte infiltration of the salivary glands that causes multiple types of peripheral neuropathy; zidovudine or corticosteroids can help. Additional laboratory tests (rheumatoid factor, anti-CCP antibodies, double-stranded DNA, anti-Sm/RNP, complement C3, C4, cryoglobulins, ANCA, ACE level) can sometimes help differentiate primary Sjögren's from other autoimmune or rheumatological conditions (e.g., lupus, sarcoidosis, ANCA- associated vasculitis) that can all cause neuropathies. If clinically indicated, screening tests for cancer, including anti-neuronal paraneoplastic antibodies, are sometimes performed to rule out malignancy (e.g., small cell lung carcinoma) as the cause of the neuropathy.

Neuroimaging studies and spinal tap are useful diagnostic tools for CNS involvement. If the history and physical examination suggest findings of brain or spinal cord involvement, MRI with contrast should be performed to identify features of demyelinating disease or vasculitis. The spinal tap may identify elevated protein, elevated white blood cells, oligoclonal bands, or a high IgG index that help document CNS inflammation. In appropriate circumstances (e.g., a patient on chronic immunosuppressive therapy), cultures and stains for bacteria, fungi, and tuberculosis will be performed on the spinal fluid to rule out a CNS infection. Formal neuropsychological testing is useful to evaluate patients with cognitive dysfunction. The results of many of the above studies do not correlate well with one another. Therefore, at the present time, an entire battery of tests is recommended for complete evaluation when clinically warranted.

When in doubt, the diagnosis of a small-fiber peripheral neuropathy can sometimes be documented by performing a skin biopsy at different levels in the leg to count nerve fiber density. In some cases a biopsy of a peripheral nerve (e.g., sural nerve near the ankle), muscle, or even brain may be indicated to look for vasculitis. Because the treatment of vasculitis involving the nervous system usually involves the use of toxic medications, this diagnosis must be documented as firmly as possible before starting treatment.

Treatment of Neurological Manifestations

The treatment of neurological manifestations of Sjögren's is always facilitated by an accurate and timely diagnosis. There are few controlled studies in Sjögren's to provide guidelines for treatment. At present most treatment decisions are made based on the clinical scenario, anecdotal reports, the physician's experience, and the knowledge of the patient's other medical problems. Additionally, the experience in treating other diseases (e.g., CNS lupus, diabetic neuropathy) is sometimes borrowed to provide a rationale for choice of therapy in Sjögren's.

Mild peripheral sensory neuropathies in Sjögren's that cause burning or tingling of the feet and hands are usually treated symptomatically with medications such as gabapentin (Neurontin) or pregabalin (Lyrica). Trigeminal neuralgia may respond to treatment with carbamazepine (Tegretol). Other classes of medications typically used for pain related due to peripheral neuropathy, such as tricyclic antidepressants (e.g., amitriptyline [Elavil]) may provide benefit but are usually avoided because they have side effects that may exacerbate the dryness symptoms of Sjögren's.

In patients who have neuropathy due to mononeuritis multiplex or who demonstrate progressive and severe sensorimotor symptoms with loss of coordination or progressive weakness, immunosuppressive therapies are warranted. Choices include corticosteroids (either oral or intravenous), azathioprine (Imuran), oral or intravenous cyclophosphamide (Cytoxan), intravenous gamma globulin (several forms), or intravenous rituximab (Rituxan). The choice of therapy at the present time is largely empirical. The gravity of the clinical situation and possible benefits of treatment must be carefully weighed against the likelihood of serious side effects.

CNS disease and true vasculitis are serious but uncommon problems. Patients with active and/or progressive disease are also treated with immunosuppressants as discussed above. Neurological tests are often repeated to assess patient response to therapy and justify continued treatment. Optic neuritis is treated in similar fashion. Life-threatening infections or low blood counts can occur as a complication of therapy and must be closely monitored.

As previously discussed, ischemic stroke can occur in Sjögren's and can be disabling or life-threatening. In some groups, strokes may occur more frequently when associated with the presence of antiphospholipid antibodies. According to guidelines laid out by the American Heart Association, a person with Sjögren's who has suffered a stroke but does not have antiphospholipid syndrome may be treated with a medicine that acts against platelets to prevent clots, such as aspirin. Platelets are one of the main components of a blood clot that causes stroke.

If a patient with Sjögren's is found to have antiphospholipid antibodies on blood work at the time of the stroke, and this is confirmed on testing 3 months later, then warfarin (Coumadin) may be necessary. Warfarin is a more potent blood thinner that acts against vitamin K to prevent blood clots. Care must be taken to follow the blood-thinning effects of warfarin by checking the International Normalized Ratio (INR). Warfarin has many interactions with other medicines as well as some foods such as green vegetables, so dietary counseling is advised. Patients must be closely monitored for bleeding side effects.

Orthostatic hypotension can be a disabling complication of an autonomic neuropathy and can cause syncope (passing-out spells) or pre-syncope. A person may complain of lightheadedness or dizziness with prolonged standing or arising from a seated position, and have low blood pressure. This can be treated with medicines used to raise blood pressure, such as midodrine (ProAmatine) and fludricortisone (Florinef).

Summing Up

Sjögren's syndrome can affect the peripheral, autonomic, and central nervous systems. A thorough neurological evaluation is necessary to document the problem. Complications are sometimes disabling and even life-threatening. However, effective treatments exist for most problems. The choice of therapy depends largely on the severity of the clinical situation and the physician's experience. Patients on immunosuppressants and blood thinners must be carefully monitored for side effects. Further research is sorely needed to document the efficacy of existing treatments and to discover new and better therapies in the future.

FOR FURTHER READING

Alexander E. Central nervous system disease in Sjögren's syndrome: new insights into immunopathogenesis. *Rheum Dis North Am.* 1992; 13(3): 637–72.

Chai J, Herrmann DN, Stanton M, et al. Painful small-fiber neuropathy in Sjögren's syndrome. *Neurology.* 2005; 65(6): 925–7.

Delalande S, De Seze J, Fauchais A, et al. Neurologic manifestations in primary Sjögren's syndrome: a study of 82 patients. *Medicine.* 2004; 83: 280–91.

Goransson LG, Bruun J, Harboe E, et al. Intraepidermal nerve fiber densities in chronic inflammatory autoimmune diseases. *Arch Neurol.* 2006; 63(10): 1410–3.

Goransson LG, Herigstad A, Tjensvoll AB, et al. Peripheral neuropathy in primary Sjögren's syndrome. A population-based study. *Arch Neurol.* 2006; 63(11): 1612–5.

Griffin JW, Cornblath DR, Alexander E, et al. Ataxic sensory neuronopathy and dorsal root ganglionitis associated with Sjögren's syndrome. *Ann Neurol.* 1990; 27(3): 304–15.

Klein CM, Vernino S, Lennon VA, et al. The spectrum of autoimmune autonomic neuropathies. *Ann Neurol.* 2003; 53(6): 752–8.

Lopate G, Pestronk A, Al-Lozi M, et al. Peripheral neuropathy in an outpatient cohort of patients with Sjögren's syndrome. *Muscle Nerve.* 2006; 33(5): 672–6.

Mellgren SI, Conn DL, Stevens JC, et al. Peripheral neuropathy in primary Sjögren's syndrome. *Neurology.* 1989; 39(3): 390–4.

Mellgren SI, Goransson LG, Omdal R, Primary Sjögren's syndrome associated neuropathy. *Can J Neurol Sci.* 2007; 34: 280–7.

Mori K, Iijuma M, Koike H, et al. The wide spectrum of clinical manifestations in Sjögren's syndrome associated neuropathy. *Brain.* 2005; 128(Pt 11): 2518–34.

Niemela RK, Hakala M, Huikur HV, et al. Comprehensive study of autonomic function in a population with primary Sjögren's syndrome. No evidence of autonomic involvement. *J Rheumatol.* 2003; 30(1): 74–9.

27

Complementary and Alternative Therapies for Sjögren's Syndrome

Paul F. Howard, MD, FACR, FACP, and C. Keith Wilkinson, ND

Complementary medicine, also referred to as "alternative" medicine or therapy, offers expanded treatment options for people with Sjögren's syndrome. Complementary therapies are best classified according to their approach (Table 27–1). Functional medicine is a broad group of treatment modalities focusing on achieving optimal health with therapies such as dietary intervention, nutritional supplementation (e.g., vitamins, minerals, amino acids, botanicals), detoxification, and intravenous therapies to influence physiological functions of the body. Mind–body medicine includes therapies of meditation, guided imagery, and counseling to address the association between mental state and physical health. Energetic-based therapies include traditional Chinese medicine, acupuncture, and homeopathy. Finally, body movement includes therapies such as exercise, physical therapy, yoga, Tai Chi, and other movement arts.

When choosing to use complementary medicine, many patients feel they are faced with an "either/or" choice of working with their conventional medical doctor or choosing an alternative practitioner. This is unfortunate since complementary medicine should not limit the care available but rather provide additional options for the patient. Ideally, patients should be actively involved in their care and seek out conventional and alternative practitioners open to working with each other.

Since one of the authors of this chapter is a naturopathic physician, the approaches discussed are guided by the naturopathic principle that the body has a remarkable ability to heal. By understanding possible imbalances surrounding diseases, naturopathic physicians work with the patient to remove the causes that prevent the body from healing and allow the body to restore itself to health. This approach often contrasts with conventional forms of treatment that sometimes focus on quick symptomatic relief but do not address the underlying cause of the disease. *The reader should be cautioned that none of the*

TABLE 27–1
Types of Complementary Therapies

Functional Medicine	Diet
	Ortho-molecular supplementation
	Environmental medicine
	Detoxification
Mind–Body	Meditation
	Guided imaging
	Biofeedback
	Hypnosis
Energetic	Reiki
	Craniosacral therapy
	Magnetic
	Pulse electric stimulation
	Therapeutic touch
	Homeopathy
	Acupuncture/traditional Chinese medicine
Body movement	Rolfing
	Reflexology
	Chiropractic
	Yoga
	Tai Chi
	Postural re-education
	Movement/exercise therapy–focused and general

modalities/supplements reviewed in this chapter has been subject to a controlled trial in Sjögren's patients. They are generally harmless, and many of our patients report subjective improvement with them. However, until evidence-based protocols document statistically significant improvement in a clinical study, Sjögren's patients should employ these approaches at their discretion in consultation with their physician.

General Treatments

DIET

The foundation of health nearly always begins with the quality of the food we eat. The primary concern with most chronic disease, including Sjögren's, is the presence of inflammation. Unfortunately, much of the food consumed in modern diets is pro-inflammatory. Foods promoting inflammation include simple or refined sugars that quickly raise blood sugar and stimulate surges of pro-inflammatory insulin. Other examples include oils that are highly refined and hydrogenated, processed grains and carbohydrates, and red meats that contain high amounts of a pro-inflammatory fat called arachidonic acid. Dairy, wheat, gluten, eggs, and citrus commonly contain food allergens that promote inflammation and artificial ingredients such as sweeteners and preservatives that can trigger immune reactions through their antigenic load.

In contrast, an anti-inflammatory diet relies on minimally processed whole foods and is more plant-based (Table 27–2).

This includes an abundance of colorful vegetables and moderate fruit consumption, minimally processed fats such as those in avocadoes, olive and coconut oils, fatty fish such as salmon and mackerel, moderate whole grains such as quinoa, amaranth, brown and wild rice, as well as moderate meat consumption such as free-range chicken, smaller non-predatory fish such as wild salmon, tilapia, anchovies, and white fish, or free-range poultry, beef, or bison. This type of diet is anti-inflammatory because:

1. Foods in their natural state tend to have a carbohydrate, fat, and protein ratio that moderates swings in blood sugar and minimizes pro-inflammatory insulin surges.
2. Minimally processed foods naturally have fewer additives that can pose an antigenic load on the immune system.
3. It eliminates many of the common food allergens mentioned above.
4. It has a higher nutrient content of vitamins, minerals, and phytonutrients.
5. It contains more essential fats that are naturally anti-inflammatory.

Because food plays such an important role in good health, implementation of an anti-inflammatory diet is nearly always a starting point of naturopathic treatment. As challenging as this may seem, significant dietary changes are often necessary. For Sjögren's patients, an anti-inflammatory diet is so important to the process of removing the contributors to inflammation that it is often pointless to proceed to more advanced or focused therapies until some basic progress is made here.

TABLE 27–2

Components of an Anti-Inflammatory Diet

- Plant-based
- Minimally processed whole foods
- High in anti-inflammatory fats
- Moderate free-range/organic meat
- Moderate in whole grains
- Low in food additives
- Low in common food allergens.
- Low in refined oils

ELIMINATION DIETS

Advanced dietary therapy can be performed with more restrictive regimens through elimination and/or fasting diets. These diets recognize that some foods, perhaps otherwise beneficial for most people, can cause a specific allergenic and pro-inflammatory reaction in others. The elimination diet restricts foods to typically steamed vegetables, whole grains, small amounts of nonrefined oils like those in the anti-inflammatory diet, and often consumption of protein shakes made from hypoallergenic protein sources such as rice or pea proteins. The elimination diet is typically carried out over several weeks.

An even more restrictive form of this diet is the medically supervised short-term water fast. This is an aggressive dietary therapy typically used in more severe cases of chronically ill people. Nevertheless, the intent of either the elimination or fasting diet is to drastically reduce the antigenic load of foods to which a person could be reacting. By removing reactive foods, symptoms can often subside. When foods are slowly reintroduced one by one and with special awareness of worsening of symptoms, the patient can often detect that foods affect their disease and select accordingly. It is best to work through these dietary changes with a practitioner trained in these therapies, such as a naturopathic physician. Numerous other resources are also available that provide more detailed information.

SUPPLEMENTS

Intensive farming, processing, and preparation yield foods of lower nutrient quality. It is believed that the nutrient content in foods alone can be insufficient for optimal health, especially for someone dealing with chronic disease. Additionally, even with the best intentions, it is often difficult to eat the most nutritious foods all of the time. Therefore, we recommend daily supplements of high-quality bioavailable broad-spectrum multivitamins, minerals, and essential fatty acids in dosages that are sufficient for optimal health, not just prevention of nutrient deficiency. Of particular concern to patients with Sjögren's and other autoimmune conditions is the need for supplements that are free of additives, fillers, binders, and colorings, which are often found in bargain wholesale and inexpensive drugstore-variety supplements.

Specific Supplements

Beyond basic supplementation is the need for two additional nutrients specific to autoimmune patients. Fish oil is high in the omega-3 unsaturated fatty acids eicosapentaenoic (EPA) and docosahexaenoic (DHA) acid. These fatty acids function as potent substrates to make hormone-like substances called prostaglandins. These prostaglandins help shift the body away from inflammation. If the diet is deficient in EPA and DHA, which is common in modern diets, the body tends to overproduce pro-inflammatory prostaglandins. Rather than "suppressing" inflammation, supplementation with EPA and DHA shifts the body away from the pro-inflammatory prostaglandin to production of the anti-inflammatory series. To more fully address the levels of systemic inflammation common in Sjögren's, the dosage of fish oil should be higher than the standard dose used for cardioprotection (1 to 2 grams/day). One must read supplement labels and consume a combined EPA + DHA dosage of 3,000 to 4,000 mg per day. Fish oil is available in capsule or liquid forms. Liquid forms are often more concentrated (i.e., higher dosage with fewer teaspoons than capsules), but both forms are suitable. It is important to use oils that have been adequately tested for contaminants such as PCBs, dioxins, and heavy metals as well as rancidity, indicating that the oils have become oxidized and spoiled.

The second supplement specific for autoimmune patients is vitamin D, well known for its benefits in calcium absorption and support of conditions such as osteoporosis. New evidence shows that vitamin D plays an important role in regulating immune function, which is often dysfunctional in autoimmune conditions. Vitamin D regulates the balance between different white blood cells, particularly T-helper and T-suppressor lymphocytes. When T-helper cells become uncontrolled due to inadequate vitamin D levels, overactive immune function can develop, leading to worsening of autoimmune conditions. Vitamin D is also responsible for inhibiting production of intracellular messengers, such as NF-kappaB, a primary initiator of systemic inflammation.

Compounding the effects of vitamin D deficiency, it is theorized that the cellular vitamin D receptors in people with autoimmune disease are less responsive to normal circulating levels of vitamin D. Therefore, we recommend maintaining vitamin D levels at 50 to 100 ng/mL, the high end of normal. Often the general Recommended Dietary Allowances (RDA) guidelines of 800 IU of supplemental vitamin D_3 (cholecalciferol) are insufficient, and it must be dosed at levels of 2,000 to 7,000 IU per day to reach optimal levels. This can be accomplished by working with a physician and monitoring blood levels of 25-hydroxyvitamin D. More information on vitamin D can be found in Chapter 28.

Treatments for Specific Health Issues

There are two areas of treatment that address specific areas of concern in Sjögren's: gastrointestinal (GI) health and use of anti-inflammatory botanicals. From a naturopathic perspective, the GI tract plays a vital role in the possible cause of autoimmune disease. The GI tract has a primary function in digestion of food and absorption of nutrients. It also plays a very important role from an immunological perspective. A common misconception is that the GI tract is "inside" the body. From an anatomical standpoint, it is actually a hollow tube that is open to the outside world at the mouth and the anus. Nothing truly gets "inside" the body until it crosses the mucosal lining of the GI tract and then into the systemic circulation. From an immunological standpoint, the GI tract forms a physical barrier that keeps foreign substances, undigested foods, pathogenic bacteria, viruses, and parasites out of the body. This barrier function plays a critical role in our understanding of immune dysregulation in autoimmune disease and restoration of immunological health.

Basic to the understanding of autoimmunity, the body has lost the ability to determine self from non-self and therefore begins an immune reaction against one's own tissue, setting off the autoimmune disease. Considering intestinal barrier function, imagine if this intestinal barrier became permeable and allowed foreign substances to leak across the gut and into the systemic circulation. Once these substances (e.g., partially digested carbohydrates and protein peptides from food, pathogens, etc.) are present in the circulation, they can appear as foreign antigens to the immune system and initiate an immune response. If there is molecular similarity between the foreign substance and one's own tissue, the immune systems can simultaneously mount a response against both substances and trigger autoimmune disease. This phenomenon is termed "leaky gut" (increased intestinal permeability) and is believed to be a common cause of autoimmune diseases. Causes of intestinal permeability include pro-inflammatory diets, loss of normal GI bacteria related to the use of a low-fiber diet or frequent oral antibiotics, parasites, overgrowth of pathogenic bacteria, decreased pancreatic function, and putrefaction of foods in the GI tract.

Treatment of intestinal permeability begins with dietary modification such as anti-inflammatory, elimination, or short-term fasting diets. Next, it is appropriate to restore gut function through specific GI supplementation. The GI tract should be repopulated with beneficial bacteria such as *Lactobacillus* and *Bifidobacterium* species of probiotics. Probiotics should be from suppliers that provide viable high-quality strains of bacteria and dosed in quantities of 15 to 100 billion bacterial units per day. To assist in the growth of these bacteria, prebiotics can be used, which function as food to feed the probiotics. Commonly used prebiotics are fructo-oligosaccharides (FOS) and inula, which can be dosed with probiotics. Supplementation of the amino acid glutamine and N-acetyl glucosamine, primary fuels used by mucosal cells to regenerate, is helpful for rebuilding the GI lining. Doses of 2 to 3 grams several times per day should be sufficient. Additionally, botanicals such as deglycerized licorice and slippery elm dosed at 0.5 to 1 grams several times per day can be used to soothe inflamed GI tissue and allow the healing process to start.

Sjögren's patients are particularly susceptible to oral ulceration and oral candidiasis (yeast). The local mucosal irritation associated with the xerostomia of Sjögren's can be treated with folic acid, a necessary nutrient for cellular regeneration. Liquid preparations of folic acid can be added to water and used as a 1-minute swish and swallow twice per day. To minimize the risk of oral candida, the anti-inflammatory diet should be followed, with a specific focus on restricting consumption of simple carbohydrates and sugars. If oral candida is detected, antimicrobial mouthwashes such as grapeseed extract, caprylic acid, gentian violet, or conventional prescription Nystatin swish and swallow can be used.

Anti-inflammatory botanicals may appear no different from conventional anti-inflammatory drugs such as prednisone or nonsteroidal anti-inflammatories (NSAIDs) that address the symptom of inflammation but not the underlying cause. However, botanicals typically have minimal side effects and can minimize or eliminate the need for more harmful prescription drugs while other efforts are being made to correct the underlying causes or aggravating factors of disease. Common botanicals are Boswellia, Curcumin, Ginger, and Harpagophytum (cat's claw). These all have mechanisms that cause decreased expression of pro-inflammatory cell signals like NF-kappaB and pro-inflammatory prostaglandins. There are many products available that provide several of these botanicals in combination or as a single supplement. Dosing depends on each botanical, type of preparation (i.e., dried plant capsule or liquid tincture forms), and combination used.

Movement and Exercise Therapy

Exercise is rarely considered to be an alternative or complementary therapy. Most commonly, it is considered a rehabilitation method for a specific or isolated problem following surgery, accidents, or hospitalization. However, the available evidence strongly suggests that exercise substantially improves the quality of life for the majority of people with Sjögren's.

People with Sjögren's have diminished cardiovascular conditioning (aerobic capacity) stamina and joint mobility. They also are impaired significantly by fatigue, anxiety, and depression. In 2003 Stombeck and colleagues studied over 50 people with Sjögren's compared to age-matched control subjects and measured their baseline aerobic conditioning by stress testing; their mobility, balance, and stamina by standardized tests; and fatigue, anxiety, and depression by self-administered questionnaires. Compared to control subjects, aerobic capacity was reduced by 11% in Sjögren's, the equivalent of adding 10 years onto a person's age. There was also a significant increase in fatigue, depression, and anxiety. They were able to estimate that nearly 50% of the fatigue experienced by Sjögren's patients was due to a combination of poor aerobic capacity, reduced functional abilities, and depression.

Since fatigue is a dominant problem in Sjögren's, exercise to improve aerobic capacity would be expected to improve fatigue. Stombeck confirmed this in a small study in 2007. Sjögren's patients who participated in an exercise program of moderate to intense activity (45 minutes per session, three times a week for 12 weeks at 60% to 80% maximum predicted heart rate) demonstrated improved aerobic conditioning and less fatigue and depression. Other studies have shown that regular conditioning programs also benefit patients with rheumatoid arthritis (RA) and systemic lupus erythematosus (SLE). The benefits of exercise programs are summarized in Table 27-3.

Cardiovascular disease, as manifested by heart attacks and strokes, is increased in inflammatory conditions such as RA and SLE. One study also suggested a possible increased risk of atherosclerotic heart disease in Sjögren's. Atherosclerosis, increased blood pressure, loss of balance and joint mobility, and reduced muscle mass and aerobic capacity are all associated with aging. As outlined in Table 27-3, exercise is a proven anti-aging program that is inexpensive and evidence-based.

Most people with rheumatic disease do not appreciate the overwhelming benefits of moderate exercise. In a survey in 21 countries, nearly 80% of people with RA did not exercise regularly and less than 14% performed light to moderate exercise 3 days per week. Factors such as fatigue, pain, and joint immobility may contribute to difficulties in adhering to an exercise program. However, better patient education, exercise modification, and a more graduated increase of exercise intensity can all help to promote compliance.

EXERCISE RECOMMENDATIONS

Both aerobic and muscle-strengthening activities are critical for healthy aging. Patients should consult with a health care professional before beginning their exercise routine. The following recommendations are based on the American College of Sports Medicine and American Heart Association 2007 guidelines for exercise in older adults over 65 or younger adults with chronic

TABLE 27–3
Effects of Moderate Exercise

Improved	Aerobic capacity
	Joint mobility
	Balance
	Muscle mass
Reduced	Fatigue
	Depression
	Anxiety
	Blood pressure
	Cholesterol
	Body fat

health conditions. The use of a heart rate monitor is recommended to help patients analyze their workout in terms of intensity level.

1. Do moderately intense aerobic exercise **30 minutes a day, five days a week** *or* vigorously intense aerobic exercise **20 minutes a day, 3 days a week.** Moderate-intensity aerobic exercise means working hard at about a level-six intensity on a scale of 10 (0 = rest, 10 = extreme exertion). You should still be able to carry on a conversation during moderate-intensity aerobic exercise and reach a heart rate 50% to 55% of maximum predicted. A simple formula for determining maximum predicted heart rate is (220 – your current age.) Intense aerobic exercise results in perspiration and shortness of breath, making it difficult to carry out a conversation (heart rate 70% to 80% of maximum predicted).
2. Do 8 to 10 strength-training exercises, 10 to 15 repetitions of each exercise, two or three times per week.
3. If you are at risk of falling, perform balance exercises.
4. Develop your physical activity plan with a health professional or physical therapist.

The activity plan identifies specific levels of physical activity for a person based on his or her health condition, risk for falls, abilities, and fitness with strategies for increasing activity gradually over time.

Yoga or Tai Chi for 1 hour could also be performed in place of the combined strengthening and balance recommendations (items 2 and 3 above). Yoga can provide many benefits to patients with rheumatic disease, including pain relief, better flexibility, improved quality of life, and normalization of the adrenal circadian production.

How to Choose an Alternative Healthcare Provider

Finding an alternative medical provider can be challenging since training, experience, certification, and familiarity with therapies may vary considerably among practitioners. Here are some basic questions that can help patients to select an alternative practitioners.

Questions to ask of an alternative medical physician or provider:

1. Do you have a current license recognized by the ruling state/national agency or jurisdiction?
2. Did you graduate with a degree from a recognized institution?
3. Do you carry malpractice insurance? (This typically provides an additional level of verification of professional credentials.)
4. Are you a member in good standing with your professional organization? Does your organization have a process of

self-regulation and ethical codes that would warrant removal if not adhered to?
5. Are the office and the practitioner's manner professional?
6. Do you provide diagnoses, treatment plans, and reasonable expectation of results and side effects?
7. Do you keep accurate records and are you willing to share them with other providers?
8. Are you willing to suggest second opinions to assess your care and judgment of my health condition?

It is not easy to choose a new healthcare provider, traditional or alternative. Therefore, a careful medical consumer should obtain advice from multiple trusted sources (current medical providers, family, friends, and certifying organizations) to make the best possible decisions.

Summing Up

Complementary and alternative medicine therapies provide additional options for Sjögren's patients that can be added to conventional treatments. Anti-inflammatory diets and dietary supplementation with vitamin D, omega-3 fatty acids, other nutrients, probiotics, and botanicals all help enhance the body's own natural healing process. Regular exercise to improve conditioning and strength not only alleviates fatigue but also provides numerous other health benefits.

FOR FURTHER READING

Ames BN, et al. High-dose vitamin therapy stimulates variant enzymes with decreased coenzyme binding affinity (increased Km): relevance to genetic disease and polymorphisms. *Am J Clin Nutrition.* 2002; 75: 616–58.

Black JK. *The Anti-Inflammation Diet and Recipe Book.* Alameda, CA: Hunter House Publishers, 2006.

Bosch P, Traustadottir T, Howard P, Matt K. Functional and physiological effects of yoga in women with rheumatoid arthritis: a pilot study. *Alternative Therapies.* 2009; 15(4): 24–31.

Deluca HF, Cantorna MT. Vitamin D: its role and uses in immunology. *FASEB J.* 2001; 15(4): 2579–85.

Fairfield K, Fletcher R. Vitamins for chronic disease in adults: scientific review. *JAMA.* 2002; 287(23): 3116–26.

Metsios GS, et al. Rheumatoid arthritis, cardiovascular disease and physical exercise: a systematic review. *Rheumatology.* 2008; 47(3): 239–48.

Strömbeck B, Ekdahl C, Manthorpe R, Jacobsson LT. Physical capacity in women with primary Sjögren's syndrome: a controlled study. *Arthritis Rheum.* 2003; 49(5): 681–8.

Strömbeck BE, Theander E, Jacobsson LTH. Effects of exercise on aerobic capacity and fatigue in women with primary Sjögren's syndrome. *Rheumatology.* 2007; 46(5): 868–71.

Vasquez A. Reducing pain and inflammation naturally. Part 4: Nutritional and botanical inhibition of NF-kappaB, the major intracellular amplifier of the inflammatory cascade. *Nutritional Perspectives Journal of the Council on Nutrition of the American Chiropractic Association*, July 2005.

Vasquez A. Reducing pain and inflammation naturally. Part 7: Rheumatoid arthritis as a prototypic pattern of inflammation. *Nutritional Perspectives Journal of the Council on Nutrition of the American Chiropractic Association*, July 2009.

28

Vitamin D and Sjögren's Syndrome
Jeffrey Wilson, MD

Background: Something Old

Until recently vitamin D deficiency has been associated primarily with metabolic bone problems. Severe deficiency indicated rickets in children and osteomalacia in adults. With the introduction of bisphosphonate treatment for osteoporosis there was renewed interest in the role of vitamin D as part of the therapeutic regimen. The accepted normal range for 25-hydroxyvitamin D levels was 8 to 50 ng/mL. This old standard accounted for an underestimation of vitamin D deficiency and insufficiency and was replaced in 2007 with the new normal range of 32 to 100 ng/mL.

With respect to Sjögren's syndrome, as recently as 2005 (third edition of the *Sjögren's Syndrome Handbook*), vitamin D was mentioned only in its role of treating osteoporosis, with special consideration for the patient on corticosteroids or the patient with conditions predisposing to osteoporosis or vitamin D deficiency (such as the autoimmune liver disease primary biliary cirrhosis). For the Sjögren's patient, as with our general patient population, vitamin D is increasingly important.

Something New

In 2003, an article was published in the *Mayo Clinic Proceedings* relating low vitamin D levels with persistent, nonspecific musculoskeletal pain. It stimulated an interest in checking vitamin D levels in all the patients in our clinic. The findings were in line with subsequent review articles by Michael Holick in *Mayo Clinic Proceedings* (March 2006) and later in the *New England Journal of Medicine* (July 2007). Vitamin D deficiency was common, affecting over 70% of the patient population, including our Sjögren's patients.

The reviews and subsequent investigations relate a wide array of diseases associated with vitamin D deficiency, including many forms of cancer, cardiovascular disease, multiple sclerosis, type 1 diabetes, psoriasis, and autoimmune disorders such lupus and rheumatoid arthritis. How can vitamin D be related to so many varied illnesses? Some researchers feel it should be considered a hormone rather than a vitamin. "Vitamin" is derived from "vital amine" and implies something from exogenous sources; it is not manufactured by our bodies. This is clearly different for vitamin D, which is produced by the skin in response to sun exposure. The discovery that most cells and tissues have vitamin D receptors and an enzyme for converting to active vitamin D suggests that the biological functions of vitamin D extend far beyond those of calcium homeostasis and bone health.

Diagnosis

The diagnosis is made by a blood test checking the 25-hydroxyvitamin D level (not the 1,25- level, which is of limited usefulness). While levels less than 32 ng/mL define vitamin D deficiency, it is less clear what constitutes insufficiency. What is a target goal of therapy? It should be no surprise after 50 years of considering deficiency to be less than 8 ng/mL that the optimal level is not yet clearly defined. A level of 50 to 60 ng/mL is currently the goal of our treatment. How do we achieve that?

Treatment

The treatment regimen includes a prescription for 50,000 IU vitamin D_2 (ergocalciferol) weekly, with 2,000 IU of over-the-counter vitamin D_3 (cholecalciferol) daily (including the day 50,000 IU is taken) for 8 to 12 weeks. A follow-up 25-hydroxyvitamin D level is checked at that time and adjustments are made in the regimen. The most common maintenance regimen is 50,000 IU vitamin D_2 every other week (we have our patients take it on the 1st and 15th day of each month to facilitate compliance) and 2,000 IU D_3 daily. Vitamin D levels are then checked every 6 months. Maintenance regimens, however, vary greatly. Most of our lupus patients have very low initial levels—often less than 7 ng/mL (with little difference according to race). They may end up taking 50,000 IU (D_2) every Monday and every Thursday, with 5000 IU (D_3) daily. On the other hand, an older osteoarthritis patient may need only 50,000 IU monthly or 5,000 IU daily. The only way to determine the proper regimen is with follow-up testing.

TOXICITY

With such widely varying treatment regimens, there is concern about possible vitamin D toxicity. However, this is extremely rare and relates to the effect of the vitamin D supplementation on the patient's serum calcium level. Researchers have suggested that daily vitamin D_2 doses of 50,000 IU for 3 months would be required to produce toxic levels. A 93-year-old nursing home patient was recently evaluated at the office taking that exact regimen due to incorrect admission orders. Her 25-hydroxyvitamin D level was 144 ng/mL, but her calcium level was normal and she had no signs or symptoms of hypercalcemia. In our practice, the finding of hypercalcemia is most often related to a developing cancer (usually breast or lung cancer) or hyperparathyroidism.

Patients on vitamin D supplementation almost universally notice that their hair, fingernails, and toenails grow faster, and their fingernails and toenails are stronger. There is often a subjective increase in strength and energy. Several patients have noted fewer seasonal allergy symptoms and fewer frequent cold and flu episodes. Long-term studies in the future will be required to determine if the hoped-for decreases in the incidence of associated cancers or cardiovascular events are realized.

Something Sjögren's

Are there special considerations regarding vitamin D supplementation and the Sjögren's patient beyond those on corticosteroids or rare patients with primary biliary cirrhosis?

Tina's story is instructive. This 56-year-old white woman had been followed since 1994 with a history of Sjögren's syndrome. 25-hydroxyvitamin D levels in 2003 (43 ng/mL) and 2004 (37 ng/mL) were normal. In November 2005 her level was less than 4 ng/mL. For over 25 years the patient had carried a diagnosis of irritable bowel syndrome. Subsequent testing included a tissue transglutaminase IgA level of more than 250 U (normal 0 to 30 U), and a small bowel biopsy confirmed the diagnosis of celiac disease. Her clinical symptoms of "irritable bowel syndrome" resolved with the usual dietary modifications for celiac disease. Her story reminds us that our patients are dynamic and vitamin D levels should be followed at least yearly. It also reminds us that most especially in our Sjögren's patients we need to remain vigilant for other autoimmune diseases developing, such as hypothyroidism, B_{12} deficiency, and celiac disease.

Antimalarial medicines such as hydroxychloroquine (Plaquenil) are a frequent part of the treatment regiment for Sjögren's patients. Vitamin D supplementation has allowed a reduction in the usual dose of Plaquenil from 200 mg twice a day to 200 mg once a day without worsening in sicca or other Sjögren's-related symptoms such as arthralgias or rash. This is not only beneficial economically but also decreases the potential for ocular toxicity.

The Future

An article in the June 2007 *Arthritis and Rheumatism* "Are We at a Stage to Predict Autoimmune Rheumatic Diseases?" raises some hopeful considerations for the future. The author writes: "The capability of prediction will be valuable only if preventive measures can be adopted. Knowledge is accumulating to recommend an avoidance of exposure to ultraviolet light, specific diet, avoidance of specific chemicals (silica, mercury, toxic oil and the like), use of specific contraceptives or vaccines, and, based on animal studies, administration of vitamin D." For the existing Sjögren's patient, beyond the general benefits of vitamin D, will supplementation prevent the development of other autoimmune disease manifestations such as B_{12} deficiency, Addison's disease, celiac disease, or hypothyroidism? With an appreciation of the familial tendency for these illnesses, perhaps there is a more intriguing question for the future: If other family members are vitamin D-deficient, will vitamin D supplementation help prevent Sjögren's or other autoimmune diseases from developing?

Summing Up

While there have been no well-designed studies of the role of vitamin D in Sjögren's, a large number of patients with lupus, scleroderma, and rheumatoid arthritis are vitamin D-deficient. Twenty percent to 30% of them have Sjögren's as well. Sjögren's patients should have 25-hydroxyvitamin D levels obtained, and if levels are low patients often benefit from replacement therapy. Low vitamin D levels are associated with musculoskeletal pain and more disease activity.

FOR FURTHER READING

Bizarro N, Tazzoli R, Shoenfeld Y, Are we at a stage to predict autoimmune rheumatic diseases? *Arthritis Rheum.* 2007; 56: 1736–44.
Holick MF, High prevalence of vitamin D inadequacy and implications for health. *Mayo Clin Proc.* 2006; 81: 353–73.
Holick MF, Vitamin D deficiency. *N Engl J Med.* 2007; 357: 266–81.
Plotnikoff GA, Quigley JM Prevalence of severe hypovitaminosis D in patients with persistent, nonspecific musculoskeletal pain. *Mayo Clin Proc.* 2003; 78: 1463–70.

29

Testing New Drugs and Future Directions
Young H. Lee, BA, E., William St. Clair, MD, and
Philip L. Cohen, MD

Sjögren's syndrome is an autoimmune disease characterized by chronic lymphocytic inflammation of exocrine glands, or glands that secrete products into ducts that lead to the external environment, notably the lacrimal and salivary glands. It is this chronic inflammation of the lacrimal and salivary glands that produces symptoms of dry eyes and dry mouth (also known as sicca symptoms), the hallmark of this disease. New therapies for Sjögren's are needed to curb the inflammatory response in these glandular tissues and restore tear and saliva flow.

Sjögren's occurs as either a primary or secondary condition. In primary Sjögren's the patient has no other known connective tissue diseases and develops sicca symptoms from an initial insult to the lacrimal and salivary glands. In secondary Sjögren's the patient has another autoimmune disease, such as rheumatoid arthritis (RA) or systemic lupus erythematosus (SLE), and subsequently develops sicca symptoms. Many patients with primary Sjögren's also develop extra-glandular disease that may affect the skin, joints, lung, kidney, nervous system, and blood vessels. These disease manifestations may cause more problems in some cases than the dry eyes and dry mouth. For example, some patients with primary Sjögren's may develop interstitial lung disease and suffer from shortness of breath that limits their physical activities. Other patients may experience rash, arthritis, vasculitis, or numbness in their feet from a peripheral neuropathy. It is expected that any new drugs developed for the treatment of primary Sjögren's would improve at least some of the extra-glandular manifestations of disease.

While currently available therapies for Sjögren's may improve some of its symptoms, they do not appear to modify the natural course and progression of this disease. Artificial tears, topical cyclosporine, and secretagogues, such as pilocarpine (Salagen) and cevimeline (Evoxac), have been shown in clinical studies to significantly reduce the symptoms of dry eyes and dry mouth. Treatment with hydroxychloroquine (Plaquenil) may be useful in combating the fatigue, rash, and joint pain of primary Sjögren's, although well-designed studies have not yet provided convincing evidence of this drug's beneficial effects for these indications. Current efforts are focused on the discovery of new drugs that can modify the disease process in primary Sjögren's and thereby reduce glandular damage and improve long-term outcomes. This future goal is analogous to the recent advances in the treatment of RA that have led to the approval of several new drugs that reduce joint inflammation and damage in this disease.

The chronic inflammation in primary Sjögren's is caused by immune cells called lymphocytes, including both B and T lymphocytes, and by secreted cytokines and chemokines (substances that regulate inflammation), which work together in concert to cause damage to the body's normal tissue. Thus, B and T lymphocytes, as well as certain chemokines and cytokines, have been considered to be attractive targets for therapy of Sjögren's. Many of these experimental approaches use drugs that are called biologics, so named because they are based on natural substances in the body. Our own natural antibodies, which help to fight off infections, form the blueprint for monoclonal antibodies—examples of which include rituximab (Rituxan) (anti-B cell) and infliximab (Remicade) (anti-cytokine), which are approved for the treatment of RA. The term "monoclonal" refers to the fact that it is a single antibody designed to uniquely recognize a specific target, such as a lymphocyte or cytokine. Monoclonal antibodies such as rituximab bind to the surface of a cell, often leading to its rapid elimination from the body. Other monoclonal antibodies, such as infliximab, recognize a cytokine, neutralizing its effects and cutting back the inflammatory response.

A host of studies has begun to explore the use of biologic treatments for Sjögren's. Neutralizing the effects of certain cytokines and chemokines may not only be a way to suppress tissue inflammation and destruction and inflammation, but these strategies may also be exploited to prevent the influx ("trafficking") of inflammatory cells into the sites of disease. In principle, therapies can be designed to block many different cytokines or their receptors, preventing B and T cells from participating in the inflammatory response. In this chapter, we will review these emerging therapies for primary Sjögren's and the way they may work to reduce inflammation and damage in this disease. Indeed, the outlook is bright for the future treatment of primary Sjögren's.

Targeting the B Cell

B cells play an active role in the inflammatory pathways involved in Sjögren's. They produce immunoglobulins, or antibodies; patients with Sjögren's commonly present with a polyclonal hypergammaglobulinemia as well as various associated autoantibodies, including rheumatoid factor (RF), anti-SSA (Ro), and anti-SSB (La) antibodies. Certain patients develop vasculitis, or blood vessel inflammation, due to deposition in blood vessel walls of immunoglobulin, especially of cryoglobulins, which develop in some individuals and which come from monoclonal B-cell populations. In this regard, monoclonal B-cell proliferation in salivary glands is seen in 20% to 30% of patients, and approximately 5% of patients develop malignant B-cell lymphomas. Due to the clear role of B cells in Sjögren's, they have been an inviting target for recent biological therapies.

B-Cell Depletion

Rituximab (Rituxan) is a chimeric mouse/human monoclonal antibody directed against CD20, a surface molecule specific to the B cell. Rituximab, originally developed for lymphoma therapy, works by profoundly depleting mature B cells of the body. Because of the prominent role of B cells in primary Sjögren's, several studies have examined the potential benefits and safety of rituximab therapy for this disease. In one study, the drug improved sicca symptoms, reduced swelling of the parotid glands, and decreased systemic symptoms, including those from joint pain and vasculitis. In another study, patients with Sjögren's experienced measurable increases in salivary secretions, recovery of some salivary gland function, and improvement in subjective sicca symptoms. Most recently, a randomized, double-blind, placebo-controlled study showed improvements in stimulated whole saliva flow rates, subjective ratings of fatigue and experience of sicca symptoms, and a reduction in RF levels following infusion with rituximab.

Rituximab has also shown efficacy in reversing some of the inflammatory effects of primary Sjögren's at the microscopic level in the tissues. In a small sample of five patients treated with rituximab, biopsies of the parotid gland showed a decrease in lymphocytic infiltration, largely a reduction of the number of B cells within the tissue, and a decrease in the number of germinal centers, which are centers where B cells mature and proliferate. These patients also showed a corresponding increase in parotid salivary flow rates and a decrease in the sodium concentration in the saliva, which indicates improved functioning of the cells within the parotid gland.

Adverse reactions from the use of rituximab in a variety of autoimmune diseases have ranged from minor infusion reactions (such as flushing, dyspnea, nausea, vomiting, blood pressure instability), to serum sickness, to the rare development of progressive multifocal leukoencephalopathy (PML), a lethal viral infection of the brain. Serum sickness is caused by the production of antibodies against rituximab, or human antichimeric antibodies (HACAs), and consists of fever, arthritis, arthralgia, myalgia, and purpuric skin lesions. Although rituximab has shown preliminary success in case studies and small clinical trials, larger studies are necessary to confirm its efficacy and safety for the treatment of primary Sjögren's.

Epratuzumab is also a human monoclonal antibody targeted against the B cell. It is directed against CD22, another B-cell surface molecule, and acts to reduce B-cell levels in the body modestly, but more importantly to reduce the state of activation of B cells. It has the theoretical advantage of being more readily reversible, as B-cell depletion is not the primary mechanism of action. The agent was tested in a study of 16 patients with primary Sjögren's, and approximately half to two thirds of the patients exhibited a clinical response to the treatment that included recovery of tear production and salivary flow as well as decreases in immunoglobulin G levels and the erythrocyte sedimentation rate (ESR), a marker of inflammation in the body. Patients also noted subjective reduction of fatigue. Adverse reactions possibly related to epratuzumab therapy were described in 10 of the patients, ranging from minor infusion reactions, headaches, and paresthesias to more severe reactions, including a transient ischemic attack with associated seizure in one patient, and an osteoporotic fracture in another. Further study of epratuzumab is needed to substantiate its efficacy and safety for the treatment of primary Sjögren's.

BAFF Inhibition

B-cell activating factor (BAFF), also known as B-lymphocyte stimulator (BLys), is a cytokine necessary for B-cell maturation and survival. BAFF levels are increased in the blood and salivary gland tissue of patients with primary Sjögren's. Blood levels of BAFF are correlated with levels of autoantibodies, including RF, anti-SSA, and anti-SSB, pointing to the possibility that BAFF stimulates the production of autoreactive B cells. Belimumab (Benlysta), a human monoclonal antibody directed against BAFF, has undergone trials in the treatment of SLE and was recently approved in the United States for this indication. Belimumab has demonstrated efficacy in reducing levels of peripheral B cells and, in one study, was able to show improvement in serologically active (ANA and/or anti-dsDNA positive) SLE patients. Belimumab is being tried in Sjögren's patients in two investigator-initiated clinical trials in Europe. It may prove to play a role in therapy for primary Sjögren's.

Targeting the T Cell

In primary Sjögren's, the chronic inflammatory infiltrates in salivary gland tissues contain abundant populations of T lymphocytes, which are among the earliest detectable cells in the natural course of this disease. T cells can stimulate the immune response and help B cells produce antibodies. Therefore,

T cells are considered to be attractive therapeutic targets in autoimmune disease, including primary Sjögren's.

Drugs Interfering with T-Cell Function

Alefacept (Amevive) is a monoclonal antibody that blocks the interaction between LFA-3 and CD2, which is necessary for the activation and proliferation of memory T cells. The net effect is depletion of CD4+ T cells. It has been used for the treatment of psoriasis and has been well tolerated thus far, with the advantage of having little association with opportunistic infection. Alefacept has not yet been tested in primary Sjögren's but may be evaluated for use in the future.

Abatacept (Orencia) is another agent that interrupts T-cell function. It blocks sites on the T cell that interact with B cells, dendritic cells, and other antigen-presenting cells, and in this way inhibits T-cell activation and production of pro-inflammatory cytokines and chemokines., Owing to the role of T cells in Sjögren's, abatacept may have some potential for its treatment. Controlled trials of abatacept in Sjögren's are needed to explore this question.

TNF-α Inhibition

Tumor necrosis factor alpha (TNF-α) is a pro-inflammatory cytokine. TNF-α and its receptors are increased in the salivary glands of patients with primary Sjögren's, forming the rationale for targeting this cytokine. There are five approved biological agents that target TNF-α: infliximab (Remicade), etanercept (Enbrel), adalimumab (Humira), golimumab (Simponi), and certilizumab (Cimzia).

In 2001, a pilot study using infliximab (Remicade) in primary Sjögren's patients found significant improvement in fatigue and both subjective and objective measurements of dry mouth and dry eyes in as little as 2 weeks. In a 1-year follow-up of these patients on a maintenance regimen, the improvement in fatigue, dry mouth, and dry eyes persisted, and symptoms completely resolved in a small minority of the study group. However, more recently, a larger randomized, placebo-controlled study failed to replicate these findings. Following treatment with infliximab, there was no statistically significant difference between placebo and treatment groups with regard to lacrimal and salivary gland function, pain, fatigue, laboratory values of ESR and C-reactive protein (CRP), and measurements of physical and mental health.

Etanercept (Enbrel) was first tested in an uncontrolled study of a group of 15 patients with primary Sjögren's and then subsequently examined in a

28-patient randomized, placebo-controlled trial. Neither study found etanercept to be efficacious for the treatment of Sjögren's. In the uncontrolled study, etanercept failed to improve sicca symptoms or objective measures of salivary or lacrimal gland function. In the randomized, placebo-controlled study, no difference in outcomes was detected between the treatment and control groups with regard to oral or ocular symptoms. The evidence to date indicates that TNF-α inhibitors are not effective for the treatment of primary Sjögren's.

Interferon Inhibition

Interferons are proteins with antiviral and immunomodulating properties. In 1993, the use of weekly intramuscular injections of interferon-alpha (IFN-α), a type I interferon, was first studied for the treatment of xerostomia (dry mouth) in primary Sjögren's. Initial studies suggested IFN-α might be a potential target for the treatment of this disease.

Patients with primary Sjögren's have been shown to exhibit increased IFN-related gene activation in salivary glands and peripheral blood. In a recent study, labial salivary gland biopsy specimens, plasma, and peripheral blood cells from patients with primary Sjögren's were examined for IFN-α–positive cells, IFN-α levels, and IFN-α gene mRNA levels, respectively. Of the 37 patients, 27 (60%) had detectable IFN-α–positive cells in the labial salivary gland biopsies, compared to 3 of 24 control specimens, and the levels of IFN-α were also higher in patient cells. Patients also had higher concentrations of IFN-α in plasma than control groups, and IFN-α mRNA levels in peripheral blood cells were upregulated in patients with primary Sjögren's.

It has been hypothesized that the production of interferons may play an important role in the autoimmune destruction of glandular cells. Therefore, agents that inhibit interferons have been considered for the treatment of primary Sjögren's and other autoimmune processes, particularly SLE.

Gene Therapy

Gene therapy is an area of scientific development that has the potential for a more permanent solution for the treatment of many diseases. More traditional treatments, including medications and biological agents, require frequent dosing to maintain drug levels in order to exert their therapeutic effects. Gene therapy has been tested only in animal models of Sjögren's thus far. However, many technical problems remain to be solved before gene therapy becomes widely used for the treatment of human autoimmune disease. Nevertheless, the results in animal models provide proof-of-concept that gene therapy may ameliorate an immune-mediated, chronic inflammatory response (Table 29–1).

Female, nonobese diabetic (NOD) mice develop spontaneous auto-immune sialadenitis resulting in loss of salivary flow. In the laboratory, they are widely used as a model of Sjögren's. Interleukin-10 (IL-10) is a cytokine with known immunosuppressive effects; it is a potent inhibitor of other pro-inflammatory cytokines. In one experiment, the human IL-10 gene was delivered to the submandibular glands in a group of NOD mice via a viral vector. When compared to controls, these mice, whether they were treated before or after the onset of sialadenitis, demonstrated increased salivary flow rates. Biopsies of the submandibular glands also showed significant reduction in inflammatory infiltrates.

In a similar study, the submandibular glands of NOD mice were treated with the vasoactive intestinal peptide (VIP) gene through viral vectors before the onset of sialadenitis. VIP is a hormone with anti-inflammatory functions. When compared to control mice, the treatment group maintained higher salivary flow rates and lower levels of several pro-inflammatory cytokines in submandibular gland extracts. Serum levels of these cytokines were not affected, and lymphocytic infiltrates into the glands remained elevated. It appears that VIP may have a rationale as a possible treatment for Sjögren's in the future.

The efficacy of gene transfer has also been examined in the lacrimal glands. In a rabbit model, the induction of autoimmune dacryoadenitis, which stimulates the inflammatory destruction of lacrimal glands, may be regulated by cytokines. IL-10 and TNF inhibitors were introduced through viral vectors into lacrimal gland epithelial cells extracted from the affected rabbits to test for an anti-inflammatory effect. IL-10 tends to exert anti-inflammatory effects, while TNF operates as a pro-inflammatory substance that may trigger cell

TABLE 29–1

Innovative Therapies Germane to Sjogren's Syndrome

Agents that target T cells: abatacept (Orencia)

Agents that target B cells

B-cell depletors: rituximab (Rituxan) has had several positive Sjögren's trials; epratuzumab (UCB) (one positive Sjögren's trial)

BAFF inhibitors: belimumab (Benylsta, Human Genome Sciences) has been approved in the United States for the treatment of lupus and is being evaluated in two initial small trials for the treatment of Sjögren's

Other BAFF inhibitors under study: atacicept (Merck Serono), A-623 (Anthera), and Lilly 2127399

Agents that block interferon activation: ronalizumab (Roche Genentech), NNC0152 (Novo Nordisk), and Medi 545 (Medimmune/Astra Zeneca), AMG 811 (Amgen)—are in lupus clinical trials

Toleragens: Laquinomod (TEVA), Rigerimod (Cephalon) are in lupus clinical trials

Cytokine antagonists inhibitors to IL-6 (tociluzumab, Actemra, Roche) on the market for RA, being studied for lupus and CNTO 311 (Centocor)

---

death and gland destruction. In the cells treated with IL-10 and TNF-inhibitor genes, lymphocyte proliferation was significantly less than in control cultures. Although these preliminary experiments in cultured cells are promising, further studies will be necessary in animal models before considering if this approach might be applicable for the treatment of human disease.

Summing Up

The development of therapies for Sjögren's trails far behind RA, another debilitating rheumatic disease. Unlike treatments for RA, disease-modifying agents have not yet been developed for the treatment of primary Sjögren's. Only recently have newer drugs used for other rheumatologic diseases undergone testing in patients with primary Sjögren's. Researchers have become increasingly aware of the complications that come with Sjögren's, and both investigators and pharmaceutical companies have begun to study the efficacies of newer agents for the treatment of Sjögren's.

Of the biological therapies discussed here, B-cell–targeted agents have demonstrated the most promise thus far. As biological agents are tested for the use in various other rheumatic diseases, their application to Sjögren's will become much clearer. Much of the work in biological agents for the treatment of Sjögren's is still preliminary, and therapies directed at T cells, cytokines, and other inflammatory mediators will most likely be studied further and refined in the years to come.

FOR FURTHER READING

Båve U, Nordmark G, Lövgren T, et al. Activation of the type I interferon system in primary Sjögren's syndrome: a possible etiopathogenic mechanism. *Arthritis Rheum.* 2005; 52: 1185–95.

Boren EJ, Cheema GS, Naguwa SM, et al. The emergence of progressive multifocal leukoencephalopathy (PML) in rheumatic diseases. *J Autoimmun.* 2008; 30: 90–98.

Calabrese LH, Molloy ES. Progressive multifocal leucoencephalopathy in the rheumatic diseases: assessing the risks of biological immunosuppressive therapies. *Ann Rheum Dis.* 2008; 67(Suppl 3): iii: 64–65.

Carson KR, Focosi D, Major EO, et al. Monoclonal antibody-associated progressive multifocal leucoencephalopathy in patients treated with rituximab, natalizumab, and efalizumab: a review from the Research on Adverse Drug Events and Reports (RADAR) Project. *Lancet Oncol.* 2009; 10: 816–24.

Devauchelle-Pensec V, Pennec Y, Morvan J, et al. Improvement of Sjögren's syndrome after two infusions of rituximab (anti-CD20). *Arthritis Rheum.* 2007; 57: 310–317.

Furie R, Stohl W, Ginzler EM, et al.; Belimumab Study Group. Biologic activity and safety of belimumab, a neutralizing anti-B-lymphocyte stimulator (BLyS) monoclonal antibody: a phase I trial in patients with systemic lupus erythematosus. *Arthritis Res Ther.* 2008; 10: R109.

Gottenberg JE, Guillevin L, Lambotte O, et al.; Club Rheumatismes, Inflammation (CRI). Tolerance and short-term efficacy of rituximab in 43 patients with systemic auto-immune diseases. *Ann Rheum Dis.* 2005; 64: 913–20.

Groom J, Kalled SL, Cutler AH, et al. Association of BAFF/BLyS overexpression and altered B cell differentiation with Sjögren's syndrome. *J Clin Invest.* 2002; 109: 59–68.

Hansen A, Lipsky PE, Domer T. Immunopathogenesis of primary Sjögren's syndrome: implications for disease management and therapy. *Curr Opin Rheumatol.* 2005; 17: 558–65.

Katsifis GE, Moutsopoulos NM, Wahl SM. T lymphocytes in Sjögren's syndrome: contributors to and regulators of pathophysiology. *Clin Rev Allergy Immunol.* 2007; 32: 252–64.

Kok MR, Yamano S, Lodde BM, et al. Local adeno-associated virus-mediated interleukin 10 gene transfer has disease-modifying effects in a murine model of Sjögren's syndrome. *Hum Gene Ther.* 2003; 14: 1605–18.

Koski H, Janin A, Humphreys-Beher MG, et al. Tumor necrosis factor-alpha and receptors for it in labial salivary glands in Sjögren's syndrome. *Clin Exp Rheumatol.* 2001; 19: 131–7.

Lodde BM, Mineshiba F, Wang J, et al. Effect of human vasoactive intestinal peptide gene transfer in a murine model of Sjögren's syndrome. *Ann Rheum Dis.* 2006; 65: 195–200.

Mariette X, Ravaud P, Steinfeld S, et al. Inefficacy of infliximab in primary Sjögren's syndrome: results of the randomized, controlled Trial of Remicade in Primary Sjögren's Syndrome (TRIPSS). *Arthritis Rheum.* 2004; 50: 1270–6.

Mariette X, Roux S, Zhang J, et al. The level of BLyS (BAFF) correlates with the titre of autoantibodies in human Sjögren's syndrome. *Ann Rheum Dis.* 2003; 62: 168–71.

Masaki Y, Susumu S. Lymphoproliferative disorders in Sjögren's syndrome. *Autoimmun Rev.* 2004; 3: 175–82.

Meijer J, Meiners P, Vissink A, et al. Effective rituximab treatment in primary Sjögren's syndrome: A randomised, double-blind, placebo-controlled trial. *Arthritis Rheum.* 2010; 62: 960–68.

Merrill JT, Neuwelt CM, Wallace DJ, et al. Efficacy and safety of rituximab in moderately-to-severely active systemic lupus erythematosus: the randomized, double-blind, phase II/III systemic lupus erythematosus evaluation of rituximab trial. *Arthritis Rheum.* 2010; 62: 222–33.

Pijpe J, Meijer JM, Bootsma H, et al. Clinical and histologic evidence of salivary gland restoration supports the efficacy of rituximab treatment in Sjögren's syndrome. *Arthritis Rheum.* 2009; 60: 3251–56.

Pijpe J, van Imhoff GW, Spijkervet FK, et al. Rituximab treatment in patients with primary Sjögren's syndrome: an open-label phase II study. *Arthritis Rheum.* 2005; 52: 2740–50.

Ramos-Casals M, Brito-Zeron P. Emerging biologic therapies in primary Sjögren's syndrome. *Rheumatology.* 2007; 46: 1389–96.

Sankar V, Brennan MT, Kok MR, et al. Etanercept in Sjögren's syndrome: a twelve-week randomized, double-blind, placebo-controlled pilot clinical trial. *Arthritis Rheum.* 2004; 50: 2240–5.

Schiemann B, Gommerman JL, Vora K, et al. An essential role for BAFF in the normal development of B cells through a BCMA-independent pathway. *Science.* 2001; 293: 2111–4.

Seror R, Sordet C, Guillevin L, et al. Tolerance and efficacy of rituximab and changes in serum B cell biomarkers in patients with systemic complications of primary Sjögren's syndrome. *Ann Rheum Dis.* 2007; 66: 351–57.

Shiozawa S, Morimoto I, Tanaka Y, Shiozawa K. A preliminary study on the interferon-alpha treatment for xerostomia of Sjögren's syndrome. *Br J Rheumatol.* 1993; 32: 52–4.

Steinfeld SD, Demols P, Appelboom T. Infliximab in primary Sjögren's syndrome: one-year followup. *Arthritis Rheum.* 2002; 46: 3301–3.

Steinfeld SD, Demols P, Salmon I, et al. Infliximab in patients with primary Sjögren's syndrome: a pilot study. *Arthritis Rheum.* 2001; 44: 2371–5.

Steinfeld SD, Tant L, Burmester GR, et al. Epratuzumab (humanised anti-CD22 antibody) in primary Sjögren's syndrome: an open-label phase I/II study. *Arthritis Res Ther.* 2006; 8: R129.

Vitali C, Bombardieri S, Jonsson R, et al., the European Study Group on Classification for Sjögren's Syndrome. Classification criteria for Sjögren's syndrome: a revised version of the European criteria proposed by the American-European Consensus Group. *Ann Rheum Dis.* 2002; 61: 554–58.

Voulgarelis M, Dafni UG, Isenberg DA, Moutsopoulos HM. Malignant lymphoma in primary Sjögren's syndrome: a multicenter, retrospective, clinical study by the European concerted action on Sjögren's syndrome. *Arthritis Rheum.* 1999; 42: 1765–72.

Wallace DJ, Stohl W, Furie RA, et al. A phase II, randomized, double-blind, placebo-controlled, dose-ranging study of belimumab in patients with active systemic lupus erythematosus. *Arthritis Rheum.* 2009; 61: 1168–78.

Zandbelt MM, de Wilde P, van Damme P, et al. Etanercept in the treatment of patients with primary Sjögren's syndrome: a pilot study. *J Rheumatol,* 2004; 31: 96–101.

Zheng L, Zhang Z, Yu C, et al. Association between IFN-alpha and primary Sjögren's syndrome. *Oral Surg Oral Med Oral Pathol Oral Radiol Endod.* 2009; 107: e12–8.

Zhu Z, Stevenson D, Ritter T, et al. Expression of IL-10 and TNF-inhibitor genes in lacrimal gland epithelial cells suppresses their ability to activate lymphocytes. *Cornea.* 2002; 21: 210–4.

PART FIVE

LIVING WITH SJÖGREN'S

30

Quality of Life and Sjögren's

Barbara M. Segal, MD

Why Study Health-Related Quality of Life?

Research designed to measure health-related quality of life has provided new understanding of what living with Sjögren's syndrome means to patients and their families. New drugs are in the pipeline for Sjögren's, so it is more important than ever to have a comprehensive picture of the effect of Sjögren's on health status. A description of the effect that a new treatment has on disease activity or progression is incomplete without an evaluation of the effect treatment might have on symptoms such as fatigue and pain that diminish a person's ability to function. Demonstration of a significant improvement in quality of life is now an important outcome measure for any new therapy.

How Quality-of-Life Research is Done

The first large community-based survey to provide a comprehensive description of health status and the impact of primary Sjögren's syndrome was conducted in 2007. Sjögren's patients who were members of the Sjögren's Syndrome Foundation and healthy controls were recruited by mail, and primary Sjögren's patients in eight rheumatology practices across the United States also were invited to participate. Survey respondents were asked to fill out extensive questionnaires about their medical history, types of health problems, and complications from Sjögren's.

Quality-of-life data also have been collected by investigators in Europe who used similar carefully designed questionnaires to assess the impact of disease on all aspects of functioning. The Medical Outcomes Survey Short Form-36 (SF-36) is a widely used measure of health-related quality of life designed for use in population surveys. Population norms are available for demographic subsets by age and gender. Normative values have been established for healthy people using data from large population samples; these are then compared with patient data to assess the impact of disease.

SF-36 scale scores provide a means to measure the effects of illness on each of eight domains of health status: physical activity, usual role functioning, pain, general health, vitality, social activity, role functioning difficulties caused by emotional problems, and mental health. The domain scores can be used to derive two summary measures of health status: physical (PCS) and mental (MCS) summary measures. Used extensively in rheumatology, the SF-36 has been applied in studies of different conditions to assess relative health status, the effectiveness of interventions, and the validity of new disease-specific questionnaires. Sjögren's researchers also frequently use the Profile of Fatigue and Discomfort (PROFAD-SSI), which is based upon descriptors used by patients with primary Sjögren's (e.g., fatigue, joint and muscle pain, and cold hands). Important aspects are the physical (needing to rest, low stamina, weak muscles) and mental experience of fatigue (difficulty concentrating and poor memory). While the PROFAD-SSI is currently the best quality-of-life measure available for use in Sjögren's, a major effort to develop outcome measures for all aspects of Sjögren's, including activity levels, is being investigated and is an evolving process. Although previous studies have shown that health quality is reduced and the functional impact of Sjögren's is similar in European and American cohorts, relatively few data are available on the impact of Sjögren's in men.

What Has Been Learned About Sjögren's and Health-Related Quality of Life?

While awareness of Sjögren's has increased, the disease still is not widely recognized by the public or the medical profession. Complexities in establishing the diagnosis and a lack of awareness of the importance of early diagnosis have contributed to lengthy delays, typically between 5 to 7 years, before the diagnosis of Sjögren's is established. As many as 50% of Sjögren's patients remain undiagnosed. Low public recognition of the impact of the disease, along with the fact that healthcare providers often have the perception that Sjögren's is a relatively benign disorder, has contributed to under-appreciation of the healthcare burden associated with Sjögren's.

Essentially nothing was known regarding the economic cost, functional impairment, or impact on work productivity associated with Sjögren's. Available data on health status were difficult to interpret because of the small size of the disease groups studied. Unlike research in diabetes, cancer, and rheumatoid arthritis, which is well supported, primary Sjögren's has attracted relatively little government-sponsored research funding. To raise public awareness and physician perception of the seriousness of Sjögren's, major gaps in our knowledge of how Sjögren's affects health and quality of life needed to be filled in.

Fortunately, a dramatic increase has occurred in Sjögren's and quality-of-life research. Not only are the systemic features and complications related to sicca better understood, but progress in the past decade has led to increased awareness of the impact of primary Sjögren's on all aspects of life. The burden of illness associated with primary Sjögren's is substantial. Studies performed worldwide show that the health status profile of people with primary Sjögren's is remarkably consistent regardless of their country of origin. Sjögren's has been shown to affect both physical and mental well-being. Comprehensive data covering a wide range of health outcomes collected in large cohorts with well-validated questionnaires demonstrate that the impact of Sjögren's is similar to that of other serious autoimmune disorders. In persons with primary Sjögren's, reduction in general health and physical and mental well-being is similar to that reported by persons with systemic lupus erythematosus (SLE) and active rheumatoid arthritis (RA). In one study carried out in the United Kingdom, primary Sjögren's patients and SLE patients rated the severity of their physical fatigue and cognitive symptoms at a comparable level but reported slightly less physical fatigue on average than patients with RA.

Oral and ocular sicca symptoms, fatigue, and pain each contribute to reduced quality of life in primary Sjögren's. Not surprisingly, patients with the most severe sicca symptoms report the greatest impact on all activities of daily life: physical activity, daily activities, social interactions, mental alertness, sexual relations, career productivity, and choice of occupation. Interestingly, in a large survey of patients with RA, non-inflammatory rheumatic disease, and fibromyalgia, the prevalence of sicca symptoms was increased in all three patient groups, and the likelihood of self-reported sicca symptoms was related to illness severity, therapy, and psychological distress. Extra-glandular features of primary Sjögren's, especially lung involvement, also contribute to poor quality of life.

The social and economic cost of primary Sjögren's to the patient and society is high. Visits to specialists, medication use, costs of dental care, and increased rates of hospitalization contribute to a significant increase in healthcare costs for patients with Sjögren's. Direct healthcare costs are more than doubled in patients with primary Sjögren's. A significant increase in work disability also has been documented in Sjögren's patients in the United States as well as in European countries. Most importantly, research on health-related quality of life has demonstrated the large unmet health needs of people with Sjögren's.

Summary of Quality-of-Life Research

The conclusions reached in more than 15 different studies of primary Sjögren's health-related quality of life in the past 20 years are strikingly in agreement.

These studies have shown, first, that Sjögren's has a global impact on health status affecting all aspects of life. Second, the prevalence of persistent abnormal fatigue is about 70% in primary Sjögren's. Fatigue and pain that arises from nerve damage, fibromyalgia, and joint inflammation are major contributors to poor physical well-being. Depression, which contributes to but accounts for less than half of the fatigue, is present in about one third of primary Sjögren's patients and is a major factor associated with reduced emotional well-being. Sicca symptoms reduce physical well-being, and social functioning is particularly affected in women with vaginal dryness. Third, the impact of primary Sjögren's on functional status is similar across disease groups in multiple countries and therefore is not culturally dependent.

One of the most complex factors contributing to diminished health quality is the coexistence of fibromyalgia and primary Sjögren's. For reasons that are not well understood, fibromyalgia often accompanies systemic autoimmune disease. Chronic widespread pain suggestive of fibromyalgia is reported in about 22% of Sjogren's patients, suggesting that allodynia and hyperalgesia, two manifestations of fibromyalgia pain that are also characteristics of neuropathic pain, may be important sources of discomfort in Sjögren's. Pain related to nerve damage and the pain of fibromyalgia are similar in that both types of pain are associated with central mechanisms and abnormal pain processing. The fact that primary Sjögren's and fibromyalgia can coexist causes difficulties in reaching a correct diagnosis and makes treatment more challenging. When patients who have fibromyalgia but do not have a diagnosis of autoimmune disease are compared to autoimmune patient groups with no fibromyalgia, the most severe reduction in quality of life is consistently related to the presence of fibromyalgia.

Fibromyalgia patients suffer frequently from anxiety, depression, and poor sleep, symptoms commonly associated with chronic pain. Sicca symptoms in fibromyalgia are also common and stem from medications used to treat pain, mood disorder, or sleep disturbance, and possibly from poorly understood neurological problems. Most fibromyalgia patients also have fatigue, so the overlap with primary Sjögren's is substantial. Fibromyalgia is believed to be associated with abnormal processing of pain signals. Pain that is not attributable to inflammation in joints or muscles is sometimes referred to as non-nociceptive pain (meaning pain not related to activation of peripheral pain receptors), which is found in about 10% to 20% of primary Sjögren's patients. A similar syndrome characterized by the presence of chronic widespread pain accompanies lupus in about 20% of patients.

The explanation for the high prevalence of fatigue and pain in Sjögren's is complex. Poor sleep quality is an important problem contributing to fatigue. Muscle pain associated with deconditioning contributes to fatigue, as does depressed mood. In patients with Sjögren's, pain can arise from nerve damage or dysfunction of nerve fibers in skin, mucosal surfaces, or cranial nerves.

Rarely, the inflammatory process involves the nerve cell body in the spinal cord, known as the dorsal root ganglion, which receives sensory input from pain fibers. Joint pain arises from inflammation of the joint lining, although interestingly there also may be an increase in osteoarthritis of large joints in primary Sjögren's. To effectively manage fatigue and improve sleep quality, pain, and especially chronic pain, must be appropriately diagnosed and effectively treated.

How Can Treatment Improve Quality of Life in Sjögren's?

In most autoimmune disorders, including primary Sjögren's, exercise has been shown to have beneficial effects on fatigue. Numerous studies also have demonstrated the association of fatigue with low mood and pain as well as the association of fatigue with pessimistic beliefs and negative feelings and beliefs about one's ability to control symptoms. Interventions designed to improve mood and coping skills can also be useful. New medications for sleep and pain that are being tested for conditions such as fibromyalgia also might be applicable to Sjögren's.

While topical therapies to protect and lubricate the ocular surface and oral cavity and medications that stimulate secretion will continue to have an important role in the treatment of primary Sjögren's, immune-modulating drugs for Sjögren's with the potential to slow or reduce damage to glands and organs are likely to be increasingly important in the management of the disorder. Drugs that target antibody-producing cells directly appear especially promising for Sjögren's. Disease-modifying therapy that promises to reduce fatigue, possibly improve sicca severity, and reduce damage to the lung and kidney likely will become available in the near future.

Summing Up

A focus on health-related quality of life in Sjögren's has been long overdue but is finally gaining attention and momentum. Recent studies demonstrate that the burden of illness in Sjögren's is significant and equates with quality-of-life studies of patients with SLE and RA. Sjögren's affects patients' daily physical, social, and mental activities and has social and economic repercussions for all societies at large.

FOR FURTHER READING

Bennett RM. Fibromyalgia: the commonest cause of widespread pain. *Compr Ther.* 1995; 21: 69–75.

Bowman SJ, Booth DA, Platts RG, UK Sjögren's Interest Group. Measurement of fatigue and discomfort in primary Sjögren's syndrome using a new questionnaire tool. *Rheumatology.* 2004; 43: 758–64.

Goodchild CE, Treharne GJ, Booth DA, Bowman SJ. Daytime patterning of fatigue and its associations with the previous night's discomfort and poor sleep among women with primary Sjögren's syndrome or rheumatoid arthritis. *Musculoskeletal Care.* 2010; 8(2): 107–17.

Karlson EW, Liang MH, Eaton H, et al. A randomized clinical trial of a psychoeducational intervention to improve outcomes in systemic lupus erythematosus. *Arthritis Rheum.* 2004; 50: 1832–41.

Meijer JM, Meiners PM, Huddleston Slater JJ, et al. Health-related quality of life, employment and disability in patients with Sjögren's syndrome. *Rheumatology (Oxford).* 2009; 48(9): 1077–82.

Ng WF, Bowman S. Primary Sjögren's syndrome: too dry and too tired. *Rheumatology (Oxford).* 2010; 49: 844–53.

Rhodus NL, Fricton J, Carlson P, Messner R. Oral symptoms associated with fibromyalgia. *J Rheumatol.* 2003; 30: 1841–5.

Segal B, Bowman SJ, Fox PC, et al. Primary Sjögren's syndrome: health experiences and predictors of health quality among patients in the United States. *Health & Quality of Life Outcomes.* 2009; 7: 46.

Segal B, Thomas W, Rogers T, et al. Prevalence, severity, and predictors of fatigue in subjects with primary Sjögren's syndrome. *Arthritis Rheum.* 2008; 59: 1780–7.

Strombeck BE, Theander E, Jacobsson LT. Effects of exercise on aerobic capacity and fatigue in women with primary Sjögren's syndrome. *Rheumatology (Oxford).* 2007; 46: 868–71.

Wolfe F, Michaud K. Predicting depression in rheumatoid arthritis: the signal importance of pain extent and fatigue, and comorbidity. *Arthritis Rheum (Arthritis Care and Research).* 2009; 61: 667–73.

Wolfe F, Michaud K. Prevalence, risk, and risk factors for oral and ocular dryness with particular emphasis on rheumatoid arthritis. *J Rheumatol.* 2008; 35: 1023–30.

31

Lifestyle Issues—Emotional

Teri P. Rumpf, PhD, and

Lynn C. Epstein, MD, DLFAPA, FAACAP

Chronic: Of diseases, etc.: Lasting a long time, long-continued, lingering, inveterate; opposed to *acute*. (*Oxford English Dictionary* online, 2010)

Until you have one, living with a chronic disease is difficult to imagine. Most episodes of illness are acute, intermittent, and of moderate duration. In contrast, the constant, habitual, and recurrent nature of a chronic illness is completely different. We are accustomed to thinking of ourselves as generally well, occasionally sick. Even after it arrives, a disease that never ends and has many different manifestations is not easy to comprehend or accept.

Chronicity: The Illness That Never Goes Away

Only with the passage of time does one begin to grasp the impact Sjögren's can have on every aspect of life. While there may be periods when patients feel well, or relatively well, this is a disease that requires adaptation and accommodation. There may be good days and bad, exacerbations or periods of relative calm, but rarely a return to the consistency of living with good health. Patients learn that there are new limits to what they can do—only to have those limits change, and change again. Since fatigue is a frequent component of Sjögren's, people struggle to predict how they will feel at a given time on a given day, which makes planning anything difficult. Instead of multi-tasking and multiple activities, Sjögren's patients find it necessary to simplify and stay focused, to break things down into baby steps, and learn to pace themselves. Unlike an acute illness with dramatic and obvious manifestations, Sjögren's is invisible and unpredictable and sometimes other people do not even believe it is there. This, in turn, creates further obstacles for patients.

With time and experience, patients learn that there are choices to be made about how to live and learn to look for opportunities to make them. Given limited energy, the most important tasks must be given priority to maintain quality of life. Eventually, a "new normal" does develop—that is, a sense of how to live with the multiple accommodations the disease necessitates.

Uncertainty and Stress

A chronic illness generates uncertainty. Many questions arise: What do these symptoms mean for me? Is the diagnosis definitive? Is this it, or will the disease change and become something else, something even worse? Will I be able to work, take care of my children, and live my life as I have been living it? What will the future look like? Will others see me differently? How does the disease change the way I view myself? Does anyone believe me? Because people with Sjögren's often look much better than they feel, they find that most people do not understand the turmoil they are going through.

The stresses and uncertainty of a chronic illness evoke a variety of emotions: sadness, depression, anxiety, loss, demoralization, confusion, and the frustration of not being able to do things as before. The losses are real. It is natural to react to them. Constant immersion in the medical system is a stressor, even as it provides the hope of finding a treatment that will improve the state of one's health. The line between being able to cope and not cope is often quite thin and may revolve around a single experience that pushes someone too far—for instance, a doctor who does not believe the person's experience or a family member who is indifferent. How people react to stress is a function of both their life histories and personal circumstances, of who they are and what is going on in their lives. Everyone reacts differently.

Emotions occur on a continuum, from manageable to overwhelming, from sadness and loss to severe clinical depression. States of clinical anxiety and depression may be part of a biological response to a stressful reality or part of the disease itself. They may be fluctuating, transitory, or enduring. When necessary, medication can be helpful. Antidepressants may do double duty since they are often used in the treatment of chronic pain.

Many years of research on the stress response have documented a strong connection between the mind and body. The acute stress response, the "fight-or-flight response," mobilizes the individual for action through the release of hypothalamic, pituitary, and adrenal hormones, leading to a temporary increase in blood sugar, heart rate, respiration, and blood pressure as well as a temporary activation of the immune response. On the other hand, with chronic stress, these levels remain elevated, upsetting the endocrine balance, increasing the release of glucocorticoids, and challenging immune system functioning. In a similar fashion, chronic stress is associated with decreasing brain levels of norepinephrine and serotonin, affecting mood and feelings of well-being.

It is important not to lose sight of who you are and what matters to you. One respondent, when asked about her reactions to Sjögren's, answered eloquently: "The two major emotions that come to mind when I'm asked about what it's like to live with Sjögren's syndrome are frustration and a sense of loss, which tend to intertwine. There's the reality of continually needing to reinvent myself as I decline physically, but at the same time trying desperately to hold onto my former self. It seems like a constant struggle, and there are times when the urge to abandon those activities that I love but lack the energy for creeps into my brain. For now, it comes in spurts of moments or days, but the need to hold onto as much as I can eventually wins out over those urges. I feel like I'm living on the edge of a precipice, wondering what will be the next symptom to put me out of action.

"There have been many losses both large and small; the loss of a career, the inability to be physically active . . . the lack of energy to do things spontaneously, little everyday things that used to be taken for granted . . . Thankfully I am a resilient person and that is what keeps me going, keeps me trying to be active in the things that matter most to me. Each day is a compromise of what I'd like to do and what I can do. I have never been a quitter, always somehow managing to rethink my goals, adapt my lifestyle around the barriers that Sjögren's creates . . . I impatiently wait for better treatments and perhaps, eventually, a cure."

Acknowledging the need to assess the impact of illness and to prioritize goals can help an individual move forward. Without erasing the illness or the accommodations required, self-evaluation can clarify what's involved and can help identify strategies for amelioration. The importance of attitude is central to the process. It is vital to find pathways to prevent overwhelming circumstances from blocking motivation. Progress may be small and incremental, but it needs to be valued. Another respondent says that she keeps a running "to do" list and takes heart from noticing the completed items, although it may take days or even weeks for each entry. Having a degree of control helps her stay focused and keeps her from feeling completely overwhelmed.

Illness and Relationships

Biological changes affect relationships. It can be difficult for family and friends to understand why a patient can no longer function the way she used to. A person who is fatigued and unwell may not feel like going out, or it may take all her energy just to arrive at a planned activity, even before she begins to participate. It can also be difficult for friends and relatives to appreciate the disparity between the way a person looks and feels. Unlike more dramatic diseases or medical crises, with an invisible chronic illness, assistance and support may not be forthcoming because other people do not recognize the need for them.

By sharing with others the ongoing challenges of living with Sjögren's, patients can further insights and help set realistic goals. The impact of Sjögren's on children (and grandchildren) is significant because children, especially young children, do not always have the vocabulary to express what they see and feel. They may feel that the illness is their fault. While some may act out in response to changes at home, others may withdraw for fear of making things worse. It is possible for the same child to act in both ways at different times. Patients need to be aware of the impact of their disease on their children and grandchildren and give words to the situation, explaining as much as is appropriate given the ages of the children involved.

Other people's reactions can either help or hinder an individual's ability to cope with chronic illness. The extent of the disease may not matter as much as the level of support. In unpublished research with breast cancer patients, one of the authors found that patients who have at least one friend or family member with whom they could communicate freely were less depressed than those who lacked such a relationship. The impact of illness on relationships is described in a variety of books that we have listed in the resource section of this chapter. When friends and family don't know what to do or say, they often do or say nothing. Sometimes this is a form of denial; sometimes it is not knowing what the right thing to do might be. Patients can help by taking the lead, by explaining the impact of the disease as clearly as possible. This is an ongoing process, not a single discussion. Friends and family learn that emotional support is often more about "being there" for the person with chronic illness than it is about "doing" something.

In a marriage or partnership, the changes of chronic illness can destabilize longstanding relational patterns. A partner, spouse, or family member may be able to offer certain kinds of help but not others. He or she may offer to take on additional physical tasks, such as cleaning or cooking or doing the laundry, but may not be able to talk about what is happening. In other words, some people are able to offer support that is instrumental but not emotional. On the other hand, patients may need both kinds of support: assistance with day-to-day living (instrumental) as well as emotional. A wide support system fills in the gaps so that an individual is not totally dependent on a spouse or adult child or children. The more people available, the broader the support system, the more likely needs are to be met.

The Role of Doctors

A relationship with a medical professional is like any other—sometimes the personalities involved work well together and sometimes they do not.

The doctor–patient relationship is extremely powerful in its ability to heal or hurt. Without any other intervention, a relationship with a physician may heal because it allows the patient to share the burden of the illness. Although the medical status remains the same, a healing interaction allows the patient to feel unburdened and lighter, which in turn makes her feel more positive and hopeful.

Location and insurance may determine the medical professionals available, but if the relationship doesn't feel right, it is appropriate to seek another opinion and make a change. Patients with Sjögren's, like those with other chronic diseases, form long-term relationships with their doctors, and it is important that the relationship be one of trust and mutual understanding. The quality of communication between doctor and patient is critical, especially in the current, ever-more-pressured medical environment. Patients need to take responsibility for what they communicate to their physicians and understand how important it is to use their time together well. A medical encounter that goes well is healing; one that does not increases a patient's sense of disappointment and frustration.

Maximize a Sense of Well-Being

Although the challenges and unpredictability of living with Sjögren's can be daunting, there are effective strategies to maximize well-being. Acknowledging the need to assess the impact of illness and to prioritize goals can help patients move forward. What do you need to do? Where to begin and how to pace yourself are key variables. While feelings of loss are not inappropriate, it is important to try and take action to keep them from reaching clinical proportions of anxiety and depression. Especially in the context of limited energy and emotional resources, it is important to assess and consciously decide how best to use the resources available. You do what you can to live as normally as possible. An important caveat is to be reasonable and not to blame yourself for setbacks.

Chronic illness means dealing with a series of overlapping and fluctuating physical, emotional, and real-life challenges. A good place to begin is by looking at what is possible now, given the physical and emotional resources that you have. A three-step approach to coping begins with a self-assessment of how you feel, followed by taking stock of what you need to do, so that you can then actively choose how best to allocate limited energy. Rather than bemoaning the inability to do everything that you did in the past, it is constructive to prioritize options so that you do what matters most. Recognizing that some responsibilities aren't optional helps you determine how you need to proceed. To move forward, it is necessary to live in the real world as it is and make alternative arrangements when necessary to meet responsibilities. If something must be done that you are no longer able to do, it is key to acknowledge this fact and get assistance or break it down into smaller components that can be done. While some aspects of chronic illness are beyond control, others are subject to how you address them. Chronic illness, by definition, will be with you for a long time. More of a marathon than a sprint, coping means doing what is possible and learning to break down complex tasks into more manageable components. Projects can be viewed as puzzles with many pieces to bring together before they can be completed.

Be Proactive: Find a New Normal

Living well in the present is facilitated by "controlling the controllable," setting priorities for how to live and what to get done. Depending on the circumstances and your preferences, this can vary from taking a nap, getting some exercise, reading a book, spending time with friends, or canceling stressful activities. Some people spread out doctors' appointments; others bunch them together and get them over with all at once. By consciously deciding how much to push, you can pace yourself and better address the responsibilities that you feel are most important. Skip feeling obliged to old priorities and labeling tasks with "should." Instead, consider the risk/benefit balance and the gain you get for the pain. An economic model of energy expenditure is appropriate in that you will have to budget yourself and focus on what matters most to you. How much to push yourself and in which arenas are choices best made consciously.

Assessment of your status and prioritizing your options are ongoing activities that are best modified according to your needs. What are your strengths at a given time? What are your vulnerabilities? What are the opportunities available to you? What are the challenges you face? Key aspects to success in these domains are to be proactive and consciously make choices from among competing options.

When you feel discouraged and overwhelmed, strive to make adjustments to reach a better place. Sharing your thoughts and feelings with friends and family can help to reduce distress and develop a plan to address challenges appropriately. What lifestyle changes do you need to make? If you have been employed, do you need to reduce your responsibilities, workload, and/or hours employed? Should you talk with your employer about working part-time or cutting back on responsibilities? Is an accommodation necessary or desirable? Is disability an option? Whatever you decide to do, actively considering your options becomes a point of reference for your self-assessment and a way of taking some control.

How can you navigate your way through your challenges and responsibilities? You can't do everything at once. However, by setting realistic goals, prioritizing the stepping stones, and making adjustments in the schedule as necessary, you can make progress and move in the right direction. Life goes on. You do what you can to take control and to provide outlets for stress. You pace yourself, consciously allocating time, energy, and focus to what matters most to you. As discussed elsewhere in this book, exercise, relaxation techniques, diet, and adequate sleep can help you maintain a constructive attitude and optimize functioning. Similarly, it can be energizing to pay attention to how the small steps you accomplish build into the larger tasks you need to do. An important goal is to find your "new normal," a point that may need to be adjusted many times with fluctuations in your status.

Life is a work in progress, and chronic illness influences practical matters related to how you function. By repeatedly assessing how you feel, managing your expectations, and choosing the best options, you can take control and help maximize your well-being.

Summing Up

If Sjögren's is complicated for the specialists who diagnose and treat it, imagine how complicated it can be for the patient. Having a chronic illness that is largely invisible to family, friends, and colleagues adds to the already difficult task of coping with physical symptoms and complications. Many strategies

---

Box 31–1
Takeaway Points

- **Chronic and invisible:** Sjögren's is a chronic, invisible illness that may vary in intensity and effect but never goes away.
- **The mismatch:** Patients with Sjögren's often look better than they feel. A mismatch occurs. Other people may not believe they are really sick.
- **Uncertainty:** A chronic illness generates stress and uncertainty. Patients do not know what will happen next and can't predict how they will feel.
- **Dealing with ongoing challenges:** Anxiety, confusion, frustration, and depression are all common concomitant emotions. They may be mild, moderate, or severe. There may be a biological component and medication can be helpful.
- **Managing relationships and coping:** Biological changes can lead to changes in relationships with family and friends. Patients must learn to communicate what they are and are not able to do. They must likewise communicate this to their physicians.
- **Self-care:** Adaptation is difficult. Physicians can help validate the changes in patients' lives and encourage them to maximize a sense of well-being.
- **Prioritizing choices to move forward:** Patients need to prioritize goals and allocate the resources to attain them.
- **Finding the "new normal":** Eventually, a new normal develops for most people. However, even after it does, the parameters shift with the disease.
- **Bottom line:** Sjögren's is more of a marathon than a sprint. It is also an uninvited guest that must be accommodated.

---

exist that can help patients cope with the cascading emotions, stress, and physical repercussions that result from such a disease and affect relationships and daily functioning (Box 31–1).

FOR FURTHER READING

Burns DD. *Feeling Good: The New Mood Therapy*. Avon Books, 1980.

Brill A, Lockshin MD. *Dancing at the River's Edge: A Patient and Her Doctor Negotiate Life with Chronic Illness*. Tucson, AZ: Schaffner Press, 2009.

Charmatz K, Paterniti D, eds. *Health, Illness and Healing: Society, Social Context and Self.* Los Angeles: Roxbury Publishing Company, 1999.

Cousins N. *Anatomy of An Illness*. New York: Basic Books, 1979.

Cousins N. *Head First: The Biology of Hope*. New York: E.P. Dutton, 1989.

Frank A. *At The Will of the Body: Reflections on Illness*. New York: First Mariner Books Edition, Houghton Mifflin, 2002.

Groopman J. *The Anatomy of Hope: How People Prevail in the Face of Illness*. New York: Random House, 2004.

Hafen B, Karren K, Frandsen K, Smith N L. *Mind/Body Health*. Boston: Allyn and Bacon, 1996.

Halpern S. *The Etiquette of Illness: What to Say When You Can't Find the Words*. New York and London: Bloomsbury, 2004.

Kleinman A. *The Illness Narratives*. New York: Basic Books, 1988.

Lown B. *The Lost Art of Healing*. Boston: Houghton Mifflin, 1996.

Ornstein R, Sobel D. *Healthy Pleasures*. Reading, MA: Perseus Books, 1989.

Piburn G. *Beyond Chaos: One Man's Journey Alongside His Chronically Ill Wife*. Atlanta: Arthritis Foundation, 1999.

Rumpf T, Hammitt K. *The Sjögren's Syndrome Survival Guide*. Oakland, CA: New Harbinger Publications, 2003.

Sternberg EM. *The Balance Within: The Science Connecting Health and Human Emotions*. New York: WH Freeman and Company, 2001.

Wells SM. *A Delicate Balance: Living Successfully with Chronic Illness*. Cambridge, MA: Perseus Books, 2000.

32

Enhancing Resilience Through Mind/Body Interactions

Margaret Baim, MS, NP

It is easy to see why living with a chronic and unpredictable condition such as Sjögren's syndrome can be a stressful experience and can add to the stress of daily life that is unavoidable for everyone, healthy or not. Any perception of threat, either real or imagined, is a trigger for stress, and Sjögren's patients can face both. Stress can come from many sources for Sjögren's patients, whether from the biological inflammation that accompanies the disease or from constantly dealing with multiple symptoms and their repercussions (including a constant sensation of dryness, pain, fatigue, and sexual dysfunction) or from living with the fear of potential complications such as developing cancer or having a baby with heart block. Stress also is exacerbated by coping with lifestyle changes brought on by Sjögren's and expectations and reactions from family, friends, and colleagues.

Although stress leads to negative feelings such as worry, fear, sadness, and frustration, this unwelcome state of mind can prompt us to heal and develop greater resilience. In this chapter we explore how stress works within the body and review findings from the new science of mind/body medicine; you will learn how the development of certain attitudes and behaviors can offset stress, making the leap from unwelcome states of mind to a greater sense of well-being.

The Stress System

Resilience is defined as the body's ability to meet a demand, mount an appropriate response, and turn off that response when it is no longer needed. The body's vast network of communication designed to perform these functions is the stress system. For example, when your body needs energy, the brain releases signals leading to hunger and food-seeking behaviors. Once this need is satisfied, those signals are replaced by other signals that lead to feelings of satisfaction. Another example is the release of signals and responses needed to run and catch a bus: blood flow is diverted from the stomach to the arms and legs, heart rate and breathing rate increase, and once the bus is either caught or determined to be a lost cause, further signals return the body to its baseline state.

The control center of the stress system is the brain. Weighing a mere three pounds, the brain requires one third of our total daily caloric requirements to perform its extensive functioning. Just think: during waking hours the brain is a constant surveyor of the world around us. Every movement and sound must be interpreted as threat or non-threat. Internally, every thought, memory, exertion, and emotion alters its activity. Repeated activity has been shown to alter its structure over time; this property is termed "neural plasticity." One notable influence on the brain's activity and subsequent neural plasticity is psychological stress. For those coping with the daily challenges and unpredictable nature of Sjögren's, periods of stress are to be expected. However, recent findings show that long periods of psychological stress can lead to changes within the brain's neural pathways that can lead to *self-perpetuating* activation of the stress system. Just as pavement wears down where wheels hit the roadway, thinking the same thoughts and experiencing the same moods day after day can create a well-worn pattern in our brains. Living in a stressful state of mind caused by fear, anxiety, worry, and sadness can lead to deeply rooted neural pathways.

However, mood is just one way that stress steals our sense of well-being. Psychological stressors activate the stress system, beginning from brain responses and terminating in certain cells within our immune system. Stress induces these cells to work harder, and this overexertion leads to a series of toxic byproducts. Collectively, these byproducts impose a new type of stress on the body: *oxidative stress*. Too much oxidative stress is damaging because the mechanisms in place for our body to cope with these toxic byproducts are overtaxed. Among the consequences of unchecked oxidative stress is the production of pro-inflammatory proteins. These proteins, in turn, interfere with the production of hormones needed to stabilize mood and support feelings of well-being. The more we activate the stress system through psychological pathways, the more demand is placed on cells and the more wear and tear our bodies suffer. Ultimately too much wear and tear leads to imbalances, experienced as mood disturbances, physical symptoms, and exacerbation of preexisting conditions and disease states.

So what is the good news? You have the power to cope with stress, thereby reducing the burden on your stress system and offsetting the effects of oxidative stress. Just as it is physiologically supportive to eat a *balanced, antioxidant-rich diet*, to engage in routine *physical activity*, and to obtain *recuperative sleep*—all of which offset oxidative stress and work to restore balance within the stress system—*attitude and state of mind* also work to restore mind/body balance and support resilience.

Perception and Cognitive Reappraisal

The way we think matters. Years of study have demonstrated how our brains and bodies change between stressed and non-stressed states of mind. We all understand what it feels like to be stressed, but this awareness is only the tip of the iceberg: beneath it rests a host of physiological processes that also play a part in the stress response. Under the influence of stress, the lower regions of our brain are most active; this is referred to bottom-up control. In non-stressed states, in contrast, the upper regions of the brain associated with higher processing are most active; this is termed top-down control. Figure 32–1 shows the differences in activity between stressed and non-stressed brains. Greater activity in the upper, prefrontal regions is associated with enhanced executive function, regulation of emotions, and positive, adaptive perspectives.

As neurobiologist Robert Sapolsky outlines in his book *Why Zebras Don't Get Ulcers*, humans, unlike other animals, remember threats. This memory can be recalled to reactivate the stress system even when the threat is no longer present. Having this ability to remember is part of our advanced development,

Prefrontal regulation during alert, non-stress conditions

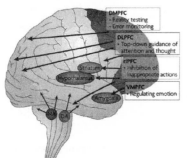

Dorsal Medial Pre Frontal Cortex (DMPFC)
- Reality testing
- Error monitoring

Dorsal Lateral PFC (DLPFC)
- Top-down guidance of attention and thought

Right Inferior PFC (RIPFC)
- Inhibits inappropriate motor actions

Ventral Medial PFC (VMPFC)
- Regulates emotion

Amygdala control during stress conditions

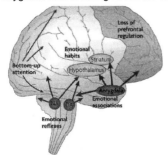

FIGURE 32–1 **From Arnsten AF.**
Stress signalling pathways that impair prefrontal cortex structure and function. *Nat Rev Neurosci.* 2009;10:410–422.

but it becomes a curse rather than a blessing if not used wisely. The perception of threats is a call to *adapt*; without adaptive coping, threats remain in memory to activate and sustain activation of the stress system long after the fact. Research on coping suggests that adaptive attitudes lead to a greater sense of well-being and longevity. Specifically, the deployment of problem-solving strategies, the acceptance of stressors beyond our control, and a general attitude of positivity correlate to feelings of well-being and longevity. Most recently, the role of these adaptive perspectives is understood to offset activation of the stress system because they lead to top-down control of the brain.

As John Milton said, "The mind is its own place and in itself, can make a Heaven of Hell, a Hell of Heaven." In cognitive theory, emotions correspond with a particular perception. For example, anger is felt in response to a perception of injustice, and sadness is felt in response to a perception of loss. Since these perceptions cause suffering and the wearing-and-tearing-down effects of oxidative stress, it is wise to see them as challenges for adaptation rather than succumbing to their grip. When a particular negative emotion is felt, we must learn to reflect on the underlying perception at work. Negative emotions focus on what we do not want, whereas adaptation works with what is. Choosing to adapt can provide an opportunity to redirect our perceptions toward those of greater service to us. Adaptive perspectives lead to positive emotions and behaviors such as compassion, wisdom, change, process, humor, gentleness, kindness, strength, patience, persistence, and influence. Positive and adaptive qualities turn off the stress system and restore top-down control of the brain. Hundreds of positive emotions and adaptive behaviors are available to counteract psychological and emotional suffering. As these perspectives and behaviors are applied to a stressful experience, the more adaptive and resilient one becomes. Over time, these perceptions and behaviors become embodied and effortless.

Three positive emotions often cited in studies on happiness and coping with chronic illness are *appreciation, positive expectation*, and *acceptance*. Each can be applied to most situations, and each originates from top-down control of the brain.

Appreciation

Two perspectives can lead to appreciation: valuing all you have, and understanding that a challenging situation could always be worse. Living in a state of appreciation can help buffer against stress. A useful practice is to begin and close each day with *appreciations*, or an accounting of the things one appreciates in life. To deepen this practice, focus on any memory of an appreciation until you relive the feeling. Generally it takes less than 30 seconds to relive an emotion evoked by a particular memory. Once the memory is recalled, its neural effect becomes strengthened and over time more accessible and easily felt. As Voltaire said, "Appreciation is a wonderful thing: It makes what is excellent in others belong to us as well."

Appreciations typically fall into three categories: appreciation of oneself, the world, and others. It is wise to practice appreciations of each type. As appreciation for oneself develops, the need to feel appreciation from others lessens. Since feeling underappreciated activates the stress response, building self-appreciation can provide an additional stress buffer. Although the world has its troubles, it also can bring countless appreciations to mind, such as its abundant resources, ever-changing beauty, or endless opportunity for creative endeavors. Finally, feeling and expressing appreciation of others enhances resilience not only for the giver but also for the receiver. In a culture where much of our communication is negative, this attitude is a welcome influence.

Positive Expectation

The placebo response is activated through positive expectation and is well known to buffer against pain and depression; it originates from upper brain regions associated with top-down control, motivation, and reward. Positive expectancy can lead to the development of desirable qualities and abilities. Ellen Langer, professor of psychology at Harvard University, has studied the influence of positive expectations. She found that even the expectation of losing weight influences weight loss; the expectation is, in a sense, a self-fulfilling prophecy. Through recent brain-mapping studies, this phenomenon is understood through two mechanisms: release of dopamine and activation of the brain's reward and motivation circuitry. A general attitude of positive expectation not only allows the brain to release mood-stabilizing chemicals but also provides the motivation necessary to accomplish what is desired. Unlike negative expectations that bring on feelings of anxiety and stress, positive expectation feels good, buffers stress, and contributes to achieving what is positively expected.

Acceptance

Resisting "what is" leads to stress. As outlined in theologian Reinhold Niebuhr's *Serenity Prayer*, wisdom is knowing when to accept what is beyond our control. Surrendering to what is beyond our control stops resistance and allows the mind to begin the process of acceptance. Acceptance empowers one to find whatever is good in the midst of a challenging situation. Patience, perseverance, strength, giving and receiving support, compassion, kindness, gentleness, and learning are only a few of the many qualities developed and expressed through acceptance. When Sjögren's patients explore problem-solving strategies and define what is possible to change, acceptance of what remains limits stress and enhances overall resilience. Given the role stress plays in promoting inflammation and in compromising the body's natural ability to heal, accepting what is unavoidable makes good therapeutic sense. As George Orwell said, "Happiness can exist only in acceptance."

Self-Perception

According to neuroscientist Joseph LeDoux, we are who we remember ourselves to be. This valuable understanding of how the brain works and how malleable the brain appears to be explains the influence our self-perceptions have on our coping. Long-held views or self-identifications can be either empowering or self-defeating. Viewing oneself as weak, victimized, or anxious is a stress-activating perception and limits the development of adaptive, positive perceptions such as learning, strength, and acceptance.

Meditation

Cultivating adaptive perspectives and healing stressful memories are made easier through meditation. In recent studies on brain function, alterations in both brain structure and activity can be measured after only 8 weeks of a daily meditation practice. These changes are consistent with greater top-down control of the brain, less stress activation, and improved mood and physical symptoms.

Meditation is a natural state of mind elicited through a focused and receptive mode of awareness. For example, drinking to quench thirst or enjoying a delicious piece of fruit can bring the mind into a meditative state. The drink or fruit is focused upon, and the accompanying enjoyment leads to a receptive and positive attitude. Much as a perception of a threat activates the stress response and leads to bottom-up control of the brain, a focused and receptive awareness elicits the body's relaxation response and leads to top-down control of the brain. In a meditative state, negative emotions triggered from remembered threats are made less prominent by activating the regions of the brain responsible for storing positive memories, positive expectations, and other adaptive perspectives. Recent studies on meditation not only demonstrate neural changes consistent with reduced stress, greater top-down control, and more positive and adaptive perspectives, but they also show changes in gene expression throughout the body that alter cellular functioning. Rather than overproducing oxidant toxins as cells do in response to stress, certain types of cells are known to reduce or even reverse their oxidative stress in response to meditation. Thus, building a meditation practice is well worth the time and effort.

BUILDING A MEDITATION PRACTICE

You already meditate. Every time you look at something or someone with a focused and receptive state of mind, you are in a meditative state. Viewing someone or something pleasing, new, and interesting naturally focuses the mind and activates top-down control of the brain. However, the ability to sustain and retain this state of mind and return to it at will when stressed requires practice. The first step toward controlling your own awareness is to build an ability to concentrate and sustain a particular focus.

The following strategies represent a few meditation methods to support your practice; although there are many ways to activate stress, there are just as many ways to activate a non-stressed, meditative state of mind (Tables 32–1 and 32–2). Any mental activity that engages the mind toward a sustained focus of receptive interest will lead to desired change. Body-based practices such as Hatha Yoga, Qigong, and Tai Chi are well-known meditation methods beyond the scope of this chapter. However, once you develop any meditation practice, expanding it through the use of other methods can bring added benefit.

SINGLE-POINTED FOCUS

Concentrating on a soothing or empowering word, phrase, or image is one method for building concentration. Aligning your single-pointed focus to a natural rhythm such as the breath often helps sustain focus.

IMAGINE A DESIRABLE SELF

The mind's influence on behavior is well known. Olympic athletes have learned to imagine themselves performing their skill perfectly. Studies on rehabilitation

TABLE 32–1
Meditation

Meditation	Focused Approach
Single-pointed	Focus on a positive word, phrase, image, or combination.
Self imagery	Imagine a well-developed and adaptive self.
Safe place imagery	Imagine a nurturing and healing environment.
Mindfulness	Hold awareness in the present, non-threatening moment.
Time travel	Focus on a positive or adaptive memory. Focus on a positive or adaptive desire.
Insight	Perceive through non-stressed, adaptive brain regions.

TABLE 32–2

How to Begin Meditating

Frequency

Practice daily! Regular and frequent practice improves neural plasticity in a cumulative fashion.

Duration

After 10 minutes of practice, physiological change is measurable. Begin with 10 to 20 minutes and slowly increase to 20 to 30 minutes.

Lifestyle

Meditating at the same time each day and in the same place helps integrate this new behavior into your normal routine. Placing a sacred or healing symbol in this environment serves as a positive reminder of this new state of mind.

Developing and maintaining a meditative state of mind throughout the day is challenging. Try meditating first thing in the morning and again at bedtime. While meditating in the morning sets the right tone for the day, meditating at bedtime reduces stress hormones and other chemicals that interfere with your ability to obtain deep, recuperative sleep.

Redirecting the Wandering Mind

Each time the mind wanders from your intended focus (commonly every few seconds), gently return to it without recrimination. Simply noticing how often the mind wanders while sustaining an attitude of interest builds focus and receptive awareness. Your mind will wander less as you develop the ability to sustain your focus. Over time, lapses in this ability may indicate the influence of greater stress or of needing more recuperative sleep.

after a stroke show greater recovery associated with imagining the use of pre-stroke abilities. If you are anxious, imagining yourself calm, balanced, powerful, and accepting is corrective. If you are inclined to feelings of sadness and depression, imagining yourself as appreciative and filled with positive expectancy brings about a more adaptive persona.

SAFE PLACE

Rest the mind on the memory or creation of a safe, nurturing place. As with any mental focus, it is important to keep the perspective positive and supportive. A pleasing memory of an old friend can conjure up the loss of that friendship, or a wishful experience can begin to feel remote or hopeless. Any stress-activating shift in perception can be instructive and useful if met with a receptive awareness. Understanding the nature of your stress is an expression of self-compassion. From the perspective of a safe place, you can ask yourself what is needed to heal. Moving your mind away from the indulgence of stress-activating thoughts to those that heal is an integral aspect of developing a meditative state of mind.

MINDFULNESS

If the mind is in the present moment, and the present moment does not pose a threat, then the brain is functioning in non-stressed, top-down control.

However, holding mental focus in a moment-to-moment awareness is challenging. To begin, pick a discrete and pleasant activity like eating an apple or drinking a cup of tea. Bringing the mind to the experience of seeing, tasting, smelling, touching, and hearing is a way to maintain present awareness. Noticing how one feels or thinks in any given moment is also part of mindfulness when accomplished with an open, receptive attitude of interest. Negative judgments or memories of stress may come to mind, but if met in mindfulness, a deeper, more adaptive awareness is likely to follow from maintaining top-down control. In this nonjudgmental state of self-awareness, clarity and wisdom are more accessible.

TIME TRAVEL

Reliving pleasant memories or focusing on a desirable outcome also frees the mind from the control of stress-activating regions. Holding awareness on the positive aspects of a memory or on a desirable expectation free of worry or negativity arouses the senses to relive the memory or begin enjoyment of an expectation. Expectations influence language and behavior, and these in turn become influences themselves. Therefore, be careful to create expectations for your own good and for the good of others.

INSIGHT

Carrying on a conversation with ourselves is common. We often ask ourselves questions such as, "Should I buy this?" or "What time do I need to get up?" If stressed, answers to these questions are likely to come from bottom-up brain processes where the brain stores memories of threats. Perceiving through these pathways can be stress-activating and can become a habitual way of sustaining stress and blocking positive or adaptive perceptions. Posing questions with an open, receptive attitude, as in a meditative state of mind, often brings new and more serviceable insights. To help sustain a positive and focused awareness, especially when asking a question whose answer can elicit stress, it is useful to first imagine a safe place. Once fully secure in this place, ask the question to an imagined wise person or a loving presence. If you prefer a particular answer, the stress response takes over and insight may be blocked.

Through the years I have taught thousands to meditate and have had the privilege of watching many heal from the stress of traumatic memories and stress imposed by chronic illness. Those with Sjögren's can use the tools described in this chapter to promote healing and cope positively with the added stress that is an inevitable part of this disease. The mind is an expression of free will; through both cognitive reappraisal and meditation, this free will can be used more wisely in support of adaptive and healing perspectives. Using psychological stress as a signal to heal enhances resilience.

Although physical limitations may continue, a growing sense of well-being can be achieved.

Summing Up

Increasing awareness of mind/body connections and taking advantage of ways to reduce stress can help Sjögren's patients cope better with the emotional and physical challenges of their disease. Meditation and cognitive strategies to ease anxieties and stress and focus on more positive feelings and perspectives can be valuable tools in a patient's struggle to develop a sense of well-being and more positive life experience.

FOR FURTHER READING

Benson H, Proctor W. *Relaxation Revolution: Enhancing Your Personal Health Through the Science and Genetics of Mind Body Healing.* Scribner, 2010.

Crum AJ, Langer EJ. Mind-set matters: exercise and the placebo effect. *Psychol Sci.* 2007; 18: 165–71.

Fontana D. *The Meditation Handbook: The Practical Guide to Eastern and Western Meditation Techniques.* Watkins, 2010.

Fredrickson B. *Positivity: Groundbreaking Research Reveals How to Embrace the Hidden Strength of Positive Emotions, Overcome Negativity, and Thrive.* Crown, 2009.

Kabat-Zinn J. *Wherever You Go, There You Are: Mindfulness Meditation in Everyday Life.* Hyperion, 2005.

Sapolsky R. *Why Zebras Don't Get Ulcers*, 3rd ed. Holt Paperbacks, 2004.

http://www.soundstrue.com/guide/meditation/ On-line guidance, books, and audio from a variety of wisdom traditions

http://www.parallax.org/ Resources from Buddhist monk, Thich Nhat Hanh, the most prolific writer on mindfulness

33

Related Topics on Living with Sjögren's

33A: SEX

Anne E. Burke, MD, MPH

Sjögren's syndrome can affect women's sexuality. Reasons for this include physical symptoms that can occur with Sjögren's, such as vaginal dryness and pelvic pain. Also, for some women, the age when they are diagnosed with Sjögren's may coincide with the early stages of menopause and its accompanying hormonal changes. But other factors, such as mood, fatigue, and the general challenges of living with a chronic illness, can also affect sexual function and sexual satisfaction for women with Sjögren's.

Like other autoimmune diseases, Sjögren's affects more women than men. This may be because hormones such as estrogen play a role in its cause. Despite this, some symptoms of Sjögren's in women were all but ignored for years, and sexual problems are an example. Sjögren's is not unique in this regard. Until about a decade ago, researchers did not pay much attention to the sexual effects of most chronic illnesses. Neither did doctors in practice: previous studies suggested that fewer than half of women with Sjögren's ever had a doctor ask them about sexual symptoms. Fortunately, this seems to be changing. While we are still learning more about Sjögren's and sexual function, there is growing recognition of these connections. In this section, we discuss some factors that can affect sex in women with Sjögren's.

Vaginal Dryness

Women with Sjögren's often experience vaginal dryness, along with dry mouth and dry eyes. Vaginal dryness is more common in women who have Sjögren's than in women who don't: as many as 75% of women with Sjögren's may have this problem. In women with Sjögren's, vaginal dryness may be caused by inflammation of the glands that would usually lubricate the vagina. The physical stress of many chronic illnesses, including Sjögren's, can contribute to vaginal dryness, too.

Hormones such as estrogen can also affect the severity of vaginal dryness. In many cases, women are in their 40s when they are diagnosed with Sjögren's. This can coincide with the start of the hormonal changes that lead into menopause. This phase, when periods become less regular and symptoms of menopause may start to come and go, is called perimenopause. During this time, hormone levels may start to follow unpredictable patterns. Along with this, women may have symptoms such as hot flashes and low sex drive in addition to vaginal dryness. Perimenopause can last for several years, but as a woman transitions into menopause, her estrogen levels decrease. This can cause symptoms to worsen. If a woman has Sjögren's and is perimenopausal or menopausal, she has two good reasons for vaginal dryness. However, even younger women with Sjögren's can suffer from vaginal dryness.

Vaginal dryness can cause problems with sexual function. Without enough lubrication, vaginal intercourse may be painful. The friction caused by having sex without enough moisture can even cause abrasions or small cuts in the vagina, which can increase pain levels. Not only can this make sex painful at the time, it can make women want to avoid sex due to fear of the pain happening again.

There are some treatment options for vaginal dryness. Over-the-counter products may be a good place to start. One of the newest products on the market is Luvena, which is glycerin- and preservative-free and uses enzymes, proteins, and a pre-biotic believed to help balance the pH. Combined, these characteristics act as antibacterial/antiyeast agents. Some products, such as Replens, contain a compound called polycarbophil. This is a vaginal moisturizer that does not contain hormones. It hydrates the epithelial cells that line the vagina, and it can last for up to 72 hours. Other water-based lubricants (such as K-Y or Astroglide) may help to increase lubrication for intercourse. There are also products that contain botanical or oil-based natural ingredients, such as aloe vera or vitamin E, though these have not been studied specifically for women with Sjögren's, and they may damage condoms.

Vaginal estrogen treatments may help with dryness. There are several forms of estrogen that can be used in the vagina. These include creams, pills, and rings. For women whose dryness is caused at least in part by low estrogen levels (such as women who have gone through menopause), these medications can improve the health of the vaginal cells and increase moisture over time. These usually require a prescription from a healthcare provider. Some women may use hormone pills or patches for a limited time, primarily if they have other symptoms such as hot flashes. "Natural" hormone treatments, such as soy supplements or black cohosh, have not been well studied in women with Sjögren's.

Sometimes lubricants and hormones do not completely fix the dryness, and a more creative approach is necessary. A couple may seek alternatives to vaginal intercourse, such as oral sex or masturbation. It may also help to talk with a partner about new ways to approach vaginal sex. Sometimes more fore-play is helpful. Women may also opt to limit vaginal intercourse to shorter periods of time to decrease painful friction. Some women with Sjögren's have also found that it helps to plan sex around times of the menstrual cycle when natural lubrication is greatest. A lot of patience from both partners can be helpful as a solution is found. Women with Sjögren's should not be afraid to discuss this with their doctors, either. While not all doctors are comfortable treating sexual symptoms, many will refer patients to someone who can.

Dry Mouth

Dry mouth is a very common symptom of Sjögren's. Women with Sjögren's may find that even kissing can be uncomfortable. Just as dry mouth can affect chewing and swallowing, it can also affect activities like deep kissing, or giving oral sex to one's partner. Treatments that improve dry mouth may also make things like deep kissing more comfortable. These can range from simple things like chewing gum (to stimulate saliva) to prescription medications. Women can discuss these options with their healthcare provider.

Pelvic Pain and Painful Sex (Dyspareunia)

Many women with Sjögren's suffer from neuropathic pain in different parts of the body. They can also experience pelvic pain and may have feelings of blad-der or urinary irritation more often than women without Sjögren's. Often these types of pain can be difficult to treat, which can be frustrating. Any of these symptoms can make sexual intercourse painful. Pain during sex is called dys-pareunia. One study reported that over 60% of women with Sjögren's com-plained of dyspareunia. However, other studies have found that if there are no other medical problems, women with Sjögren's may not have dyspareunia any more frequently than other women.

Dyspareunia can either be deep (felt with deep vaginal penetration) or superficial (felt with initial vaginal penetration). There can be many causes of dyspareunia and/or pelvic pain that are not related to Sjögren's. Causes of deep dyspareunia can include ovarian cysts, endometriosis, infection, or scarring from any previous surgeries. Vaginal dryness or vulvar pain can cause superficial dyspareunia. Therefore, if a woman with Sjögren's is having problems with sex due to pelvic pain, she should have an evaluation to make sure there are no other causes. If another cause is found, that should be treated appropriately. Sometimes no obvious cause is found for the pain, and it may be related to Sjögren's.

Dyspareunia can be very challenging. Women may feel like they should "put up with the pain" to please their partner. Over time, this can start to have a negative effect on the relationship. Further, the presence of dyspareunia can make a woman want to avoid sex, for obvious reasons. Persistent dyspareunia can also cause involuntary tension to develop in the pelvic muscles, so that sex becomes even more painful over time. This too can start to affect a woman's relationship with her partner. In some cases, partners may try to avoid sexual activity so as not to cause pain, and this can hurt satisfaction and self-esteem on both sides.

Dyspareunia and pelvic pain can be difficult to "cure," especially when there is no clear, fixable cause. However, there are some treatment strategies that can help. Couples can start with things like trying different positions to find those that are most comfortable. Treating vaginal dryness may also help. Women with chronic pain may also benefit from pelvic physical therapy (PT). This involves spending several sessions with a physical therapist trained in pelvic rehabilitation. Some pelvic PT techniques include biofeedback, electrical stimulation, physiotherapy, and vaginal dilator therapy. With a physician's prescription, insurance will often cover several pelvic PT sessions. Therapists may also discuss techniques that women can use at home after the PT sessions end. Some women may benefit greatly from cognitive therapy that focuses on improving sexual function, especially if such therapy is part of a larger treatment approach. Dealing with any psychological effects of the pain through counseling and learned coping skills can be helpful for many women as well.

Fatigue, Mood, and Quality of Life

As most women know, "sex" is not just about the pelvic organs. The quality of a woman's sex life is affected by what is going on in the rest of her life, and a condition like Sjögren's can certainly play a big role. Many factors common to other chronic illnesses can also affect those with Sjögren's. The systemic inflammation that occurs with Sjögren's and other illnesses can itself lead to diminished libido. Further, fatigue or depressed mood can affect sexual function. Fatigue may be due to the illness itself or to medication side effects. Either way, when fatigue makes it difficult just to get through the day, sex can become a low priority.

Many women with Sjögren's have problems with depression. This may be due to the stress of dealing with illness. In some cases, too, women had symptoms of Sjögren's for some time before it was actually diagnosed. Years of not knowing what was wrong, dealing with frustrating symptoms, or worrying that symptoms were all in one's head can contribute over time to depressed mood. Decreased self-esteem and depression can also result when Sjögren's-related disability prevents a woman from fulfilling the roles she is used to. Whatever the cause, depression can make it difficult to have a satisfying sex life.

When depression is properly treated, its effects on sexual function may lessen.

That being said, some treatments for depression may affect sexual function and behavior. A commonly used type of antidepressant is an SSRI (selective serotonin reuptake inhibitor). Medications such as fluoxetine (Prozac), sertraline (Zoloft), and paroxetine (Paxil) are examples of SSRIs, and these can be associated with a higher incidence of sexual problems than some other medications. If one of these medications may be affecting a woman's sexual function, options include trying a different medication or maybe just lowering the dose. It is important, though, that any changes in medication don't cause depression to worsen.

Chronic conditions like Sjögren's can affect overall quality of life, which can in turn affect sexual function and satisfaction. Issues like physical disability, stiffness, chronic pain, emotional stress, and altered self-image all can have a negative impact on a woman's quality of life and in turn on her sex life. This can be something of a vicious cycle: the resulting problems with sexual functioning may in turn result in worse quality of life, which can further impair sexual relationships, and so on.

Problems like fatigue or depression may not go away easily. Sometimes the answer is to work around them. Some women with Sjögren's have found that it helps if they plan when they are going to have sex. Rather than acting as spontaneously as they may have in the past, they may need to prioritize time for sexual activity. This can include "scheduling" times with a partner and allowing more time for foreplay. For women who suffer from fatigue, it may help to target times of the day or days of the week when the fatigue is likely to be less severe. Pain or stiffness may require that couples try different techniques to minimize discomfort. Women who take medications for depression or anything else should consider asking their healthcare providers if a change may lessen any sexual side effects without causing other problems. In any case, it is important that women not hesitate to raise their sexual concerns with their healthcare providers. Many factors can have a real effect on sexuality, and there is no shame in admitting this. Seeing a healthcare provider or counselor with specific expertise in sexual health may also be beneficial.

Partnerships

A woman's relationship with her partner is an important contributor to sexual function and satisfaction. This can be especially true for women with conditions like Sjögren's. The fatigue and physical symptoms caused by Sjögren's can take a toll on the relationship. Forcing oneself to "be strong" for one's partner can cause resentment or a feeling of isolation. This can be true whether the "sick" partner is trying to be strong for the "healthy" partner or vice versa.

Further, a woman with Sjögren's may feel inadequate or burdensome to her partner, while the partner may feel resentful and stressed about the illness. Or she may feel so overwhelmed by Sjögren's that she pays less attention to her relationship with her partner. Fortunately, these feelings do not occur in all couples, but they can happen. And when they do, sexual problems and lack of affection can be common.

It is important to acknowledge such feelings, whether or not a couple is experiencing sexual difficulties. Open communication is important to any healthy partnership. It becomes even more important when a chronic illness like Sjögren's is present, because that can color the relationship for both partners. It may also be helpful for partners to understand that there are physical reasons for Sjögren's to affect women's sexual functioning, and thus some problems may be nobody's "fault." Counseling can be helpful for many couples who are having difficulties in their partnerships due to Sjögren's.

Sexual Well-Being

Sexual *function* should be differentiated from sexual *well-being*. Sexual function refers to a woman's ability to engage in sexual activity, whereas sexual well-being is a more subjective measure of satisfaction with one's sexuality. Women with Sjögren's may experience changes in sexual function for the reasons described above or perhaps other reasons as well. For some women, the changes caused by Sjögren's will make it difficult or impossible to return to a previous "sexual status quo." Women with Sjögren's may have physical or psychological reasons to have sex differently or less frequently. However, many other women with Sjögren's continue to enjoy similar levels of sexual activity and satisfaction compared to "healthy" women. Even with the limitations of Sjögren's, women and their partners can maintain a state of sexual well-being if both are able to accept a "new normal" in their sexual relationship. This may require more patience, effort, and creativity as well as altered expectations if the disease progresses over time. But it can be done, and women with Sjögren's can still enjoy a satisfying sex life.

Summing Up

Sexual well-being is important to quality of life, and those living with Sjögren's often face more challenges than their "healthy" counterparts. Symptoms associated with Sjögren's can interfere with a positive sex life and include vaginal dryness, pain (pelvic, muscle, joint, and neuropathic pain), fatigue, dry mouth, and depression. In addition to Sjögren's, perimenopause, menopause, and/or medications can add to sexual difficulties in a partnership, exacerbating dryness and contributing to low libido.

In addition to treating the disease as a whole to improve Sjögren's symptoms, over-the-counter lubricating products, prescription hormones, and specialized physical therapy can make a difference. Good communication with one's partner, sometimes with the help of a counselor, as well as using tools to improve one's quality of life overall can help enhance sexual well-being.

FOR FURTHER READING

Basson R. Sexual function of women with chronic illness and cancer. *Womens Health*. 2010; 6(3): 407–29.

Glazer HI, Rodke G. *The Vulvodynia Survival Guide: How to Overcome Painful Vaginal Symptoms & Enjoy an Active Lifestyle*. Oakland: New Harbinger Publications, 2002.

Lehrer S, Bogursky E, Yemini M, et al. Gynecologic manifestations of Sjögren's syndrome. *Am J Obstet Gynecol*. 1994; 170(3), 835–7.

Schoofs N. Caring for women living with Sjögren's syndrome. *J Obstet Gynecol Neonatal Nurs*. 2003; 32(5): 589–93.

Tristano AG. The impact of rheumatic diseases on sexual function. *Rheumatol Int*. 2009; 29(8): 853–60.

Verschuren JE, Enzlin P, Dijkstra PU, et al. Chronic disease and sexuality: a generic conceptual framework. *J Sex Res*. 2010; 47(2): 153–70.

H. Kenneth Fisher, MD, FACP, FCCP

Problems with sleep are seen in more than 70% of U.S. adults with rheumatic disorders. The main sleep complaint reported by primary Sjögren's patients is that their sleep is nonrestorative: about two thirds report they are fatigued, both physically and mentally. Depression is not the principal cause, though it is often present as well. The characteristics of disabling fatigue in primary Sjögren's are indistinguishable from those of patients with rheumatoid arthritis (RA) or systemic lupus erythematosus. Sleep disturbances are rated moderate or severe in 75% of patients with primary Sjögren's, more than is found in RA alone, RA with sicca symptoms, or osteoarthritis. Among patients with primary Sjögren's, those who also have fibromyalgia symptoms have especially severe sleep complaints.

What Sleep Characteristics Do Sjögren's Patients Experience?

The somatic fatigue of Sjögren's patients is different from sleepiness and is commonly progressive during the day. Mental fatigue is also progressive during the day, and both symptoms are associated with poor nocturnal sleep and physical discomfort during the night. Nocturnal awakenings due to musculoskeletal pain, anxiety, and other sleep-disturbing symptoms are all associated with daytime fatigue.

Besides daily progressive daytime fatigue, daytime sleepiness self-measured by the Epworth Sleepiness Scale is also common in Sjögren's patients. Bladder irritability and urinary urgency are seen more often in primary Sjögren's patients than in osteoarthritis patients and may play a role in poor sleep quality.

What Causes Poor Sleep in Sjögren's?

It seems unlikely that inflammation by itself explains the disturbed sleep of Sjögren's patients. When compared with both healthy controls and RA patients,

Sjögren's patients differ in several ways that might result in worse sleep quality. They have more muscle tension at bedtime, more symptoms of restless legs syndrome, and more pains during the night. Not surprisingly, they have a larger sleep deficit. More frequently than those in the comparison groups, Sjögren's patients do not feel rested after sleep and complain of daytime fatigue and sleepiness.

Full overnight polysomnograms (sleep studies) have been reported in only a small number of Sjögren's patients, but these provide objective data that support the subjective complaints. Although sleep architecture is generally normal, time awake after sleep onset is considerably greater among Sjögren's subjects and reduces sleep efficiency from 94% in healthy controls to 70% among Sjögren's subjects. Half the Sjögren's subjects demonstrate alpha brain wave activity intruding into delta (deep) sleep, an anomaly seen commonly in fibromyalgia patients who also suffer from prominent daytime fatigue.

The exact links between disturbed nocturnal sleep and daytime fatigue are not yet known, but one hint that the autonomic nervous system may be involved comes from the observation that those primary Sjögren's and fibromyalgia patients with the greatest levels of daytime fatigue are also the ones with the lowest diastolic blood pressures.

Knowledge that the surface tension of airway-lining fluids in Sjögren's patients is abnormally high led to speculation that some of the daytime fatigue and sleepiness might be caused by increased risk of obstructive sleep apnea due to airway collapse. However, recent studies have found no increased airway collapsibility in patients with primary Sjögren's.

Can Commonly Coexisting Conditions and Medications Affect Sleep?

Dryness, musculoskeletal and chronic pain, neuropathies, and sensitivity to cold and heat are all commonly seen in Sjögren's and can interfere with sleep. Keeping inflammation, pain, and the patient's disease under control will improve sleep. If depression is part of the patient's medical picture, recognize that this condition can add to sleep problems.

In addition, coexisting fibromyalgia and autoimmune thyroid disorders can complicate the clinical picture. Up to 25% of Sjögren's patients have autoimmune thyroid disease, which can occur as hypothyroidism (Hashimoto's thyroiditis) or hyperthyroidism (Graves' disease). While these conditions would seem to have opposite impacts on sleep, both can interfere with the quality of sleep. Hashimoto's can add to the joint and muscle pain and stiffness already experienced by many Sjögren's patients, and the anxiety and restlessness that occur in Graves' can diminish sleep quality. Thyroid disease often is underdiagnosed, and thyroid function should be checked in Sjögren's patients.

Medication lists should be checked for side effects that include interference with sleep. Prednisone, especially when taken in the evening, can cause some patients to become nervous and have difficulty sleeping.

Before trying medications for troubled sleep, basic rules of sleep hygiene should be followed. Regular exercise can increase a sense of well-being, can help with depression if it exists, and can improve sleep; however, patients should avoid exercise in the few hours before bedtime. Finally, relaxation techniques can help before bedtime and if a patient awakens in the middle of the night.

What Can Be Done for Sjögren's Patients with Fatigue Induced by Poor Sleep?

Now that we understand more about the nature of the disabling fatigue in primary Sjögren's patients, what can we do about it? Only very tentative answers are available so far. Exercise has been shown to improve both aerobic capacity (as expected) and also fatigue levels. Six months' use of a disease-modifying agent (the monoclonal antibody rituximab [Rituxan]) has also been shown to reduce fatigue. Other biological agents under investigation to treat Sjögren's and related autoimmune disorders may prove useful as well.

If we allow ourselves to look further afield, we might draw hope from studies of patients with fibromyalgia who have very similar pain, sleep, and fatigue complaints to those seen in Sjögren's. Treatment with sodium oxybate (Xyrem) (a natural substance found in all of us) reduced nighttime alpha intrusion, pain, and daytime fatigue in one study and improved sleep quality and level of symptoms in another. While this drug was found to be effective for some sleep disorders, it has not undergone clinical trials specifically in Sjögren's and was not recommended for FDA approval for use in fibromyalgia as recently as August 2010; physicians and patients also will want to keep in mind that it is expensive and requires a difficult schedule for taking the drug. Given the similarity of symptoms in fibromyalgia and primary Sjögren's, it is reasonable to anticipate that primary Sjögren's patients also might benefit from medications used in this condition. So far no such studies have been reported.

Most Sjögren's patients do not require sleep medication, and if they do their choice is limited by the drying properties of commonly used agents such as tricyclics and antihistamines. However, Zolpidem (Ambien), melatonin derivatives (e.g., Rozeram), certain herbal preparations (e.g., valerian root, Calmes Forte), and benzodiazepines (e.g., clonazepam [Klonopin], lorazepam [Ativan], temazepam [Restoril]) may be appropriate in selected circumstances.

Summing Up

Sleep problems are common in Sjögren's patients, with the most frequent complaint being nonrestorative sleep. Sleep efficiency and time spent in deep sleep appear reduced in many Sjögren's patients. Those with both Sjögren's and fibromyalgia have the severest complaints. The causes of sleep problems in Sjögren's are unknown, but autonomic nervous system involvement is suspected of playing a role. While few studies have been done, medications under investigation for use in Sjögren's and other autoimmune disorders or on the market for sleep problems in fibromyalgia patients might prove useful.

FOR FURTHER READING

Abad VC, Sarinas PS, Guilleminault C. Sleep and rheumatologic disorders. *Sleep Med Rev.* 2008; 12: 211–28.

d'Elia HF, Rehnberg E, Kvist G, et al. Fatigue and blood pressure in primary Sjögren's syndrome. *Scand J Rheumatol.* 2008; 37: 284–92.

Goodchild CE, Treharne GJ, Booth DA, Bowman SJ. Daytime patterning of fatigue and its associations with the previous night's discomfort and poor sleep among women with primary Sjögren's syndrome or rheumatoid arthritis. *Musculoskeletal Care.* 2010; 8(2): 107–17.

Gudbjornsson B, Broman JE, Hetta J, Hallgren R. Sleep disturbances in patients with primary Sjögren's syndrome. *Br J Rheum.* 1993; 32: 1072–6.

Hilditch CJ, McEvoy RD, George KE, et al. Upper airway surface tension but not upper airway collapsibility is elevated in primary Sjögren's syndrome. *Sleep.* 2008; 31: 367–74.

Russell IJ, Perkins AT, Michalek JE. Sodium oxybate relieves pain and improves function in fibromyalgia syndrome. *Arthritis Rheum.* 2009; 60: 299–309.

Scharf MB, Baumann M, Berkowitz DV. Effects of sodium oxybate on clinical symptoms and sleep patterns in patients with fibromyalgia. *J Rheum.* 2003; 30: 1070–4.

Segal B, Thomas W, Rogers T, et al. Prevalence, severity and predictors of fatigue in primary Sjögren's syndrome. *Arthritis Rheum.* 2008; 59(12): 1780–7.

Strombeck BE, Theander E, Jacobsson LT. Effects of exercise on aerobic capacity and fatigue in women with primary Sjögren's syndrome. *Rheum (Oxford).* 2007; 46(5): 868–71.

Theander L, Strombeck B, Mandl T, Theander E. Can we detect treatable causes of tiredness in primary Sjögren's syndrome? *Rheumatol (Oxford)* 2010; 49(6): 1177–83.

Tishler M, Barak Y, Paran D, Yaron M. Sleep disturbances, fibromyalgia and primary Sjögren's syndrome. *Clin Exp Rheum.* 1997; 15: 71–74.

33C: SURGERY
Lynn M. Petruzzi, RN, MSN

Surgery is a stressor even for healthy patients. For patients with Sjögren's syndrome, the psychological and physical stresses related to surgery can exacerbate patients' symptoms and/or lead to a flare of the disease process. The most common postoperative problems for patients with Sjögren's include increase in sicca symptoms, skin irritation, sore throat, corneal abrasion, and exacerbation of extra-glandular manifestations. The goals of surgery are to identify, manage, and treat the first three of these problems and prevent the final two.

These problems may occur for a number of reasons. The operating room is kept low in humidity and cool to meet the standards of regulatory agencies and to ensure that the sterility of packaged items remains intact. Patients may experience increased dryness of the eyes and mouth due to the environment and the fact that anesthesia and pain medications are also drying. Skin may be irritated by the product used to clean the skin prior to surgery and from the stick on pads placed on the patient's body to monitor, for example, heart and oxygen levels. A sore throat is a frequent patient complaint, especially if a breathing tube was used.

The most effective way for patients to prevent an increase in symptoms and/or a flare is to educate themselves about surgery and anesthesia and to make sure that all members of the surgical team are knowledgeable about Sjögren's and the most common problems associated with Sjögren's and surgery. Patients also should increase the use of their oral and ocular products 1 to 2 weeks prior to surgery to ensure that their ocular surface and oral mucosa are in the best condition possible. Use of nasal saline is encouraged, even if not routinely used, to moisturize the nasal passageways. While discussion and other tips included in this chapter are written for the patient, healthcare professionals can use these tips as well to guide their communication with patients.

Discussion with Your Rheumatologist

As soon as you are aware that you are having surgery, inform your rheumatologist. He or she will communicate with your surgeon regarding your medical condition and will advise you about medications that can or cannot be continued through surgery. If you are on steroids, they will need to be continued, and your rheumatologist will make recommendations regarding dosing. Hydroxychloroquine (Plaquenil) can be continued but other immunosuppressive agents will be discontinued. Your rheumatologist will determine when to discontinue these medications prior to surgery and when they may be restarted after surgery.

Discussion with Your Surgeon

Sharing knowledge with the surgical team begins with your appointment with your surgeon. Be prepared to discuss the following:

1. Understand the type of surgery you are having.
2. Learn about the different types of anesthesia and identify your preference(s). Ask whether general anesthesia is required or if another type of anesthesia is an option.
3. Bring a complete list of your medications, including over-the-counter products, vitamins, herbals, and anti-inflammatories (e.g., Advil, Motrin). Some medications, such as vitamin E and anti-inflammatories, may need to be discontinued 5 to 7 days prior to surgery, as they may cause increased bleeding. If you are dependent on anti-inflammatories (over-the-counter or prescription) to control pain, you may want to request another type of pain medication to use before surgery.
4. If you take brand-name medications or medications that the hospital most likely will not stock or will substitute with a generic (i.e., Nexium), inform your doctor that you will bring these medications to the hospital and ask the doctor to write an order stating this (Box 33–1).

Box 33–1

Example of a Potential Doctor's Order

Patient may take own medications:

Plaquenil—brand only—200 mg bid
Nexium 40 mg qd
Salagen 5 mg 4 times/day

Box 33–2
Example of a Potential Doctor's Order

Patient may use own oral/ocular products:
TheraTears 1 gtt each eye 4 times/day and prn
Genteal gel each eye at bedtime

5. Bring a copy of your oral and ocular regimen with you, including product name, dosage (if applicable), and frequency of use. Again, inform the doctor that you will bring these items to the hospital and ask the doctor to write an order stating this (Box 33–2).
6. Bring all of your medications and over-the-counter products in their original packaging. Most hospitals require any drugs brought from home to be sent to the pharmacy for verification prior to administration. Bring only the amount of medication you anticipate needing (i.e., 2 or 3 days). This will prevent a costly loss in the event the medication is misplaced.
7. Verify on the day of surgery that your surgeon has the list of medications and over-the-counter products you will bring from home. Have an extra copy of this information with you in case it is not in your chart.
8. Discuss your extra-glandular manifestations of Sjögren's, such as arthritis, pulmonary problems, skin issues, or fatigue, that may affect your surgery.
9. Discuss with your surgeon the necessity of being the first or second surgery scheduled to decrease the length of time you will need to be NPO (nothing by mouth). It may be possible that your surgeon operates only in the afternoon. In this case you will be allowed to drink clear liquids until a specific time.

Discussion with the Preoperative Nurse

Most patients arrive at the hospital on the day of surgery. However, you will receive a phone call from a nurse prior to surgery. It is imperative that you

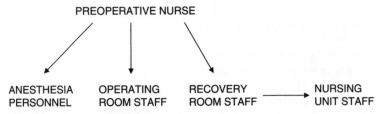

FIGURE 33C–1 **Chain of Communication**

discuss your Sjögren's with this nurse, including your medications and oral and ocular routines. Also inform him or her of any arrangements you have made with your surgeon about bringing medications and over-the-counter products from home. He or she will disseminate this information to the surgical team members. The chain of communication works like this:

Offer to bring information about Sjögren's to the nurse in the preoperative area before or on the day of your surgery. The preoperative nurse will give you preoperative instructions that include:

1. The time you should arrive at the hospital on the day of surgery
2. Approximate surgery time
3. When to stop eating and drinking before your surgery
4. What medication you should take the morning of your surgery. You will probably be told to take any medication for gastroesophageal reflux. Ask the nurse to check with the anesthesiologist whether you can take pilocarpine (Salagen) or cevimeline (Evoxac) the morning of surgery.
5. Any preparation for the surgical area (i.e., washing with a special soap)

Make sure you have important phone numbers in case you need to provide or obtain additional information before your surgery. Don't forget to bring all of your medications and eye and oral products to the hospital the day of surgery.

Discussion with the Anesthesiologist

You will speak to an anesthesiologist the day of surgery or earlier. He or she will review your health history and discuss your type of anesthesia. It is important to understand the types of anesthesia that are available.

Local anesthesia numbs a small part of the body. A shot of a local anesthetic is given directly into the surgical area to block pain. It is used for minor procedures. For either local or regional anesthesia, you may be awake during the procedure or may receive medicine to help you relax or sleep.

Regional anesthesia blocks pain to a larger area of the body. The anesthetic is injected around major nerves or the spinal cord. The major types of regional anesthesia are peripheral nerve blocks and epidural and spinal anesthesia. Peripheral nerve blocks involve a shot of anesthesia near a specific nerve or group of nerves and block pain in the part of the body supplied by the nerves. This type of anesthesia is used most often for procedures involving the hands, arms, feet, legs, and face. Epidural and spinal anesthesia involves a shot of anesthesia near the spinal cord and the nerves that connect to it. It blocks pain in an entire region of the body, such as the abdomen, hips, or legs.

General anesthesia affects the brain as well as the entire body. You may receive it through an intravenous line or breathe it in through a mask or

326 The Sjögren's Book

breathing tube. You will be completely unaware of your surgery and will not feel any pain. General anesthesia may also cause you to forget the surgery and the time right after it. General anesthesia is more drying than other types of anesthesia for several reasons: it decreases tear production, the anesthetic gases are drying, and the breathing system absorbs moisture.

The type of anesthesia you will receive depends on several things: your past and current health history, the reason for your surgery, the type of surgery, specific test results, and physician preference. In some cases you may be able to choose what type of anesthesia you have, in collaboration with your anesthesiologist. The anesthesiologist has the ultimate say in what anesthesia is used based on you as an individual and your type of surgery. His or her decision will also be based on what is the safest form of anesthesia for you.

Other issues that are important to discuss with your anesthesiologist include any arthritis in your neck or jaw and any problems with your teeth. These conditions may affect the insertion of a breathing tube if general anesthesia is planned or in the event one is required during another type of anesthesia. Request that anticholinergic medications (medications that create dryness) not be given unless necessary. Ask if a humidifier can be added to the oxygen delivered in the operating and recovery rooms. Inform the anesthesiologist if you have Raynaud's; the temperature in the operating room can be increased. Give your eye drops to the anesthesiologist and ask that he or she lubricate your eyes every 30 minutes during the procedure and pass them to the recovery room nurse after the procedure.

In the Recovery Room

You will be taken to the recovery room once your surgery is complete. You may or may not remember much about the recovery room. The nurses in this area will monitor you closely as you wake from your anesthesia. Once you are awake enough to control your swallowing, you may be offered ice chips. You will probably want the entire cup but can have only a minimal amount to prevent nausea. Once you have had some ice chips, ask the nurse if you can have your pilocarpine (Salagen) or cevimeline (Evoxac). Also ask for your eye drops and lip moisturizer at this time. Your nurse will ask if you are having pain. If so, allow him or her to give you pain medication. It will probably be a narcotic and cause increased dryness, but your comfort is important and will aid in your recovery.

On the Nursing Unit

After you recover from anesthesia you will be transferred to a nursing unit or hospital floor. Make sure your nurse is aware that you have Sjögren's.

Educate him or her if necessary and bring Sjögren's Syndrome Foundation brochures to share. He or she will be happy to have the information and will place it in the nurse's station for all staff. Give your nurse your prescription medications to be sent to the pharmacy. They may be left at your bedside for you to take or may need to be administered by the nurse, depending on hospital policy.

Request that ice chips or liquids be kept at your bedside at all times. Inform your nurse of the scheduled times you take pilocarpine (Salagen) or cevimeline (Evoxac) and ask if this schedule can be adhered to as closely as possible. You or your family should place your over-the-counter oral and ocular products and nasal spray in a convenient location that you can independently access. Use them frequently and more often than usual. Bring your moisture chamber glasses, goggles, rice sacks, and other items you use for comfort to the hospital for use if necessary. If you routinely use a humidifier, ask if your family can bring it to the hospital. If you experience pain, bleeding, or other symptoms in your eyes, mouth, or nose, notify your nurse immediately. He or she can assess the area and notify your doctor.

Take your pain medication even if it causes dryness, as it will help you be more mobile, increase your comfort, promote healing, and improve your sleep. Try a non-narcotic pain medication a day or two after surgery. If it controls your pain, take it instead of the narcotic. If you take a sleeping pill at home, definitely request one at bedtime. Fatigue and a general feeling of achiness after surgery are common. Your fatigue and musculoskeletal pain and stiffness may be increased. These issues, coupled with pain medication, may require you to need assistance when getting out of bed. Do not hesitate to ask for help from the nursing staff.

Be sure to bring any specific products you use (such as lotion, soap, toothpaste, mouthwash) with you to the hospital. If the hospital does provide toiletries, they most likely will not meet your needs. Ask your nurse to help you check to make sure all stick-on items not in use are removed from your body and to wash off excess adhesive residue and surgical soap or prep solutions around your dressing or incision. Apply your normal lotion or other products to the area, but avoid application to your incision. If you develop any skin irritation, inform your nurse. Most hospitals have hypoallergenic linens, which you may need if your skin is particularly sensitive.

Rest as much as you can in the hospital and once you are discharged home. Follow your postoperative instructions and keep all follow-up appointments. Surgery will increase your dryness; expect and be prepared for it. Appropriate planning with your rheumatologist, surgeon, and surgical team will prevent complications or identify them early, increase your comfort, and decrease your stress. We hope this information will enable you to have a positive surgical experience.

Summing Up

Surgery can exacerbate dryness, musculoskeletal pain, and fatigue in Sjögren's patients. It also can cause skin irritation and sore throat and contribute to flares in Sjögren's symptoms. Being prepared for these possible complications and knowing what information to share with your physicians and surgical team and what items to bring to the hospital will all contribute to a better surgical and recuperative experience.

FOR FURTHER READING

Cloe A. Sjögren's syndrome & general anesthesia. Available at: http://www.ehow.com/about_5052167_sjogrens-syndrome-general-anesthesia.html?sms_ss=email&at_xt=4de7c13c8172064d%2C0. Accessed March 18, 2010.

Donlon JV. Anesthetic management of patients with Sjögren's syndrome. Chapter 24. In Carsons S, Harris EK, eds. *The New Sjögren's Handbook*. New York: Oxford University Press, 1998.

Petruzzi LM, Vivino FB. Sjögren's syndrome–implications for perioperative practice. *AORN J*. 2003; 77(3): 612–21.

Rea C. Anesthesia. Available at: http://health.yahoo.com/pain-overview/anesthesia/health wise—tp17798.html. Accessed March 18, 2010.

Zheng K, John BU. Prevention of corneal abrasions in patients with autoimmune eye disease. Available at: http://www.anesthesia-analgesia.org/content/108/1/385.full. Accessed March 18, 2010.

33D: VACCINATIONS
Richard D. Brasington, Jr., MD

One of the most important aspects of "preventive health care" is receiving the appropriate vaccinations. This is particularly important for patients with Sjögren's syndrome and other autoimmune diseases with compromised immune function, especially when immunosuppressive medications are used. We can think of vaccinations in three broad categories: (1) those that everyone should receive; (2) those that are particularly appropriate for patients with autoimmune diseases; and (3) those that may be dangerous for such patients and therefore should be avoided.

Nowadays, the "standard" vaccinations are administered during the pre-school and elementary school years and include mumps, measles, rubella, tetanus, diphtheria, and so forth. For purposes of this discussion, we will assume that all patients who are ultimately diagnosed with Sjögren's have received all of the appropriate childhood immunizations. All adults need to remember that at least every 10 years they should receive a tetanus and diphtheria "booster." In reality, this booster is often administered when a question arises as to whether tetanus immunity is current; if there is no documentation of a Td booster in the previous 10 years, it is given at that point.

Patients with autoimmune disorders such as Sjögren's generally are considered to have some compromise of the immune system and increased susceptibility to infection. A simple way to think of this is to consider that if the immune system is "misdirected" toward self, it probably is not doing an ideal job of protecting against infectious agents. Obviously, someone with mild Sjögren's who does not have pronounced systemic disease will not be as susceptible to infection as a patient with systemic disease requiring prednisone and/or immunosuppressive agents such as azathioprine (Imuran, Azasan), methotrexate, or cyclophosphamide (Cytoxan).

While some patients fear that vaccines can activate the immune system and cause systemic flares, no scientific evidence exists to indicate that this is the case. In fact, studies in systemic lupus erythematosus do not suggest disease activation with pneumococcal vaccine (Pneumovax). Vaccines need to be avoided only when a previous reaction has occurred, and a reaction to one vaccination does not mean that all future vaccinations should be avoided.

The annual "flu shot" each fall is familiar to everyone. This vaccine is different each year and must be given every year. The vaccine for a given flu season is developed based on scientists' best predictions of which strains of the influenza virus will be dominant that particular year. Hence, immunity one year does not necessarily carry over until the next year. Even when vaccination does not prevent the occurrence of influenza in those who were vaccinated, it is likely that the illness will not be as severe in those who were vaccinated.

The "pneumonia shot" specifically protects against one kind of bacterial pneumonia, known as pneumococcal pneumonia, and covers 23 serotypes. Those who are elderly or chronically ill are particularly at risk of developing severe, even fatal, infections. Standard practice is to administer the pneumococcal vaccine only once, with the success rate being approximately 75% to 80%. However, in some seriously ill patients, repeat immunizations may be considered.

For patients on chronic steroids, keep in mind that doses of prednisone higher than 30 mg a day may alter antibody production. Ideally, vaccines should be administered at the lowest possible steroid dose. For patients on rituximab (Rituxan), vaccines should be given at least 3 weeks before the infusion to optimize antibody production. Similarly, vaccines should be given prior to a course of cyclophosphamide (Cytoxan), which also can suppress B-lymphocyte function. IVIg should not pose a problem and, in fact, may provide what is known as passive immunity to many microbes.

The third category of vaccines to consider is the "live virus" vaccines. The vaccines discussed above are made of killed viruses or bacteria and pose no risk of infection. However, vaccination with a live virus does pose some risk of infection, and in someone with an autoimmune disease on immunosuppressive medication, this may be quite dangerous. One such live attenuated vaccine is FluMist, which is administered as a nasal spray. FluMist should not be given to immunosuppressed patients. The definition of immunosuppressed is open to interpretation but clearly includes patients taking prednisone or immunosuppressive agents such as azathioprine (Imuran, Azasan), methotrexate, cyclophosphamide (Cytoxan), or mycophenolate (CellCept).

A relatively new live attenuated vaccine, Zostavax, is appropriate for the prevention of shingles (herpes zoster infection) in patients over the age of 60 years. However, because of the theoretical risk of infection with the herpes zoster virus, patients taking immunosuppressive agents should not receive this vaccine. Whether it would be appropriate to administer this vaccine to a patient with mild, stable Sjögren's should be considered on a case-by-case basis.

TABLE 33–1
Vaccinations and Sjögren's Patients

Killed Vaccines (Recommended if indicated)	Live Vaccines (Not advised except in special circumstances)
Pneumococcus (Pneumovax)	Polio (Sabin)
Influenza	Influenza (FluMist)
Meningitis	Herpes zoster/shingles (Zostavax)

The vaccine most recently in the news is Gardasil, which protects against human papilloma virus infection and the complication of cervical cancer. Experience with this vaccine in young women with Sjögren's is limited; there is too little evidence to recommend its routine use.

For patients who are traveling to locations where special immunizations are recommended, visit http://wwwnc.cdc.gov/travel/yellowbook/2010/chapter-8/immunocompromised-traveler.aspx and scroll down to Table 8–01 for the latest list of killed (inactivated) and live vaccines.

Summing Up

Before vaccinations are given to a Sjögren's patient, current medications should be taken into consideration and live virus vaccines avoided. Otherwise, a standard immunization schedule should be maintained. All patients with Sjögren's should have the pneumococcal pneumonia vaccine, yearly influenza vaccine, and a tetanus-diphtheria booster at least every 10 years. Live virus vaccines such as FluMist and Zostavax should be avoided except in special circumstances to be determined by the physician (Table 33–1).

FOR FURTHER READING

Butler J, Breiman R, Campbell J, et al. Pneumococcal polysaccharide vaccine efficacy: An evaluation of current recommendations. *JAMA.* 1993; 270: 1826.

CDC's Advisory Committee on Immunization Practices (ACIP) recommends universal annual influenza vaccination. Available at: http://www.cdc.gov/media/pressrel/2010/r100224.htm. Accessed May 16, 2010.

Centers for Disease Control and Prevention. Influenza, pneumococcal and tetanus toxoid vaccination of adults—United States, 1993–1997. *MMWR Morb Mortal Wkly Rep.* 2000; 49(SS-9): 39.

Centers for Disease Control and Prevention. Healthy People 2010: Objectives for Improving Health.

Fiore AE, Shay DK, Broder K, et al. Prevention and control of seasonal influenza with vaccines: recommendations of the Advisory Committee on Immunization Practices (ACIP), 2009. *MMWR Recomm Rep.* 2009; 58: 1.

Gardner P, Eickhoff T, Poland GA, et al. Adult immunizations. *Ann Intern Med.* 1996; 124: 35.

Hornberger J, Robertus K. Cost-effectiveness of a vaccine to prevent herpes zoster and postherpetic neuralgia in older adults. *Ann Intern Med.* 2006; 145: 317.

Kroger AT, Atkinson WL, Marcuse EK, Pickering LK. General recommendations on immunization: recommendations of the Advisory Committee on Immunization Practices (ACIP). *MMWR Recomm Rep.* 2006; 55: 1.

Markowitz LE, Dunne EF, Saraiya M, et al. Quadrivalent human papillomavirus vaccine: Recommendations of the Advisory Committee on Immunization Practices (ACIP). *MMWR Recomm Rep.* 2007; 56: 1.

Oxman MN, Levin MJ, Johnson GR, et al. A vaccine to prevent herpes zoster and postherpetic neuralgia in older adults. *N Engl J Med.* 2005; 352: 2271.

34

Disability and Sjögren's

Thomas D. Sutton, Esq, and
Katherine Morland Hammitt, MA

Autoimmune diseases affect as many as 23.5 million Americans, appear to be on the rise, and in 2003 were estimated to cost about $100 billion annually in direct costs in the United States alone, an amount that most likely has increased. This group of interrelated diseases includes 80 to 100 clinically distinct disorders, with Sjögren's being the second most common autoimmune connective tissue disease. The chronic and serious nature of these diseases poses a major burden on patients, their families, and society as a whole.

Sjögren's: A Potentially Disabling Disease

A recent Sjögren's Syndrome Foundation survey found that Sjögren's patients were likely to suffer from a poor quality of life compared to healthier peers. The 2007 "Burden of Illness and General Health-Related Quality of Life in a U.S. Sjögren's Syndrome Population" survey carried out by Harris Interactive emphasizes the many ways in which Sjögren's patients' lives are burdened by their disease (Box 34-1). For example, on a scale of one to four, with one being the highest, patients in this study reported the greatest impact of Sjögren's on physical activities (2.1 to 2.9) followed by intimacy (2.5 to 2.9) and career (2.2 to 2.7). This chapter focuses on the potential disability Sjögren's can cause

Box 34-1
Burden of Illness in Sjögren's Evidence Demonstrated by the Following:

- Range and severity of symptoms
- Diagnostic delays experienced by most patients (on average 6–7 years)
- High utilization of health care and associated high costs
- Use of a wide range of treatments
- Poor quality of life and functioning that affects all aspects of a patient's life

Sjögren's Syndrome Foundation 2007 survey carried out by Harris Interactive.

and, for those in the United States, offers tips and elucidates recent changes in the Social Security Administration (SSA) Disability Listings for those who wish to apply for disability compensation.

The High Cost of Having Sjögren's

The latest studies on costs incurred specifically in Sjögren's were carried out in the United Kingdom and published in 2007 and 2010. Led by Simon Bowman, PhD, FCRP, and colleagues at the University of Birmingham Medical School, the studies concluded that both direct and indirect costs in Sjögren's were about two thirds to four fifths of the costs incurred in rheumatoid arthritis (RA) and four to five times higher than healthy controls. Thus, a very real cost is associated with having Sjögren's (Table 34–1).

Direct costs include those incurred for doctor and other healthcare provider visits, hospitalization, and medications (although the cost of biological therapies was not included in Bowman's study). Indirect costs include much harder to measure costs such as loss of wages because of lack of employment or the need to work fewer hours, time lost from work on the part of others who must take care of the Sjögren's patient, and the need for the patient to hire household or other assistance. In addition, patients and their families face potential loss of health insurance or excessively high premiums; may have more difficulty than their healthy counterparts securing life, health, or disability insurance; and because of their unpredictable health and employment status may face difficulty securing loans such as mortgages.

Can Sjögren's Patients Work?

Many Sjögren's patients hold full- or part-time jobs, but for some who want to work, symptoms and complications of the disease prevent them from doing so.

TABLE 34–1
Annual Indirect and Direct Costs of Sjögren's Syndrome, Rheumatoid Arthritis, and Controls

	Indirect Costs		Direct Costs	
	Low Range	High Range	Not Including Cost of Biological Agents	Total Costs
Control group	£892 (~US$1,418)	£3,382 (~US$5,353)	£949 (~US$1,509)	£1,841–£4,331 (~US$2927–$6,886)
Sjögren's patients	£7,677 (~US$12,150)	£13,502 (~US$16,530)	£2,188 (~US$3,479)	£9,865–£15,690 (~US$15,685–$24,947)
Rheumatoid arthritis patients	£10,444 (~US$16,530)	£17,070 (~US$27,016)	£2,693 (~US$4,282)	£13,137–£19,763 (~US$20,887–$31,423)

Table reprinted from the *Sjögren's Quarterly*, Summer 2010. U.S. comparables added.

Any one of the many symptoms included in this book and/or listed under the U.S. Social Security Administration Listing of Impairments for Sjögren's Syndrome discussed in this chapter can interfere with regular activities and result in disability. For example, fatigue, joint and muscle pain, numbness and nerve pain, gastrointestinal problems, vasculitis, cognitive issues ("brain fog"), or sleep problems can each interfere with one's ability to work. Symptoms that wax and wane can prevent a patient from committing to a set schedule. Dry mouth can lead to difficulty speaking and swallowing and cause loss of teeth and oral pain and infection, problems that might interfere with some jobs. Dry eye can hinder computer use, reading, and working under bright lights. Few studies have examined Sjögren's symptoms in relation to work, but one such investigation published in 2002 by investigators at Schepens Eye Research Institute found that 37.5% of employed Sjögren's patients reported that their dry eye symptoms interfered with their work. The same study found that 60% of Sjögren's patients reported that dry eye symptoms interfered with leisure activities and lifestyle. A work environment also can aggravate symptoms and impairment through low humidity, fluorescent lights, drafts, and fumes (Box 34–2).

Sjögren's patients who need to go on disability should keep in mind that doing so might have unintended consequences. For example, rheumatic disease disability studies have documented that some recipients have faced loss of material possessions (e.g., a car), support of friends or family, and recreational activities. Others have experienced a decreased standard of living, disconnection with intimate partners, loss of hobbies, and reduced self-esteem,

---

Box 34–2
What Can You Do to Improve Your Ability to Stay Employed?

- Take care of yourself, and see your healthcare professionals regularly.
- Understand your skills and the value you can offer an employer.
- Be positive about your ability to contribute to an organization.
- Know your limitations. (If you are exhausted and make a serious mistake, your boss is more likely to remember this than another time when you "saved the day.")
- Be honest about what you can and cannot do.
- Recognize that your employer has specific goals to accomplish. Make sure you understand your employer's needs so you can suggest ways that you can help meet them.
- Talk with your employer to see if accommodations can be made that satisfy both your and your employer's requirements. For example, can tasks or schedules be modified and at the same time meet your employer's needs?
- Know your rights. Familiarize yourself with or talk to a lawyer specializing in the Americans with Disabilities Act.
- Consider investigating private disability insurance in case you reach a point at which you can no longer work.
- If your current or prospective job will not allow the flexibility or changes you need, try to find other positions and careers that will.

---

independence, and socialization with friends from the workplace. When patients go on disability, there is often a concomitant decrease in physical activity that likely compounds the problem. These issues should be anticipated at the time of a disability filing, and if another job is not appropriate in a patient's situation, mitigations should be strategized in advance to prevent emotional and physical repercussions. Remember, Sjögren's patients may or may not be disabled but are "differently abled" in any event.

U.S. Social Security Disability

Despite the fact that Sjögren's is the second most common autoimmune rheumatologic disorder in the United States, its disabling aspects have not historically been well recognized by the Social Security Administration. Indeed, until 2009, Social Security regulations did not contain any disability criteria specific to Sjögren's (the fact that Social Security finally published a Listing of Impairments for Sjögren's Syndrome in 2009 is due in no small part to the advocacy of the Sjögren's Syndrome Foundation). While the regulations now include a Listing of Impairments for Sjögren's, it is still not that familiar to most of the decision makers in the Social Security system. As a result, individuals who suffer from Sjögren's and the attorneys who represent them must be prepared to offer not only thorough medical records but also a thorough presentation regarding the many facets of the disease process and its effects on the individual's ability to function in a workplace.

For most Americans, the disability insurance programs administered by Social Security are the only source of income available when medical problems result in an inability to work. (Some individuals also have private disability insurance, either as a benefit provided by an employer or as the result of an individually purchased policy. The definitions of disability in such policies may differ somewhat from the standard of the public disability programs administered by Social Security and should be carefully consulted before a claim is made.)

There are two disability programs, each of which uses the same statutory definition of disability: the inability to engage in substantial gainful activity (SGA) because of medically determinable impairment(s) that have lasted for 12 months or are expected to last for 12 months or to result in death (42 U.S.C. § 416(i)). Disabled individuals with substantial work histories in covered employment are eligible for Disability Insurance Benefits (DIB) and, following a statutory waiting period, Medicare. In addition, the dependents of individuals found eligible for DIB may receive auxiliary benefits. Individuals without substantial work in covered employment may be eligible for Supplemental Security Income (SSI) if they meet not only the medical standard for disability but also income and resource limitations.

At press time for this publication, the Social Security Administration was considering the addition of Sjögren's to its list of diseases that may be fast-tracked for SSA disability. The Sjögren's Syndrome Foundation (SSF) in 2011 was invited to provide oral and written testimony during the SSA Compassionate Allowances Hearings. Contact the SSF for updates.

The Evaluation Process

When an individual applies for disability benefits from Social Security, a sequential evaluation process is followed in every case. At Step 1, the question is whether the claimant is performing SGA, a term defined somewhat differently for employees and self-employed individuals. If the claimant is performing SGA, the claim is denied; if not, the process continues.

At Step 2, the question is whether the claimant has a medically determinable impairment that is severe, a term Social Security has defined to mean an impairment that is more than slight and has more than a minimal effect on the claimant's ability to perform physical and/or mental work-related activities. The severity test is intended only to screen out obviously unmeritorious claims of disability at an early stage and should not be an obstacle for most Sjögren's patients. There are numerous examples of functional limitations caused by Sjögren's: xerostomia can seriously interfere with the ability to communicate due to lack of saliva; sicca symptoms may cause significant impairment of vision; fatigue may be as severe as that caused by illnesses such as lupus or chronic fatigue syndrome. These and many other symptoms of Sjögren's may result in more than minimal functional limitations, so that Sjögren's should rarely, if ever, be dismissed as a non-severe impairment at Step 2. If there is at least one severe impairment, the process continues.

At Step 3, the claimant may be found disabled if his or her condition meets or is clinically equivalent to the criteria set forth in the Listing of Impairments, found at 20 C.F.R. Part 404, Subpart P, Appendix 1. In § 14.00, the preface to the immune system disorders listings, Social Security states the following regarding Sjögren's syndrome:

a. *General.* (i) Sjögren's syndrome is an immunomediated disorder of the exocrine glands. Involvement of the lacrimal and salivary glands is the hallmark feature, resulting in symptoms of dry eyes and dry mouth, and possible complications, such as corneal damage, blepharitis (eyelid inflammation), dysphagia (difficulty in swallowing), dental caries, and the inability to speak for extended periods of time. Involvement of the exocrine glands of the upper airways may result in persistent dry cough.

(ii) Many other organ systems may be involved, including musculoskeletal (arthritis, myositis), respiratory (interstitial fibrosis), gastrointestinal (dysmotility, dysphagia, involuntary weight loss), genitourinary (interstitial cystitis, renal tubular acidosis), skin (purpura, vasculitis), neurologic (central nervous system disorders, cranial and peripheral neuropathies), mental (cognitive dysfunction, poor memory), and neoplastic (lymphoma). Severe fatigue and malaise are frequently reported. Sjögren's syndrome may be associated with other autoimmune disorders (for example, rheumatoid arthritis or SLE); usually the clinical features of the associated disorder predominate.

b. *Documentation of Sjögren's syndrome.* If you have Sjögren's syndrome, the medical evidence will generally, but not always, show that your disease satisfies the criteria in the current "Criteria for the Classification of Sjögren's Syndrome" by the American College of Rheumatology found in the most recent edition of the Primer on the Rheumatic Diseases published by the Arthritis Foundation.

The Listing for Sjögren's Syndrome is found at § 14.10 of the Listing of Impairments:

14.10 *Sjögren's syndrome.* As described in 14.00D7. With:

A. Involvement of two or more organs/body systems, with:
  1. One of the organs/body systems involved to at least a moderate level of severity; and
  2. At least two of the constitutional symptoms or signs (severe fatigue, fever, malaise, or involuntary weight loss).
OR
B. Repeated manifestations of Sjögren's syndrome, with at least two of the constitutional symptoms or signs (severe fatigue, fever, malaise, or involuntary weight loss) and one of the following at the marked level:
  1. Limitation of activities of daily living.
  2. Limitation in maintaining social functioning.
  3. Limitation in completing tasks in a timely manner due to deficiencies in concentration, persistence, or pace.

For purposes of the Listing of Impairments, constitutional symptoms or signs "means severe fatigue, fever, malaise, or involuntary weight loss. Severe fatigue means a frequent sense of exhaustion that results in significantly reduced physical activity or mental function. Malaise means frequent feelings of illness, bodily discomfort, or lack of well-being that result in significantly reduced physical activity or mental function." §12.00(C). In addition, § 12.00(I) of the Listing defines the functional criteria for disability from immune system disorders as follows:

To satisfy the functional criterion in a listing, your immune system disorder must result in a "marked" level of limitation in one of three general areas of functioning: Activities of daily living, social functioning, or difficulties in completing tasks due to deficiencies in concentration, persistence, or pace. Functional limitation may result from the impact of the disease process itself on your mental functioning, physical functioning, or both your mental and physical functioning. This could result from persistent or intermittent symptoms, such as depression, severe fatigue, or pain, resulting in a limitation of your ability to do a task, to concentrate, to persevere at a task, or to perform the task at an acceptable rate of speed. You may also have limitations because of your treatment and its side effects (see 14.00G).

When "marked" is used as a standard for measuring the degree of functional limitation, it means more than moderate but less than extreme. We do not define "marked" by a specific number of different activities of daily living in which your functioning is impaired, different behaviors in which your social functioning is impaired, or tasks that you are able to complete, but by the nature and overall degree of interference with your functioning. You may have a marked limitation when several activities or functions are impaired, or even when only one is impaired. Also, you need not be totally precluded from performing an activity to have a marked limitation, as long as the degree of limitation seriously interferes with your ability to function independently, appropriately, and effectively. The term "marked" does not imply that you must be confined to bed, hospitalized, or in a nursing home.

Activities of daily living include, but are not limited to, such activities as doing household chores, grooming and hygiene, using a post office, taking public transportation, or paying bills. We will find that you have a "marked" limitation of activities of daily living if you have a serious limitation in your ability to maintain a household or take public transportation because of symptoms, such as pain, severe fatigue, anxiety, or difficulty concentrating, caused by your immune system disorder (including manifestations of the disorder) or its treatment, even if you are able to perform some self-care activities.

Social functioning includes the capacity to interact independently, appropriately, effectively, and on a sustained basis with others. It includes the ability to communicate effectively with others. We will find that you have a "marked" limitation in maintaining social functioning if you have a serious limitation in social interaction on a sustained basis because of symptoms, such as pain, severe fatigue, anxiety, or difficulty concentrating, or a pattern of exacerbation and remission, caused by your immune system disorder (including manifestations of the disorder) or its treatment, even if you are able to communicate with close friends or relatives.

Completing tasks in a timely manner involves the ability to sustain concentration, persistence, or pace to permit timely completion of tasks commonly found in work settings. We will find that you have a "marked" limitation in completing tasks if you have a serious limitation in your ability to sustain concentration or pace adequate to complete work-related tasks because of symptoms, such as pain, severe fatigue, anxiety, or difficulty concentrating, caused by your immune system disorder (including manifestations of the disorder) or its treatment, even if you are able to do some routine activities of daily living.

If the claimant meets or equals in clinical severity all of the criteria set forth above, he or she will be found disabled at Step 3. If not, the sequential evaluation process continues.

At Step 4, the question is whether the claimant is able to perform past relevant work, either as he or she performed it or as it is generally performed in the national economy. At this point in the evaluation, Social Security evaluates the claimant's residual functional capacity (RFC) for work, which is what he or she can still do despite the effects of all medical impairments in combination. Under the regulations, work performed in the past 15 years that was SGA and lasted long enough to learn how to perform it is generally considered relevant. The claimant has the burden to show that his or her medically determinable impairment(s) preclude the performance of all past relevant work. If the claimant is found able to perform any of his or her past relevant work, the claim is denied; if not, the process continues.

At Step 5, the question is whether the claimant is able to perform any other work in the national economy, taking into account age, education, work experience, and RFC. At this step, Social Security has the burden of demonstrating that jobs within the parameters of the claimant's RFC exist in significant numbers. For claimants over the age of 50, a finding of disability may be directed by the regulations if exertional limitations reduce the RFC to sedentary or light work. However, for claimants under the age of 50, with few exceptions, a finding of disability will be made at Step 5 only if the individual proves that he or she is incapable of performing any kind of work on a regular and continuing (i.e., full-time) basis. If the claimant proves such inability, disability will be found; if not, the claim will be denied at this final step of the evaluation.

Social Security Evaluation Process

If the claimant meets the requirements in one step, he or she then moves onto the next step for consideration (Table 34–2).

THE ROLE OF THE TREATING PHYSICIAN

As is obvious from the foregoing description, the evaluation process followed by Social Security is detailed and exacting. Sjögren's patients should review the

TABLE 34–2

Steps of the Disability Evaluation Process

Step 1	Is the claimant performing "substantial gainful activity" (SGA)?
Step 2	Does the claimant have a medically determinable impairment that can be defined as severe?
Step 3	Does the claimant's condition meet or is clinically equivalent to the criteria set forth in the Social Security Administration Listing of Impairments?
Step 4	Is the claimant able to perform past relevant work?
Step 5	Is the claimant able to perform any other work, taking into account age, education, work experience, and "residual functional capacity" (RFC)?

2009 listing criteria with their rheumatologists and should also review the criteria for other immune system disorders (e.g., lupus) if they, like many Sjögren's patients, also suffer from those disorders. Great care should be taken to document involvement in every relevant organ or body system, constitutional signs such as severe fatigue and weight loss, and functional impact on daily activities, social functioning, and task completion. The opinion of a treating physician (especially that of a rheumatologist) regarding the nature and severity of the Sjögren's, particularly if it is well supported by treatment notes, clinical findings, and laboratory tests, should be accorded great weight in the disability determination process.

If it is not clear that the Sjögren's alone meets all of the criteria of the Listing, all of the claimant's impairments in combination must be considered in determining whether he or she has the RFC to sustain employment. Sjögren's, along with other physical impairments that may be present (e.g., diabetes with neuropathy, arthritis, chronic heart failure), may cause such limitations in exertion (i.e., ability to walk, stand, sit, lift, carry, push and pull) that the claimant is found disabled from a physical standpoint.

In addition, all nonexertional limitations must be considered, including mental, vision, manipulative, speech and hearing, postural, and environmental limitations. For example, Sjögren's may cause central nervous system effects similar to those seen in cases of lupus cerebritis, and cognitive dysfunction may be so severe as a result of this (or from a comorbid condition such as depressive disorder) that the claimant is unable to perform the mental functional requirements of work (e.g., ability to concentrate, focus, deal with stress, accept criticism from supervisors, etc.). When all of the claimant's exertional and nonexertional limitations resulting from all of his or her impairments in combination are considered, disability may be found where the claimant cannot perform past relevant work or sustain alternative employment on a regular and continuing basis. Thus, a claimant's failure to meet or equal the criteria of the Listing of Impairments is by no means fatal to his or her disability claim.

CLAIMANTS' RIGHTS

Individuals whose applications are denied have the right to a hearing with an Administrative Law Judge and to review of adverse hearing decisions by Social Security's Appeals Council. Claimants who are administratively denied at every level of appeal may institute civil actions against Social Security in the federal courts, which have been receptive to claims from Sjögren's patients in the past.

Several appellate opinions contain helpful discussions of the impact of Sjögren's on disability claimants, including Phillips v. Barnhart, 357 F.3d 1232 (11th Cir. 2004) (claimant with Sjögren's and fibromyalgia) and Swindle v. Sullivan, 914 F.2d 222 (11th Cir. 1990) (claimant with Sjögren's and lupus), which required Social Security to obtain Vocational Expert testimony because the claimant's impairments could reasonably cause pain and other nonexertional limitations. In Beusching v. Bowen, 1988 U.S. Dist. LEXIS 15756 (C.D. Cal. 1988), the court ruled that Sjögren's and degenerative joint disease could explain the claimant's pain and swelling in her fingers, and ordered an award of benefits despite the fact that she did not have lupus and that her peripheral vascular disease had been surgically resolved. In Mack v. Secretary of HHS, 747 F.Supp. 1208 (E.D. La. 1990), the court awarded benefits to a claimant whose Sjögren's caused corneal inflammation, eye infection, mucus accumulation, light sensitivity, and blurred vision, where the Vocational Expert testified that if she had to frequently apply medication to her eyes she could not sustain work. In Steen v. Astrue, 2008 WL 4449602 (N.D. Cal. 2008), the court awarded benefits where the treating rheumatologist diagnosed Sjögren's complicated by a monoclonal gammopathy and fibromyalgia, with problems including xerostomia with dysphagia and a host of extra-exocrine gland problems, keratoconjunctivitis sicca, and "overwhelming constitutional symptoms," and concluded that "the totality of her disease associated symptoms render her disabled."

On the other hand, in Mansfield v. Barnhart, 2005 WL 1476370 (S.D. Ind. 2005), the court affirmed a denial of benefits where the claimant's testimony about severe fatigue and inability to function resulting from her Sjögren's and rheumatoid arthritis were belied by her daily activities, her improvement with methotrexate (Trexall, Rheumatrex) injections, physical therapy, and hydroxychloroquine (Plaquenil), and her own treating rheumatologist's opinion that she had the capacity to lift 50 pounds and sit throughout an 8-hour workday.

TIPS FOR THE APPLICANT

These cases illustrate the fact that it is not necessarily easy to succeed with a disability claim, even where a serious illness like Sjögren's is involved. Sjögren's patients are well advised not only to report all of their symptoms at each physician visit, but also to keep a personal daily journal of problems from the onset of inability to work (Box 34-3). For example, if doing normal housework for one day results in being effectively bedridden for the next two to three days due to excessive fatigue or pain, the individual should document this in his or her journal. Of course, Sjögren's patients should have regular visits with a rheumatologist experienced in the treatment of this disease, and should make certain that primary physicians receive copies of all treatment notes and test reports. Finally, patients who suffer from Sjögren's who have become unable to work should retain the services of an attorney experienced in Social Security disability law early in the application process in order to facilitate communication with the physicians and proper presentation of the evidence of disability at every stage of the adjudication process. Attorneys who practice extensively in the disability arena can be quite helpful in obtaining favorable determinations at the early stages of the process, and where claims are denied their services are essential to improve the odds of prevailing on appeal, whether before a Social Security Administrative Law Judge or the federal courts.

With the help of caring professionals in medicine and law, individuals disabled by Sjögren's should be able to obtain the disability benefits provided by the Social Security Act, which are necessary to ensure at least partial replacement of lost work income and medical coverage to enable them to maintain as normal a life as possible while fighting this devastating illness.

Summing Up

Sjögren's can result in a high financial cost to patients and their families. As a potentially disabling disease, some patients who want to work or simply handle daily household tasks cannot do so. Before applying for social security disability, Sjögren's patients in the United States need to learn about the specific

Box 34-3
Quick Tips for Claimants

- Visit your rheumatologist regularly.
- Report all symptoms at each physician visit.
- Make sure your physician documents involvement of every relevant organ or body system, constitutional signs, and impact on daily activities.
- Keep your own personal daily journal, noting symptoms and how they affect your ability to perform tasks.
- Make sure that primary physicians receive copies of all treatment notes and test reports.
- Retain the services of an attorney experienced in Social Security disability law early in the application process.

For more tips, visit the Sjögren's Syndrome Foundation website at www.sjogrens.org and download the "Fact Sheet on Tips on Obtaining Disability Benefits from the Social Security Administration."

requirements and processes set by the Social Security Administration, consult with an experienced attorney, and make use of the many tips offered here for presenting a better case. Sjögren's is now included in the Listing of Disabilities following recent efforts by the Sjögren's Syndrome Foundation, facilitating the process for obtaining social security disability.

FOR FURTHER READING

http://www.niaid.nih.gov/topics/autoimmune/documents/adccfinal.pdf. U.S. Department of Health and Human Services, National Institutes of Health, National Institute of Allergy and Infectious Diseases, "Progress in Autoimmune Diseases Research," Report to Congress, March 2005.

http://www.socialsecurity.gov/disability/professionals/bluebook/14.00-Immune-Adult.htm#14_01. Social Security Disability Guidelines for Immune System Disorders in Adults.

http://www.socialsecurity.gov/disability/professionals/bluebook/114.00-Immune-Childhood.htm#114_01. Social Security Disability Guidelines for Immune System Disorders in Children.

http://www.socialsecurity.gov/compassionateallowances. Social Security Disability Compassionate Allowances for fast-tracking disability decision-making for specific diseases.

http://www.sjogrens.org/home/about-sjogrens-syndrome/brochures-and-fact-sheets. Sjögren's Syndrome Foundation Brochures and Fact Sheets.

http://www.aarda.org/autoimmune_statistics.php. American Autoimmune Related Diseases Association, Inc. Autoimmune Statistics. Autoimmune Disease Fact Sheet.

http://www.ada.gov. U.S. Department of Justice. Americans with Disabilities Act.

Bowman SJ. Estimating indirect costs in Sjögren's. *Sjögren's Quarterly.* 2010; 5(2).

Bowman SJ, St Pierre Y, Sutcliffe N, et al. Estimating indirect costs in primary Sjögren's syndrome. *J Rheumatol.* 2010; 37(5): 1010–5.

Callaghan R, Prabu A, Allan RB, et al. UK Sjögren's Interest Group. Direct healthcare costs and predictors of costs in patients with primary Sjögren's syndrome. *Rheumatology (Oxford).* 2007; 46(1): 105–11.

Meijer JM, Meiners PM, Huddleston Slater JJ, et al. Health-related quality of life, employment and disability in patients with Sjögren's syndrome. *Rheumatology (Oxford).* 2009; 48(9): 1077–82.

Segal B, Bowman SJ, Fox PC, et al. Primary Sjögren's syndrome: health experiences and predictors of health quality among patients in the United States. *Health & Quality of Life Outcomes.* 2009; 7: 46.

Sullivan RM, Cermak JM, Papas AS, et al. Economic and quality of life impact of dry eye symptoms in women with Sjögren's syndrome. *Adv Exp Med Biol.* 2002; 506(PtB): 1183–8.

35

Web, Print, and Media Resource Manual

Editor's note: Please consult the Sjögren's Syndrome Foundation website at www.sjogrens.org for updates.

When searching for information on Sjögren's, we advise you to know your source: information is only as good as the expertise of those who provide it. The motivation of those supplying information is important, too; for example, ask yourself if the source is trying to sell you something. Credibility is key, and that is why our highest recommendation for a resource on Sjögren's is the Sjögren's Syndrome Foundation (SSF). Remember, too, that your own health-care team is a critical resource for your questions and needs.

In offering a list of resources, we advise you on several points:

1. We cannot include every publication, organization, or other potential resource. We have selected some of those with which we are familiar and include these as a starting point for your search for additional information and support.
2. The resources provided are for information purposes only. We cannot guarantee the accuracy of information provided by other sources.
3. Recognize that websites and phone numbers change frequently and that new resources constantly are being created. By joining the SSF and taking advantage of its many offerings (including a subscription to *The Moisture Seekers* newsletter, patient conference discounts, and access to the members-only side of the SSF website), you will be informed of new opportunities and resources as they become available.

Organizations

SJÖGREN'S SYNDROME FOUNDATION

www.sjogrens.org
Tel: (800) 475-6473 or (301) 530-4420
The SSF is the only nonprofit group specifically geared to helping Sjögren's patients and their healthcare providers in the United States and around

the world. The SSF is the most credible resource for information and education, and its Medical and Scientific Advisory Board is composed of top international clinicians and researchers in Sjögren's.

INTERNATIONAL SJÖGREN'S NETWORK

www.sjogrens.org/home/get-connected/isn

Facilitated by the SSF, the International Sjögren's Network was created in 2009 during the International Symposium on Sjögren's Syndrome in Brest, France, to bring patient advocacy groups from around the world together to share information and increase international awareness and advocacy.

Organizations for Related Diseases

AMERICAN AUTOIMMUNE RELATED DISEASES ASSOCIATION (AARDA)

www.aarda.org

Tel: (586) 776-3900

AARDA is dedicated to the eradication of autoimmune disease. This nonprofit group serves all of those connected to autoimmune disease and focuses on autoimmune disease as an interrelated group of more than 100 diseases, including Sjögren's. The SSF partners with AARDA on advocacy issues and serves on the National Coalition of Autoimmune Patient Groups led by AARDA.

ARTHRITIS FOUNDATION

www.arthritis.org

Tel: (800) 283-7800

While the Arthritis Foundation primarily focuses on osteoarthritis and rheumatoid arthritis (which can occur with Sjögren's), information on Sjögren's and related rheumatic diseases is also provided.

LUPUS FOUNDATION OF AMERICA

www.lupus.org

Tel: (202) 349-1155

LUPUS RESEARCH INSTITUTE

www.lupusresearchinstitute.org

Tel: (212) 812–9881

S.L.E. LUPUS FOUNDATION

www.lupusny.org
Tel: (800) 745-8787 or (212) 685-4118 (NY) or (310) 657-5667
(Los Angeles)

SCLERODERMA FOUNDATION

www.scleroderma.org
Tel: (800) 722-4673 or (978) 463-5843

FEDERAL GOVERNMENT RESOURCE AND TREATMENT CENTER

Sjögren's Syndrome Clinic
National Institute of Dental and Craniofacial Research
National Institutes of Health
Bethesda, Maryland
http://www.nidcr.nih.gov/Research/NIDCRLaboratories/
MolecularPhysiology/SjogrensSyndrome/default.htm

Printed Materials on Sjögren's

SSF brochures and pamphlets can be downloaded at www.sjogrens.org, or call
the SSF at (800) 475-6473 or (301) 530-4420 for copies. Medical professionals
can request complimentary copies to distribute in their offices.

SSF BROCHURES

- *What is Sjögren's Syndrome?*
- *Dry Eyes: A hallmark symptom of Sjögren's syndrome*
- *Dry Mouth: A hallmark symptom of Sjögren's syndrome*
- *Research—Our Hope for the Future*
- *Questions to Ask Your Doctor About Sjögren's Syndrome and Dry Eye*

SSF PAMPHLETS

- *Products Used by People with Sjögren's Syndrome*
  Updated in 2010, this SSF pamphlet lists prescription and over-the-
  counter drugs and products for common symptoms of Sjögren's, the
  company that produces each item, and how to contact manufacturers.
- *Sjögren's Syndrome Self-Help: Tips for More Comfortable Living*
  This SSF pamphlet offers helpful ideas for living with Sjögren's and
  coping with symptoms. It is written by Dona Frosio and the SSF
  Publications Committee and is updated regularly.

SSF NEWSLETTERS

¤ *The Moisture Seekers Newsletter*
Join the SSF and receive the newsletter, *The Moisture Seekers*, which is published 11 times a year and features articles from leading medical professionals, tips for living with Sjögren's, and answers to some of the most popular questions about Sjögren's.

¤ *Sjögren's Quarterly*
Designed for the professional audience this newsletter also is available by subscription to patients and others with an interest in Sjögren's who want more in-depth medical and scientific information. Call the SSF to subscribe.

OTHER PAMPHLETS

¤ *Questions and Answers about Sjögren's Syndrome,* a publication of the U.S. Department of Health and Human Services, National Institutes of Health, National Institute of Arthritis and Musculoskeletal and Skin Diseases (NIAMS), updated 2010. NIH Publication No. 01–4861.
The SSF assisted NIAMS in compiling this Q&A booklet, which includes answers to common questions about Sjögren's, including symptoms, causes, diagnosis, and treatment. This pamphlet also is available in Spanish. Copies may be downloaded or ordered from NIAMS at http://www.niams.nih.gov/Health_Info/Sjogrens_Syndrome/default.asp.

¤ *Dry Mouth (Xerostomia),* a publication of the National Institutes of Health (NIH), National Institute of Dental and Craniofacial Research (NIDCR), 2002, NIH Publication No. 02–3174.
This pamphlet discusses the causes of dry mouth and the importance of saliva to oral health, provides steps to follow to relieve dryness, and includes information on Dry Mouth, Sjögren's and the Sjögren's Syndrome Clinic at the NIDCR. The publication also is available in Spanish. Copies may be downloaded or ordered from NIDCR at http://www.nidcr.nih.gov/OralHealth/Topics/DryMouth/DryMouth.htm.

Other Media

¤ A DVD for newly diagnosed patients, *Sjögren's Syndrome: A Place to Begin,* is available for viewing on the SSF website at www.sjogrens.org. Medical professionals can request a supply of DVDs to give out free-of-charge to their patients. Contact the Sjögren's Syndrome

Foundation office at (800) 475-6473 or (301) 530-4420 to learn more. This program introduces viewers to three Sjögren's patients who share their journey and Sjögren's experts who discuss the causes, treatments and manifestations of Sjögren's. The DVD provides patients with a place to begin as they develop a partnership and treatment plan with their physician.

¤ Audiotapes from SSF patient conferences also are available from the SSF through www.sjogrens.org or (800) 475-6473.

Websites for Information and Support

¤ www.sjogrens.org: The SSF website offers a wealth of information on Sjögren's, ways to connect with Sjögren's patients (for example, through support groups), participate in activities to raise awareness, and join in educational opportunities (for example, patient conferences)

¤ www.facebook.com/SjogrensSyndromeFoundation: Connect with the SSF on Facebook. Check out SSF photos, upcoming events and connect with other patients.

¤ www.livingwithdryness.com: Created by Daiichi-Sankyo, the makers of Evoxac, this website was launched in 2010 as a resource for patients on dry mouth and dry eye.

¤ www.sjogrensforum.com: Created by a patient–physician team and entitled, "Sjögren's Forum–Living Well with Sjögren's," this forum provides information on Sjögren's symptoms, tests, and medications and gives patients the opportunity to ask questions of the rheumatologist.

¤ www.dry.org: This site was created by a Sjögren's patient to offer support and information through access to articles, an e-mail list-serv (SS-L) for informational and medical questions and discussion, and a second e-mail list-serv (TalkSjo) for more socially oriented interaction and support.

¤ www.sjogrensworld.org: This internet community was created by two Sjögren's patients to support patients by offering live chats, message forums, and particularly information on neurological involvement in Sjögren's.

Registries

International Sjögren's Syndrome Registry, University of California, San Francisco
http://sicca.ucsf.edu/intl-usa.html
Tel (415) 476-0535; e-mail sicca@dentistry.ucsf.edu,

This collaboration involving nine international sites is known as the Sjögren's International Collaborative Clinical Alliance (SICCA). Funded by the National Institutes of Health, SICCA collects, processes, and stores clinical data and biospecimens from Sjögren's patients, family members, and healthy controls to promote Sjögren's research. The nine sites are University of Buenos Aires/German Hospital, Buenos Aires, Argentina; Peking Union Medical College Hospital, Beijing, China; Rigshospitalet, Copenhagen, Denmark; Kanazawa Medical University, Kanazawa, Japan; Aravind Eye Hospital, Madurai, India; Kings College London Dental Institute, London, United Kingdom; Johns Hopkins University, Baltimore, Maryland; University of California, San Francisco; and University of Pennsylvania, Philadelphia.

Sjögren's Genetics Network (SGENE)
Oklahoma Medical Research Foundation
Tel (405) 271-2534
The SGENE network is collecting DNA samples and associated clinical data for well-designed genetic studies through an international collaborative group of researchers and clinicians.

Multiple Autoimmune Disease Genetics Consortium (MADGC)
The Feinstein Institute for Medical Research
http://www.madgc.org
Tel 877-698-9467; e-mail madgc@nshs.edu
This consortium is striving to identify and understand the genes that autoimmune diseases have in common. While the major focus is on rheumatoid arthritis, multiple sclerosis, lupus, autoimmune thyroid disease, and type I diabetes, information about Sjögren's concurring in conjunction with these related diseases or in family members is included.

National Databank for Rheumatic Diseases
Arthritis Research Center Foundation
http://www.arthritis-research.org
Tel (316) 263-2125 or (800) 323-5871
This patient-reported research data bank collects information on rheumatic diseases, including Sjögren's.

Research Registry for Neonatal Lupus
NYU Medical Center
http://www.neonatallupus.com
Tel (212) 263-2255
This database was established in 1994 and provides an invaluable resource for clinicians and researchers on neonatal lupus, which can occur in babies born to mothers who are positive for anti-SSA (Ro) and/or anti-SSB (La).

Clinical Trials

http://clinicaltrials.gov
The ClinicalTrials.gov site is compiled and overseen by the federal
government agency the National Institutes of Health (NIH) and
contains federally and privately supported clinical trials conducted in
the United States and around the world in a searchable database.
http://www.ciscrp.org
The Center for Information and Study on Clinical Research Participation
(CISCRP) is a nonprofit organization dedicated to educating and
informing the public, patients, medical/research communities, the
media, and policy makers about clinical research and the role each
party plays in the process.

Select Books

BOOKS SPECIFICALLY ON SJÖGREN'S

The Sjögren's Syndrome Survival Guide, by Teri P. Rumpf and Katherine
Morland Hammitt. New Harbinger Publications, 2003.

This invaluable resource on Sjögren's provides the latest medical information, research results, and treatment methods available as well as effective
self-help strategies. Patients learn how to improve their quality of life by
taking an active role in their care and developing true partnerships with their
doctors. Hammitt compiles clear answers to questions she and many other
Sjögren's patients long found inaccessible, while Rumpf, a clinical psychologist, covers aspects of relationships, work, and finding informed and supportive medical care.

A Body Out of Balance: Understanding and Treating Sjögren's Syndrome, by
Ruth Fremes and Nancy Carteron. Avery/Penguin Putnam, 2003.

Fremes, a Sjögren's patient, discusses Sjögren's symptoms, while her doctor,
Dr. Carteron, explains the biological process, diagnosis, and treatment.
Another invaluable resource, this book provides readers with a comprehensive
guide to the wide array of symptoms of Sjögren's, traditional and complementary treatments, and coping mechanisms for patients to devise their own holis-
tic personal treatment plan.

*The Official Patient's Sourcebook on Sjögren's Syndrome: A Revised and
Updated Director for the Internet Age,* edited by James N. Parker and Philip M.
Parker. ICON Group International, 2002.

In addition to providing basic information on Sjögren's syndrome, the
authors explain how to search for and find practical information. Directions
focus on Internet use and include instructions on finding information about

clinical trials, research studies on Sjögren's, medications, alternative medicine, nutrition, medical libraries, and insurance rights.

PRACTICAL GUIDES AND BOOKS ON SYMPTOMS OCCURRING IN SJÖGREN'S

2010 Drug Guide, Arthritis Today. Arthritis Foundation. Updated annually. http://www.arthritistoday.org/treatments/drug-guide/index.php.

Disability Workbook for Social Security Applicants, by Douglas M. Smith, Physicians' Disability Services, Inc., 7th ed., 2008. http://www.disability facts.com.

Women, Work and Autoimmune Disease, by Rosalind Joffe and Joan Friedlander. Demos Medical Publishing, 2008.

Chronic Pain for Dummies, by Stuart S. Kassan, Charles J. Vierck, and Elizabeth Vierck. Wiley Publishing, Inc. 2008.

Peripheral Neuropathy: When the Numbness, Weakness, and Pain Won't Stop, by Norman Latov. An American Academy of Neurology Press Quality of Life Guide, Demos Medical Publishing LLC, 2007.

You Can Cope with Peripheral Neuropathy: 365 Tips for Living a Full Life, by Mims Cushing and Norman Latov. Demos Medical Publishing LLC, 2009.

Nuances of Nasal & Sinus Self-Help, by Susan F. Rudy. Trafford Publishing, 2003.

The Vulvodynia Survival Guide: How to Overcome Painful Vaginal Symptoms & Enjoy an Active Lifestyle, by Howard I. Glazer and Gae Rodke. Oakland: New Harbinger Publications, 2002.

The Woman's Book of Sleep: A Complete Resource Guide, by Amy J. Wolfson. New Harbinger Publications, 2001.

The Memory Bible: An Innovative Strategy for Keeping Your Brain Young, by Gary Small. Hyperion, 2002.

The Balance Within: The Science Connecting Health and Emotions, by Esther M. Sternberg. W. H. Freeman and Company, 2001.

I-Can't-Chew Cookbook: Delicious Soft Diet Recipes for People with Chewing, Swallowing, and Dry-Mouth Disorders, by J. Randy Wilson. Hunter House Publishers, 2003.

Eating for Acid Reflux: A Handbook and Cookbook for Those with Heartburn, by Jill Sklar and Annabel Cohen. Marlowe and Co., 2003.

Dry Mouth—The Malevolent Symptom: A Clinical Guide, Leo M. Sreebny and Arjan Vissink, editors. Blackwell Publishing, John Wiley & Sons, Inc., 2010. *Note:* Geared toward clinicians and allied healthcare givers but also written with the hope that patients will want to read and learn from this book. www.wiley.com/go/sreebny.

BOOKS ON COPING WITH CHRONIC ILLNESS

Dancing at the River's Edge: A Patient and her Doctor Negotiate Life with Chronic Illness, by Alida Brill. Schaffner Press, 2009.

A Delicate Balance: Living Successfully with Chronic Illness, by Susan Milstrey Wells. Perseus Publishing, 1998.

Living Well with Autoimmune Disease: What Your Doctor Doesn't Tell You That You Need to Know, by Mary J. Shomon. Harper Collins, 2002.

Thriving with Your Autoimmune Disorder: A Woman's Mind-Body Guide, by Simone Ravicz. New Harbinger, 2000.

Sick and Tired of Feeling Sick and Tired: Living with Invisible Chronic Illness, by Paul J. Donoghue and Mary E. Siegel. W. W. Norton & Company, 2000.

Finding the Way Home: A Compassionate Approach to Illness, by Gayle Heiss. QED Press, 1997.

Beyond Chaos: One Man's Journey Alongside His Chronically Ill Wife, by Gregg Piburn. Arthritis Foundation, 1999.

The Chronic Illness Workbook: Strategies and Solutions for Taking Back Your Life, by Patricia A. Fennell. New Harbinger Publications, 2001.

BOOKS ON RELATED AND OVERLAPPING CONDITIONS

The Autoimmune Connection: Essential Information for Women on Diagnosis, Treatment, and Getting On with Your Life, by Rita Baron-Faust and Jill P. Buyon. McGraw-Hill/Contemporary Books, 2003.

The Lupus Book: A Guide for Patients and Their Families, by Daniel J. Wallace. Oxford University Press, 2009.

Coping with Lupus, by Robert Phillips. Avery, 2001.

Lupus: Everything You Need to Know, by Robert G. Lahita and Robert H. Phillips. Avery, 1998.

Lupus, My Doctor, and Me: A Sacred Diaglogue, by Anita A. Fricklas and Stuart S. Kassan, Astute Press, 2010.

All About Fibromyalgia: A Guide for Patients and Their Families, by Daniel J. Wallace and Janice Brock Wallace. Oxford University Press, 2002.

The Scleroderma Book: A Guide for Patients and Families, by Maureen D. Mayes. Oxford University Press, 2005.

The Interstitial Cystitis Survival Guide: Your Guide to the Latest Treatment Options and Coping Strategies, by Robert M. Moldwin. New Harbinger, 2000.

Coping with Chronic Fatigue Syndrome: Nine Things You Can Do, by Fred Friedberg. New Harbinger, 1995.

All About Osteoarthritis: The Definitive Resource for Arthritis Patients and Their Families, by Nancy E. Lane and Daniel J. Wallace. Oxford University Press, 2002.

Resources Available in Spanish

An information sheet in Spanish on Sjögren's is available from the U.S. Department of Health and Human Services, National Institutes of Health, National Institute of Arthritis and Musculoskeletal and Skin Diseases. In addition, both pamphlets produced by the NIH and cited under "Brochures and Pamphlets" are available in Spanish.

See also *Síndrome de Sjögren,* by Juan-Manuel Anaya, Manuel Ramos-Casals, Mario Garcia Carrasco; Corpóracion Para Investigaciones Biológicas, Medellin, Colombia, 2001, and (for professionals) *Síndrome de Sjogren,* edited by Manuel Ramos-Casals, Mario Garcia-Carrasco, Juan Manuel Anaya, Joaquim Coll, Ricard Cervera, Josep Font, Miguel Ingelmo; Masson, Barcelona, 2003.

For Professionals

SJÖGREN'S QUARTERLY

This newsletter is geared toward clinicians and researchers in Sjögren's and is billed as the professionals' resource on Sjögren's. Published by the SSF, professionals may receive a complimentary subscription. Inquiries may be sent to sq@sjogrens.org.

DRY EYE VIDEOS

Clinical videos covering diagnosis and management of dry eye are now available from the Tear Film and Ocular Surface Society (TFOS). The videos are based on the 2007 Dry Eye Workshop (DEWS) sponsored by TFOS. This workshop brought international experts together to focus on developing an evidence-based report on the definition, classification, diagnosis, and management of dry eye. The videos are available at http://www.tearfilm.org/podcast.php.

SJÖGREN'S BLOG ON MEDSCAPE

Robert Fox, MD, PhD, maintains a blog and encourages rigorous discussion on issues related to Sjögren's for physicians on Medscape. *Rheum With a View* provides a forum for physicians to share patient cases and learn together about this condition. Visit http://boards.medscape.com/forums/.29f13a88/?@901. dYAya5mtcum to read and post comments. First-time users will need to complete a short registration, but otherwise access to the entire site is free. Please note that the discussion portion of the blog is limited to physicians, and physician status will be verified through the American Medical Association.

SSF WEBSITE

The SSF website (www.sjogrens.org) offers sections providing information and opportunities specifically for healthcare providers and researchers.

Professional Societies

RHEUMATOLOGY/IMMUNOLOGY

American College of Rheumatology (ACR): www.rheumatology.org
European League Against Rheumatism (EULAR): www.eular.org
Federation of Clinical Immunology Societies (FOCIS): www.focisnet.org

OCULAR

American Academy of Ophthalmology (AAO): www.aao.org
Contact Lens Association of Ophthalmologists (CLAO): www.clao.org
Tear Film and Ocular Surface Society (TFOS): www.tearfilm.org
Association for Research in Vision and Ophthalmology (ARVO):
   www.arvo.org
American Optometric Association (AOA): www.aoa.org
American Academy of Optometry (AAO): www.aaopt.org

ORAL

American Dental Association (ADA): www.ada.org
American Association for Dental Research (AADR): www.aadronline.org
International Association for Dental Research (IADR): www.iadr.org
American Dental Education Association (ADEA): www.adea.org
Academy of General Dentistry (AGD): www.agd.org
American Dental Hygienists' Association (ADHA): www.adha.org

GLOSSARY

achlorhydria: Gastric acid deficiency.

acini: One of the small saclike dilations composing a compound gland.

American College of Rheumatology (ACR): A professional association of U.S. rheumatologists.

acupuncture: The procedure of inserting and manipulating needles into various points on the body to relieve pain or for therapeutic purposes.

adaptive immunity: Normally is functionally triggered after activation of the innate immune system by foreign pathogens.

adenopathy: A swelling of the lymph nodes. In Sjögren's, this usually occurs in the neck and jaw region.

albumin: A protein that circulates in the blood and carries materials to cells. Decreased in chronic disease.

allodynia: Pain due to a stimulus that does not normally produce pain.

alopecia: Hair loss.

alveoli: Small air sacs in the bronchi.

amylase: An enzyme present in saliva; another form of amylase is produced by the pancreas.

analgesic: A drug that alleviates pain.

androgen: A steroid hormone produced from cholesterol in the adrenal cortex, which is the primary precursor of natural estrogens.

anemia: Low numbers of red cells.

anhedonia: Loss of interest or pleasure in doing things.

anosmia: Loss of smell.

antibody: Substance in the blood that is normally made in response to infection and is produced against one's own tissues in autoimmune disease. Also referred to as immunoglobulins such as IgG and IgM which are often elevated in Sjögren's. Antibodies to SSA (Ro) and SSB (La) are associated with Sjögren's.

anticardiolipin antibody: An antiphospholipid antibody.

anticentromere antibody: Antibodies to a cell nucleus associated with scleroderma.

anticholinergic: A class of medications that inhibit parasympathetic nerve impulses by selectively blocking the binding of the neurotransmitter acetylcholine to its receptor in nerve cells. A variety of these medications have side effects with resulting dry eyes and dry mouth.

anti-DNA (anti–double-stranded DNA): Antibodies to DNA; seen in half of patients with lupus.

antigen(s): A chemical substance that provokes the production of antibody. In tetanus vaccination, for example, tetanus is the antigen injected to produce antibodies and hence protective immunity to tetanus.

357

antimalarial drugs: Quinine-derived drugs, which were first developed to treat malaria and can manage Sjögren's, such as hydroxychloroquine (Plaquenil).

antimitochondrial antibodies (AMA): antibodies (immunoglobulins) formed against mitochondria, primarily mitochondria in cells of the liver found in Sjögren's patients with biliary cirrhosis.

anti-muscarinic receptor antibody: This antibody is thought to block the action of the nerves that go to the salivary and lacrimal glands, thereby reducing the production of saliva and tears.

antinuclear antibodies (ANA): Autoantibodies directed against components in the nucleus of the cell. Detection of these antibodies are used to screen for Sjögren's, lupus and other connective tissue diseases. The majority of Sjögren's patients are positive for ANA, but a negative ANA test does not exclude the diagnosis of Sjögren's. The ANA test typically involves immunofluorescent staining; a speckled or homogeneous pattern is most frequently identified with Sjögren's.

antiphospholipid antibody syndrome (APS): Thromboembolic (when a blood clot causes a blockage) events in a patient with antiphospholipid antibody.

antiphospholipid antibody: Antibodies to a constituent of cell membranes seen in Sjögren's and other connective tissue diseases. In the presence of a cofactor, these antibodies can alter clotting and lead to strokes, blood clots, miscarriages, and low platelet counts. Also detected as the lupus anticoagulant.

anti-RNP: Antibody to ribonucleoprotein. Seen in lupus and mixed connective tissue disease.

anti-Sm: Anti-Smith antibody; found only in lupus.

antispasmodic drugs: Medications that quiet spasms. Usually used in reference to the gastrointestinal tract.

anti-SSA (Ro antibody): Associated with Sjögren's, sun sensitivity, neonatal lupus, and congenital heart block.

anti-SSB (La antibody): Almost always seen with anti-SSA.

apoptosis: Process by which a cell is programmed to self-destruct.

aqueous-deficient dry eye: Disruption of the tear film because of inadequate secretion of tears or because arteries become swollen and damaged.

arachidonic acid: An unsaturated fatty acid found in animal fats that is essential in human nutrition and is a precursor in the biosynthesis of some prostaglandins which mediate inflammation.

arteriole: A very small artery.

arthralgia: Pain in a joint.

arthritis: Inflammation of a joint.

ascites: An abnormal fluid that collects in the abdomen due to certain liver and other disorders.

atelectasis: A collapse of lung tissue affecting part or all of one lung.

atrophic gastritis: Autoimmune destruction of acid-producing parietal cells of the stomach. May lead to vitamin B_{12} deficiency and pernicious anemia. Up to 20% of Sjögren's patients may have antibodies against parietal cells.

atrophic rhinitis: Symptoms are a foul smell, crusts, and even nasal bleeding. As secretions become thick and occasionally foul-smelling, secondary infection may appear.

atrophic vaginitis: A condition characterized by dryness and inflammation of the vagina with thinning of the epithelial lining due to estrogen deficiency.

atrophy: A thinning of the surface; a form of wasting.

autoantibody: Antibody that attacks the body's own tissues and organs as if they were foreign.

autoimmune hepatitis: Inflammation of the liver that occurs when immune cells mistake the liver's normal cells for harmful invaders and attack them.

autoimmune pancreatitis: An increasingly recognized type of chronic pancreatitis; it can be difficult to distinguish from pancreatic carcinoma but it responds to treatment with corticosteroids, particularly prednisone. Rare complication of Sjögren's.

autoimmune thyroiditis: Disease of the thyroid gland due to autoimmunity in which the patient's immune system attacks and damages the thyroid.

autoimmunity: A state in which the body inappropriately produces antibodies against its own tissues. The antigens are components of the body.

autonomic neuropathy: Nerve dysfunction or damage that affects the autonomic nervous system, which controls digestive, bladder, bowel, cardiac, and sexual function.

B cell or B lymphocyte: A white blood cell that makes antibodies.

BAFF (B-cell activating factor of the TNF family, also called BLyS): A powerful driver of B-cell development.

basal (resting) rate: Unstimulated (used in reference to both tears and salivary flow).

biological therapies: Treatment to stimulate or restore the ability of the immune (defense) system to fight infection and disease.

blepharitis: Common, persistent, and sometimes chronic inflammation of the eyelids, resulting from bacteria that reside on the skin.

bolus: A morsel of food, already chewed, ready to be swallowed.

brain fog: Impaired concentration and memory; can be due to various causes.

bronchi: Branches of the trachea.

buffer: A mixture of acid or base that, when added to a solution, enables the solution to resist changes in the pH that would otherwise occur when acid or alkali is added to it.

calcification: A process in which tissue or non-cellular material in the body becomes hardened as the result of deposits of insoluble calcium salts.

Candida: A yeast-like fungal organism.

candidiasis: A condition affecting the skin or oral mucosa caused by overgrowth of the common yeast (fungus) *Candida*. Formerly called moniliasis.

cariostatic: Having the ability to help prevent dental caries.

cartilage: Tissue material covering bone. The nose, outer ears, and trachea consist primarily of cartilage.

celiac spruce: An inherited, autoimmune disease in which the lining of the small intestine is damaged from eating gluten and other proteins found in wheat, barley, rye, and possibly oats. Also known as gluten enteropathy. May be 10 times more prevalent in Sjögren's patients than in general population.

central nervous system: The brain, spinal cord and optic nerve.

cheilitis: Sores at the corners of the mouth (angles of the lips).

chemokines: One of a large group of proteins that act as lures and were first found attracting white blood cells.

chronic active hepatitis: A disorder that occurs when viral hepatitis proceeds in an active state beyond its usual cause.

chronic fatigue syndrome: Best defined as a low-energy state characterized by physical or mental weariness.

collagen vascular disease: *See* connective tissue disease.

complement: A protein involved in clearing immune complexes. Levels may be decreased in Sjögren's; when complement is low, inflammation may be higher.

complementary medicine: Nonprescription use of products found in nature to treat medical conditions. Also includes noninvasive mind/body techniques such as biofeedback, acupuncture, yoga.

complete blood count (CBC): A blood test measuring the amount of red cells, white cells, and platelets in the body.

congenital heart block: A dysfunction of the rate/rhythm conduction system in the fetal or infant heart caused by antibodies to SSA or SSB.

conjunctiva: The mucous membrane covering the outside of the eyeball and the inner lining of the eyelids.

connective tissue disease: A disorder marked by inflammation of the connective tissue (joints, skin, muscles) in multiple areas. In most instances, connective tissue diseases are associated with autoimmunity.

constitutional symptom: A symptom that affects the general well-being or general status of a patient. Examples include weight loss, shaking, chills, fever, and vomiting.

contrast sialography: This test assesses the structure of the major salivary glands.

cornea: The central transparent part of the eyeball that helps focus the entering light rays. The clear "watch crystal" structure covering the pupil and iris (colored portion of the eye). It is composed of several vital layers, all of which are functionally important. The surface layer, or epithelium, is covered by the tears, which lubricate and protect the surface.

corticosteroid: A hormone produced by the adrenal cortex gland. Natural adrenal gland hormones have powerful anti-inflammatory activity and are often used in the treatment of severe inflammation affecting vital organs. The many side effects of corticosteroids markedly curtail their use in mild disorders.

costochondritis: An irritation of a rib and adjoining cartilage, causing chest pain.

C-reactive protein (CRP): This test measures systemic inflammation. Produced by the liver. The level of CRP rises when there is inflammation throughout the body.

CREST syndrome: A limited form of scleroderma characterized by calcium deposits under the skin, Raynaud's phenomenon, esophageal dysfunction, sclerodactyly (tight skin), and a rash called telangiectasia.

crossover syndrome: An autoimmune process that has features of more than one rheumatic disease.

cryoglobulinemia: A condition whereby protein complexes circulating in the blood are precipitated during cold weather. Those with cryoglobulineamia have a higher incidence of Raynaud's phenomenon, peripheral neuropathy, vasculitis (inflammation of blood vessels) and B cell lymphoproliferative disorder.

cryptogenic cirrhosis: Liver disease of unknown etiology (origin) in patients with no history of alcoholism or previous acute hepatitis.

cytokine: A group of chemicals that signals cells to perform certain actions.

demineralization: This process refers to the removal of hard minerals (calcium) from the tooth surface leading to dental caries.

demyelination: Areas of damage to the coatings of the nerve fibers.

dendritic cells: Immune cells that form part of the mammalian immune system.

dental caries: A process in which the tooth is gradually dissolved (demineralized) by acids from bacteria attached to the surface, which leads to progressive cavitation. If the caries process is allowed to continue without treatment, it will progress through the tooth into its pulp (containing the nerve of the tooth). Also known as dental decay or cavity.

dermatomyositis: An autoimmune process directed against muscles associated with skin rashes.

diuretics: Medications that increase the body's ability to rid itself of fluids.

docosahexaenoic (DHA): An omega-3 fatty acid.

double-blind study: One in which neither the physician nor the patient knows whether the patient is receiving the active ingredient being tested or a placebo (an inactive substance).

dysorexia: Impaired or deranged appetite.

dyspareunia: Painful sexual intercourse.

dyspepsia: Can be defined as painful, difficult, or disturbed digestion, which may be accompanied by symptoms such as nausea and vomiting, heartburn, bloating, and stomach discomfort (upset stomach).

dysphagia: Difficulty in swallowing. In Sjögren's, this may be attributable to several causes, among them a decrease in saliva, infiltration of the glands at the esophageal mucosa, or esophageal webbing.

dyspnea: Air hunger resulting in labored or difficult breathing, sometimes accompanied by pain.

dysuria: Pain on urination.

ecchymosis: A purplish patch caused by oozing of blood into the skin; ecchymoses differ from petechiae in size.

edema: Swelling caused by retention of fluid.

eicosapentaenoic (EPA): An omega-3 fatty acid found in fish oils.

electromyography (EMG): A technique for evaluating and recording the electrical activity produced by skeletal muscles.

endoscopy: A procedure in which a small, flexible tube called an endoscope is used to view the esophagus, stomach, and duodenum.

enzyme-linked immunosorbent assay (ELISA): A very sensitive blood test for detecting the presence of autoantibodies. ELISA is an extractable nuclear antibody test (ENA) often used to detect the presence of anti-SSA (Ro) and anti-SSB (La) that are associated with Sjögren's.

epigenetics: An emerging field that studies how these heritable modifications that do not involve changes in the nucleotide sequence lead to altered gene expression.

epistaxis: Nosebleed or hemorrhaging from the nose, which may be caused by dryness of the nasal mucous membrane in Sjögren's.

epithelial: The outside layer of cells that covers all the free, open surfaces of the body including the skin, and mucous membranes that communicate with the outside of the body.

erythema: A medical term for a red color, usually associated with increased blood flow to an inflamed area, often the skin.

erythrocyte sedimentation rate (ESR): Measures the degree to which whole blood, collected in tubes containing a chemical that prevents clotting (anticoagulant), separates into plasma (the upper layer) and packed red cells (the lower layer) over the course of one hour. Elevated with inflammation.

erythrocyte: Red blood cell.

esophageal dysmotility: Muscular incoordination of the esophagus. May affect up to one third of Sjögren's patients with dysphagia.

esophagitis: Prolonged reflux of acid results in chronic irritation of the esophagus.

esophagus: A canal (narrow tube) with muscular walls allowing passage of food from the pharynx, or end of the mouth, to the stomach.

estrogens: Any of several steroid hormones produced chiefly by the ovaries and responsible for promoting estrus and the development and maintenance of female secondary sex characteristics.

etiology: The cause(s) of a disease.

eustachian tube: The tube running from the back of the nose to the middle ear.

exocrine glands: Glands that secrete outside the body (e.g., lacrimal, salivary, or sweat glands).

exocrinopathy: Disease related to the exocrine glands.

extractable nuclear antibodies (ENA): Autoantibodies that can be detected to test for specific rheumatic diseases. The ENA panel is similar to the ANA but more specific and identifies antigens responsible for an elevated ANA. ELISA is an ENA test used to distinguish Sjögren's from other related disorders. Tests that are positive for ant-SSA and anti-SSB are identified with Sjögren's, anti-Sm with lupus, anti-RNP with lupus or mixed connective tissue disease and Scl-70 with scleroderma.

extra-glandular: Outside of the glands.

fibromyalgia: A pain amplification syndrome that can occur alone and also is seen in Sjögren's patients. This medical condition is characterized by chronic widespread pain and tender points and is linked to fatigue and sleep problems.

fibrosis: Abnormal formation of fibrous tissue.

filamentary keratopathy: Mucus strands stick to the cornea at sites of focal desiccation and surface cells extend onto the strand, making it very adherent to the cornea and causing discomfort or even pain when blinking pulls on the strand.

fissure: A crack in the tissue surface (skin, tongue, etc.).

fluorescein stain: A dye that stains areas of the eye surface in which cells have been lost.

focal lymphocytic sialoadenitis: A characteristic pattern of inflammation.

gastritis: Stomach inflammation.

gastroesophageal reflux disease (GERD): Muscle tone in the wall of the esophagus is reduced and gastric juice moves up the esophagus, producing a burning sensation behind the breastbone (heartburn) and chest pain.

gene therapy: A method of treating disease by introducing normal DNA directly into cells to correct a genetic defect that is causing the disease.

gene transfer: The insertion of unrelated genetic information in the form of DNA into cells.

genes: Control the physical traits that are passed from parents to their offspring.

genetic factors: Traits inherited from parents, grandparents, and so on.

genetics: Broadly refers to the study of genes.

genome: All of the genetic information, the entire genetic complement, all of the hereditary material possessed by an organism.

genome-wide association study (GWAS): Allows the scientist to rapidly scan the complete set of DNA, or genome, of individuals to find genetic variations associated with a complex disease, such as Sjögren's.

gingiva: The gums.

gingivitis: Inflammation of the gums.

globulin: A protein whose levels increase in inflammation.

glomerulonephritis: Inflammation of the kidney; seen in 10% of patients with Sjögren's.

goblet cell: Any of the specialized epithelial cells found in the mucous membrane of the stomach, intestines, and respiratory passages that secrete mucus.

granulocyte: A type of white blood cell.

granuloma: A nodular, inflammatory lesion.

Graves disease: A form of autoimmune thyroid disease.

halitosis: Bad breath.

Hashimoto's thyroiditis: The most common form of thyroiditis and the most frequent cause of hypothyroidism.

Helicobacter pylori: A common chronic bacterial infection of the stomach. Associated with increased risk of gastrointestinal (MALT) lymphoma.

hepatitis C virus: Not associated with Sjögren's but can present with sicca symptoms mimicking Sjögren's.

hepatitis: Inflammation of the liver; seen in Sjögren's patients who have biliary cirrhosis.

HLA: The human leukocyte antigen (HLA) group of genes play a major role in the recognition of "self" and are clearly associated with Sjögren's.

homeopathy: A method of treating disease with small amounts of remedies that, in large amounts in healthy people, produce symptoms similar to those being treated.

hormone replacement therapy (HRT): Therapy with estrogen and progesterone that is commonly used in menopause for severe hot flashes, disrupted sleep, and in some cases mild depressive symptoms.

hormones: Chemical messengers—including thyroid, insulin, steroids, estrogen, progesterone, and testosterone—made by the body.

human leukocyte antigens (HLA): A group of genes that governs the ability of lymphocytes, such as T cells and B cells, to respond to foreign and self substances.

hydroxychloroquine: Anti-inflammatory drug (trade name Plaquenil) used in the treatment of autoimmune conditions such as rheumatoid arthritis, Sjögren's, and lupus erythematosus.

hyperalgesia: An extreme reaction to a stimulus that is not normally painful.

hypergammaglobulinemia: A medical condition with elevated levels of gamma globulin.

hypergammaglobulinemic purpura: A type of skin rash, which is a purple-brown color.

hypokalemia: Low potassium levels.

hypothyroidism: A condition in which the thyroid gland does not make enough thyroid hormone.

idiopathic: Of unknown cause.

immunogenetics: The study of genetic factors that control the immune response.

immunoglobulin E (IgE): Antibody associated with allergies.

immunoglobulins (gamma globulins): The protein fraction of serum responsible for antibody activity. Measurement of serum immunoglobulin levels can serve as a guide to disease activity in some patients with Sjögren's.

immunomodulators: Medications that affect the body's immune system.

immunosuppressive agents. Drugs used in the chemotherapy of malignant disease and in the prevention of transplant rejection inhibit the activity of the immune system and occasionally are used to treat severe autoimmune disease.

incisal: Cutting edge (of a tooth).

indigestion (dyspepsia): A painful or burning feeling in the upper abdomen, usually accompanied by nausea, bloating or gas, a feeling of fullness, and sometimes vomiting.

innate immunity: Primitive responses to bacteria and viruses via a pattern-recognition mechanism.

interferon: A protein activated by the immune system and made to protect the body from infection but that is overactive in Sjögren's.

interstitial: Involving the supporting structure of the substance of an organ or tissues.

interstitial cystitis: Inflammation of the bladder; can cause urinary discomfort, urgency and frequency and occur in Sjögren's.

interstitial lung disease: Inflammation of the lung ; can lead to scarring of the lung tissue and occur in Sjögren's.

interstitial nephritis: Inflammation of the connective tissue of the kidney. Interstitial nephritis may be associated with Sjögren's.

interstitial pneumonitis: an inflammation of the supporting tissue around the alveoli (air sacs) of the lungs caused by the autoimmune process.

intraoral: Inside the mouth.

intrathoracic: Within the cavity of the chest.

irritable bowel syndrome: Spastic colitis or irritable bowel.

IV immunoglobulin or IVIg: A blood product made from the plasma component of blood pooled from thousands of donors. It contains immunoglobulins, which interact with the immune system in order to suppress it.

jaundice: Yellowing of the skin.

keratoconjunctivitis sicca: Also called dry eye.

lacrimal glands: Two types of glands that produce tears. Smaller accessory glands in the eyelid tissue produce the tears needed from minute to minute. The main lacrimal glands, located just inside the bony tissue surrounding the eye, produce large amounts of tears.

lacrimal: Relating to the tears.

laryngopharyngeal reflux (LPR): reflux of gastric contents and acids to the level of the throat; can lead to symptoms of hoarseness, chronic cough, throat clearing, mild pharyngeal dysphagia, or globus sensations (sensation of a lump or foreign body in the throat).

laryngotracheobronchitis: An acute respiratory infection involving the larynx, trachea, and bronchi. Also called *croup*.

larynx: Voice box.

latent: Not manifest but potentially discernible.

leukopenia: Low numbers of white cells.

leukorrhea: A whitish, viscid discharge from the vagina and uterine cavity.

lip biopsy: Incision of approximately 1 cm is made on the inside surface of the lower lip and minor salivary glands are removed for microscopic examination and analysis. Considered the gold standard for diagnosing the salivary component of Sjögren's.

lissamine green: A vital stain with dyeing quality similar to that of Rose Bengal but causes less discomfort. It stains dead or degenerated epithelial cells green and is used to facilitate the diagnosis of keratoconjunctivitis sicca, xerophthalmia, etc.

lymph: A fluid collected from the tissues throughout the body, flowing through the lymph nodes and eventually added to the circulating blood.

lymphadenopathy: Abnormally enlarged lymph nodes. Commonly called "swollen glands."

lymphocyte: A type of white blood cell concerned with antibody production and regulation. Promotes chronic inflammation. Collections of lymphocytes are seen in the salivary glands of Sjögren's patients.

lymphoma: A proliferation (increase) of abnormal (malignant) lymphocytes; a cancer involving the lymphatic cells of the immune system. About 5% to 10% of Sjögren's patients will develop one of the many types of lymphoma. The most common type of lymphoma in Sjögren's is MALT (mucosa-associated lymphoid tissue) lymphoma (also called extranodal marginal zone lymphoma), which is very slow–growing.

lymphoproliferation: Excessive production of lymphocytes.

macrophage: A cell that kills foreign material and presents information to lymphocytes.

mucosa-associated lymphoid tissue (MALT): Associated with the mucosa, the moist lining of some organs and body cavities. MALT refers to the most common type of lymphoma in Sjögren's.

manometry: The diagnosis of dysmotility is made by measuring the pressure inside the wall of the esophagus during swallowing.

matrix: The section of the tooth enamel that holds calcium and phosphate minerals.

meibomian glands: Fat-producing glands in the eyelids that produce an essential component of tears. Meibomian gland dysfunction frequently co-exists with dry eye.

MHC: Major histocompatibility complex or MHC is a group of genes that help the immune system recognize foreign substances. This group also is called the human leukocyte antigen (HLA) system in humans. A clear association exists between Sjögren's and the HLA genes.

mixed connective tissue disease: A connective tissue disease that manifests as an overlap of other connective tissue disorders.

monoclonal: A single antibody designed to uniquely recognize a specific target, such as a lymphocyte or cytokine.

mononeuritis multiplex: Inflammation of multiple nerves.

mucin: Thinnest layer of the tear film; layer closest to the cornea.

mucolytic agents: Medications that tend to dissolve mucus. Most patients with dry eye complain of excess mucous discharge. Some patients may benefit from these medications if other tear-film–enhancing drops are not very effective. Mucolytic agents also may be used to break up thick mucus in the throat that develops from dryness.

myalgia: Muscle pains.

necrosis: Tissue death.

neonatal lupus syndrome: A rare autoimmune disorder that is present at birth in patients with anti-SSA or -SSB; usually manifests itself with a rash or heart block.

nephritis: Inflammation of the kidneys.

nerve conduction study: A test commonly used to evaluate the function, especially the ability of electrical conduction, of the motor and sensory nerves of the human body.

neutrophil: A granulated white blood cell involved in bacterial killing and acute inflammation.

nonspecific: Caused by other diseases or multiple factors.

nonsteroidal anti-inflammatory drugs (NSAIDs): Anti-inflammatory agents that block the action of prostaglandins; used to treat pain that occurs in rheumatoid arthritis and other connective tissue disorders. Examples include ibuprofen (Motrin, Advil) and naproxen (Aleve).

norepinephrine: A hormone and neurotransmitter secreted by the adrenal medulla and the nerve endings of the sympathetic nervous system to cause vasoconstriction and increases in heart rate, blood pressure, and the sugar level of the blood.

olfactory: Relating to the sense of smell.

ophthalmologist: A physician who specializes in diseases and surgery of the eye.

optic neuritis: Inflammation of the optic nerve; may cause a complete or partial loss of vision.

oral soft tissue: Tongue, mucous lining of the cheeks, and lips.

orthostasis: Maintenance of an upright standing posture.

otalgia: Ear pain.

otitis: Inflammation of the ear, which may be marked by pain, fever, abnormalities of hearing, deafness, tinnitus (a ringing sensation), and vertigo. In Sjögren's, blockage of eustachian tubes due to infection can lead to conduction deafness and chronic otitis.

otolaryngology: The medical specialty that deals with diseases of the ear, nose, and throat.

palpable purpura: Rashes, particularly small red raised eruptions on the extremities that can cause skin changes in Sjögren's patients.

pancreatitis: Acute inflammation of the pancreas.

parasympathetic nervous system: The part of the autonomic nervous system whose functions include constriction of the pupils of the eyes, slowing of the heartbeat, and stimulation of certain digestive glands. These nerves originate in the midbrain, the hindbrain, and the sacral region of the spinal cord; impulses are mediated by acetylcholine.

parasympathomimetic agents: Systemic agents that are capable of stimulating salivary output.

paresthesias: Abnormal sensations such as tingling, constriction, and discomfort.

parotid gland flow: An empirical quantitative measure of the amount of saliva produced over a certain period of time. Normal parotid gland flow rate is 1.5 mL/min. In Sjögren's, the flow rate is approximately 0.5 mL/min, with diminution of the flow rate correlating inversely with the severity of disease.

parotid glands: One of the three pairs of major salivary glands.

parotid scintigraphy: A nuclear medicine test that evaluates the function of the parotid and submandibular glands.

pathogenesis: The development of a disease.

peptides: Any of various natural or synthetic compounds containing two or more amino acids linked by the carboxyl group of one amino acid to the amino group of another.

perforation: A hole.

pericarditis: Inflammation of the lining around the heart (the pericardium).

perimenopause: A variable time of irregular menses beginning a few years before the menopause.

periodontitis: Inflammation of the gums and soft tissue and bone surrounding and supporting the teeth.

peripheral nerves: Nerves outside the central nervous system.

peripheral neuropathy: A problem with the nerves that carry information to and from the brain and spinal cord. This can produce pain, loss of sensation, and an inability to control muscles and involve the autonomic nervous system. Common manifestations of peripheral neuropathy in Sjögren's include sensory changes and burning and tingling in the feet, legs, hands and arms.

pernicious anemia: A blood disorder caused by inadequate vitamin B_{12} in the blood.

petechia: A small, pinpoint, nonraised, perfectly round, purplish red spot caused by intradermal or submucosal hemorrhaging.

phagocytic cells: Cells, such as white blood cells, that engulf and absorb waste material, harmful microorganisms, or other foreign bodies in the bloodstream and tissues.

pharynx: Throat.

photosensitivity: Sensitivity to ultraviolet light. Present in most patients with antibodies to SSA (Ro).

placebo: An inactive substance used as a "dummy" medication.

plaque: A thin, sticky film that builds up on the teeth, trapping harmful bacteria.

plasma: The fluid portion of the circulating blood.

plasmapheresis: Filtration of blood plasma through a machine to remove proteins that may aggravate Sjögren's.

pleura: A sac lining the lung.

pleurisy: Inflammation of the lining around the lung.

polychondritis: Inflammation and destruction of the cartilage of various tissues of the body.

polyclonal: Derived from different cells.

polymyositis: A connective tissue disorder characterized by muscle pain and severe weakness secondary to inflammation in the major voluntary muscles.

polysomnography: Sleep study.

primary biliary cirrhosis (PBC): Impairment of bile excretion secondary to liver inflammation and scarring. Can occur in Sjögren's.

probiotics: The administration of "good" bacteria that kills "bad" gut bacteria.

progestins: Any one of a group of steroid hormones that have the effect of progesterone.

prostaglandins: Substances produced by the body that are responsible for features of inflammation, such as swelling, pain, stiffness, redness, and warmth.

protein: A collection of amino acids. Antibodies are proteins.

proteinuria: Excess protein levels in the urine (also called albuminuria).

proteomics: The study of proteins.

pruritus: Itching.

pulse steroids: Very high doses of corticosteroids given intravenously over several days to critically ill patients.

puncta: Small holes in the eyelids that normally drain tears. Patients with severe dry eye benefit from punctal closure, which allows maximum tear preservation.

punctal plugs: Inserted in the puncta to increase the volume of tears retained on the surface of the eye.

purpura: A condition characterized by hemorrhage into the skin, appearing as crops of petechiae (very small red spots).

radioactive isotope: Radioactive material used in diagnostic tests.

radionuclide studies: A technique in which radioactive isotopes, such as radiolabeled human serum albumin, are injected into an organ. A gamma scintillation camera, coupled with a digital computer system and a cathode ray display, reads the radioactive emissions. Areas of perfusion will show marked radiographic emissions; areas of obstruction will show no activity.

Raynaud's phenomenon: Painful blanching of the fingertips on exposure to cold. This may be seen alone or in association with a connective tissue disease such as Sjögren's.

reflux: Regurgitation due to the return of gas, fluid, or small amount of food from the stomach.

regulatory immunity: Needed to evolve to facilitate termination of a no-longer-needed adaptive response and to limit responses to "self" (auto) antigen.

remineralization: The process of restoring minerals (calcium and phosphate) to the tooth surface.

renal tubular acidosis: Damage to the tubules of the kidney; lowers pH and is associated with renal damage. Can occur in Sjögren's.

renal: Relating to the kidneys.

restless legs syndrome: Characterized by unpleasant sensations in the limbs, usually the legs, that occur at rest or before sleep; relieved by activity such as walking.

rheumatoid arthritis (RA): An autoimmune disease and form of arthritis characterized by inflammation of the joints, stiffness, swelling, synovial hypertrophy, and pain. Sjögren's frequently occurs in conjunction with RA.

rheumatoid factor: An autoantibody whose presence in the blood usually indicates autoimmune activity.

rheumatologist: A physician skilled in the diagnosis and treatment of rheumatic conditions including Sjögren's.

Ro antibody: *See* anti-SSA.

rosacea: A chronic dermatitis of the face, especially of the nose and cheeks, characterized by a red or rosy coloration with deep-seated papules and pustules and caused by dilation of capillaries. Can be mistaken for lupus or anti-SSA–associated rashes.

Rose Bengal: A dye that stains abnormal cells on the surface of the eye. It has been generally replaced by the less-irritating dye, lissamine green, for the diagnosis of dry eye (keratoconjunctivitis sicca).

salicylates: Aspirin-like drugs.

salivary flow rate: The amount of saliva naturally produced by the salivary glands.

salivary glands: Exocrine glands (parotid, submandibular, and sublingual) with ducts that produce saliva.

salivary scintigraphy: Measurement of salivary gland function through intravenous injection of radioactive material.

sarcoidosis: A systemic disease with granulomatous (nodular, inflammatory) lesions involving the lungs and, on occasion, the salivary glands, with resulting fibrosis.

Schirmer test: The standard objective test to diagnose dry eye. Small pieces of filter paper are placed between the lower eyelid and eyeball and soak up the tears for 5 minutes. The value obtained is a rough estimation of tear production in relative terms. Lower values are consistent with dry eye.

scleroderma: A connective tissue and autoimmune disease characterized by thickening and hardening of the skin. Sometimes internal organs (intestines, kidneys) are affected, causing bowel irregularity and high blood pressure. Sjögren's is not uncommon in patients with scleroderma.

sclerosing cholangitis: A chronic disorder of the liver in which the ducts carrying bile from the liver to the intestine, and often the ducts carrying bile within the liver, become inflamed, thickened, scarred (sclerotic), and obstructed.

sclerosing sialedenitis: Swelling and inflammation of the salivary glands with scarring.

secretagogue: A medication that can stimulate salivary flow.

serotonin: A chemical produced by the brain that functions as a neurotransmitter. It plays a part in the regulation of mood, sleep, learning, and constriction of blood vessels (vasoconstriction).

serum protein electrophoresis: A laboratory test that examines specific proteins in the blood called globulins. Those of clinical interest in Sjögren's are gamma globulins, which are those that produce antibodies, including immunoglobulin G, M and A (IgG, IgM and IgA.

serum sickness: An immune system reaction to medications that can include fever, swollen lymph nodes and itching.

serum: The fluid portion of the blood (obtained after removal of the fibrin clot and blood cells), distinguished from the plasma in the blood.

sialochemistry: Measurement of the constituents in saliva.

sialography: X-ray examination of the salivary duct system by use of liquid contrast medium. Radiologically sensitive dye is placed into the duct system, outlining the system clearly.

sicca: Dry. Sicca symptoms are common in Sjögren's in which symptoms of dry eye and dry mouth as well as dryness throughout the body are prominent.

signs: Changes that can be seen or measured.

sinusitis: Sinus inflammation.

Sjögren's antibodies: Abnormal antibodies found in the sera of Sjögren's patients. These antibodies react with the extracts of certain cells, and a test based on this principle can be helpful in the diagnosis of Sjögren's. *See also* SSA and SSB.

Sjögren's syndrome: A systemic multiorgan autoimmune disease that generally has a chronic or progressive course and is characterized by secretory dysfunction. It may occur alone or precede or follow the occurrence of other autoimmune diseases in the same patient.

SSA: Sjögren's syndrome-associated antigen A (anti-Ro). About 40%-60% of Sjögren's patients are positive for anti-SSA.

SSB: Sjögren's syndrome-associated antigen B (anti-La). About 20%-30% of Sjögren's patients are positive for anti-SSB.

steatorrhea: Passage of large amounts of fat in the feces, as occurs in pancreatic disease and the malabsorption syndromes.

steroids: Cortisone-derived medications.

subacute cutaneous lupus (SCLE): A unique set of photosensitive rashes, originally described in patients with lupus. May occur in Sjögren's and common in patients with anti-SSA (Ro) and anti-SSB (La) antibodies.

sublingual glands: One of the three pairs of major salivary glands. They are located in the floor of the mouth under the tongue.

synovitis: Inflammation of the tissues lining a joint.

synovium: Tissue that lines a joint.

systemic: Any process that involves multiple organ systems throughout the body.

systemic lupus erythematosus (SLE): An autoimmune disease that is closely related to Sjögren's syndrome, occurs frequently in conjunction with Sjögren's, and, similar to Sjögren's, can damage any body organ or system.

T cell: A lymphocyte (white blood cell) responsible for immunological memory.

tear breakup test: Measurement of tear breakup time is a standard part of the evaluation of dry eye since instability of the tear film is a characteristic of both aqueous-deficient and evaporative dry eye.

tear osmolarity test: Tear osmolarity testing measures the concentration of the tear film, which can be elevated in either aqueous-deficient or evaporative dry eye.

temporomandibular joint (TMJ): The joint of the lower jaw where the ball-and-socket arrangement is formed by the condyle of the lower jaw (the ball) and the fossa of the temporal bone (the socket). The joint space is filled with synovial or lubricating fluid. This joint and the surrounding synovial tissues may become inflamed inSjögren's.

thrombocytopenia: Low platelet counts.

thrush: A form of candidiasis. Infection of the oral tissues with *Candida albicans*.

thymus: A gland in the neck responsible for immunological memory.

thyroiditis: A disease in which autoantibodies cause immune system cells (lymphocytes) to destroy the thyroid gland.

tinnitus: Ringing in the ears.

titer: Test showing the strength or concentration of a particular volume of a solution. Usually refers to amounts of antibody present.

tolerance: Failure to make antibodies to an antigen.

Toll receptor: A pattern-recognition feature of the innate immune system.

trachea: Windpipe.

tracheobronchial tree: The windpipe and the bronchi into which it subdivides.

trigeminal nerve: The chief nerve of sensation for the face and the motor nerve controlling the muscles of mastication (chewing).

tumor necrosis factor (TNF): a cytokine produced primarily by monocytes and macrophages that promotes inflammation.

ultraviolet light (UV light): A spectrum of light that is found in sunlight and fluorescent and LED lighting and can affect one's health. Sjögren's patients who are positive for anti-SSA and/or have overlapping lupus are at increased risk of reacting to UV light.

undifferentiated connective tissue disease (UCTD): Features of autoimmunity such as inflammatory arthritis or Raynaud's in a patient who does not meet the ACR criteria for lupus, rheumatoid arthritis, or other disorders.

urinalysis: Examination of urine under a microscope.

urticaria: Hives.

vasculitis: Inflammation of a blood vessel.

venous thromboses: Clots in veins of the of the lower extremities and less frequently the lungs.

venule: A very small vein.

viscera: The organs of the digestive, respiratory, urogenital, and endocrine systems, as well as the spleen, heart, and great vessels (blood and lymph ducts).

vitamin B_{12} deficiency: A reduction in vitamin B_{12} from inadequate dietary intake or impaired absorption. Vitamin B_{12} deficiency is a frequent finding in autoimmune disease.

vitamin D: A fat-soluble vitamin that enhances the absorption of calcium and phosphorus from the intestine and promotes their deposition onto the bone. Vitamin D deficiency is common in autoimmune disease and has been associated with musculoskeletal pain and increased disease activity.

vitiligo: An autoimmune disease resulting in white patches on the skin due to loss of pigment.

WBC: White blood cell.

xerophthalmia: Dry eyes.

xerosis: Abnormal dryness of the skin (xeroderma), of the conjunctiva of the eye (xerophthalmia), or of the mucous membranes such as dry mouth (xerostomia).

xerostomia: Dryness of the mouth. It is usually associated with decreased salivary secretion but may occur in some individuals with normal secretion. It can be caused by many different prescription drugs, Sjögren's, radiation therapy, uncontrolled diabetes, and other diseases.

xylitol: An acceptable sweetener that has been shown to reduce dental caries.

Appendix: Products for Sjögren's Patients

The Sjögren's Syndrome Foundation offers a *Product Directory* as one of its many resources for Sjögren's patients and those who serve them. The *Directory* contains a listing of products that might be helpful for symptoms such as dry eye, dry mouth, dry nose, dry skin, dry and itchy ears, and dry vagina; footwear for neuropathy pain; and humidifiers. It also lists websites and toll-free numbers for the companies that produce the products.

The *Directory* cannot include every product available and does not signify endorsement on the part of the SSF for the extensive number of products that are included.

Products change continually, so the reader is encouraged to visit the SSF website at www.sjogrens.org for the latest listing. By joining the SSF, you will receive a copy of the *Directory* and may also view and download the *Directory* from the members-only area of the SSF website.

To join the SSF, call 800-475-6473 or 301-530-4420, e-mail ssf@sjogrens.org, or visit the website at www.sjogrens.org and click on the link "Join Now."

INDEX

Page numbers followed by "*f*" or "*t*" refer figures or tables, respectively.

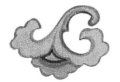

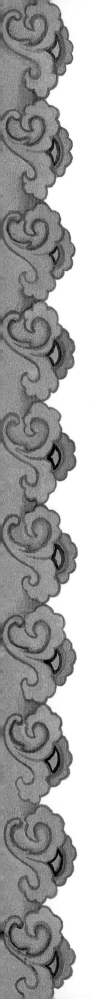

FOREWORD

Buddhism has its origins in the life and teachings of the Buddha, formerly Prince Siddhartha. His father, who reigned in northern India during the sixth century BCE, was king of the powerful Sakya tribe. As a young man, Siddhartha escaped from his father's palace by stealth and set forth on a search for the true meaning and purpose of life. After many years of meditation accompanied by extreme practices such as prolonged fasting, Siddhartha abandoned the tortures of asceticism for the middle way: a balance between all extremes. His meditation then bore fruit. In Bodh Gaya, now the modern Indian state of Bihar, Siddhartha attained enlightenment sitting in meditation beneath the Bodhi tree. Thus he became the Buddha, 'the awakened one'.

Seven weeks after his enlightenment, the Buddha began to teach others, forming a community of monks and nuns. Their teachings soon spread beyond India: south to Sri Lanka, Myanmar, Thailand, Laos, Cambodia and Indonesia; north to China, Vietnam, Korea, Japan, Mongolia, Russia, Tibet, Bhutan and Nepal. For many centuries, Buddhism flourished in these Asian countries, though the twentieth century has seen a decline in some places. Since the Second World War, however, Buddhism has found a new home in the West, and it is currently a fast-growing religion in Europe and the USA.

The tales in this collection, which are taken from several Asian cultures, illustrate various aspects of Buddhist thought. Since Buddhism is a non-theistic religion, its expression is to a great extent simply basic human wisdom. Though traditional tales from Buddhist cultures are often alive with gods, goddesses, and lesser spirits and ghosts, these are not regarded as independent entities but rather in essence as virtues and powers of mind. In the Chinese tale 'The Living Kuan Yin', the hero's generosity and kindness naturally lead him to connect with a deeper level of compassion in himself (personified by the goddess Kuan Yin), which truly has the power to answer questions and grant wishes. The theme of self-sacrificing generosity leading to the acquisition of a feminine power recurs in 'Goodheart and the Goddess of the Forest', which comes from Myanmar (formerly Burma). In this story, ensuing developments show how the ego is threatened by the supernormal abilities goodness has gained, and seeks to regain its control. The shoe is on the other foot in 'The Conch Maiden', a Tibetan tale, where the initial virtue takes a feminine form and finds fruition in a semi-divine male principle. Conch is pure white, yet flashes with all the colours. In contrast with gold and silver, it represents a wealth that is more than just the riches of this world: the wealth that lies in the true nature of the mind itself.

One of the fundamental Buddhist values is humour, which views life as real but also somewhat transparent. Hardly a better example of Buddhist humour in the Tibetan mould can be found than in 'The Foolish Boy'. Meditators young and old will readily recognise the boy's romping, guileless gullibility as a representation of the lively movements of our own thought patterns. Happily, the boy has a kind of natural sweetness, which attracts capable caretakers like his mother and wife. We also see here how simple-mindedness sometimes comes close to genius, for both break the rule of concept.

The genius of no-concept is also evoked in 'The Wisdom of the Crows', where we learn that once awareness is allowed to settle into a concept, it becomes fixed and predictable, and is easily defeated. This is one of Buddhism's key insights, one which lies at the centre of training in Buddhist meditation and the martial arts.

Humour also comes to the fore in others of the short Zen tales that have been included. In stories like 'Useless Work' or 'Where Are You Going?' we find the art of the punchline that packs a mind-lifting zap. 'The Stone Ape', a longer tale from China, is a light-hearted story that also has a shocking punchline, but in this case it involves a sobering leap of perspective, in which we see that no matter how far we go, our mind always goes along with us.

'The Man Who Didn't Want to Die', from Japan, is an engaging and provocative dance illustrating two typically Buddhist concerns — the capricious nature of desire and the ego's fear of death. Finally, the Indian tale 'Angulimala the Brigand', in which the hero becomes a holy man, is one of the best-known canonical stories of the Buddha's life.

These stories reflect many profound truths of the Buddha's teaching, but no matter how profound, the truth is always simple and can usually be grasped by young children at least as easily as adults. Life 'as the Buddha taught' is like a dream; we must not trifle with it, but we must not take it too seriously either. In these stories, just as in our own, there is always a certain lightness, changeability and play that makes it easy for fundamental warmth, intelligence and humour to come shining through.

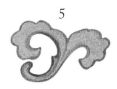

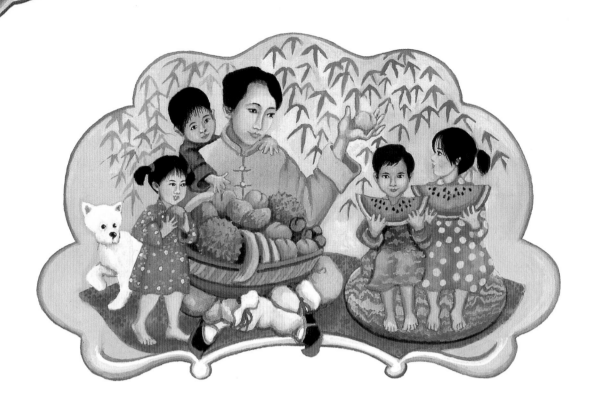

THE LIVING KUAN YIN

Once, long ago, in China, there was a young man named Chin Po-wan. His name fitted him well because in Chinese, *chin* means 'gold' and *po-wan* means 'million', and Po-wan's family had more golden coins than they could count.

Because of his name and family fortune, Po-wan thought he would always be rich, so he spent his money very freely — but not on himself. Feeling truly sorry for the poor and needy, he could never refuse them help. A poor man had only to hold out his hand and Po-wan filled it with gold. If he heard of a widow with hungry children, he made sure that they had a place to live and food for the rest of their lives. Po-wan gave unselfishly to all who were poor and without hope.

But finally, even Po-wan's huge fortune was not enough. He gave away so much that he became a poor man himself. When at last he himself had only a little food, he continued to give food to those with even less. One day, as he was sharing his bowl of rice with a beggar, he suddenly felt very sad that he had so little to give.

'Why am I so poor?' he asked himself. 'I have never done anything to harm anyone, and I have never spent much money on myself. How can it be that I don't have more to give this poor man than a handful of rice?'

This question preoccupied him for days and nights, and still no answer came to him. Then at last he had an idea. He would go to see the living Kuan Yin, the beautiful goddess of mercy and kindness to whom all people looked for comfort, especially those who were in trouble. 'Kuan Yin knows both the past and the future,' he thought. 'Surely she can answer my question.'

So Chin Po-wan set out for the South Sea where Kuan Yin lived. He travelled through many strange lands, until one day he came to a broad, rushing river. He was standing on the bank wondering how he could possibly get across, when he heard a deep, rumbling voice coming from the cliff above him.

'Chin Po-wan,' the voice said, 'if you are going to the South Sea, would you ask the living goddess Kuan Yin a question for me?'

Po-wan had never refused anything to anybody in his whole life. Besides, he knew the goddess allowed each person who came to her three questions, and he only had one of his own. So he replied, 'Yes, yes; all right, I shall.'

Turning around, he looked up to see who the voice had come from. To his amazement, towering above him he saw a huge snake, whose body was as thick as a temple pillar and twice as long. Po-wan was frightened, and he was glad that he had been quick to agree.

'Then please ask her why I am not yet a dragon, even though I have practised kindness and self-control for a thousand years,' said the big snake.

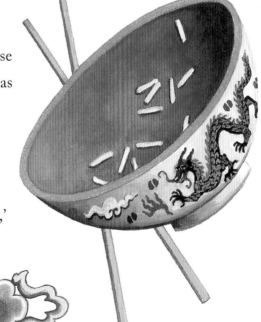

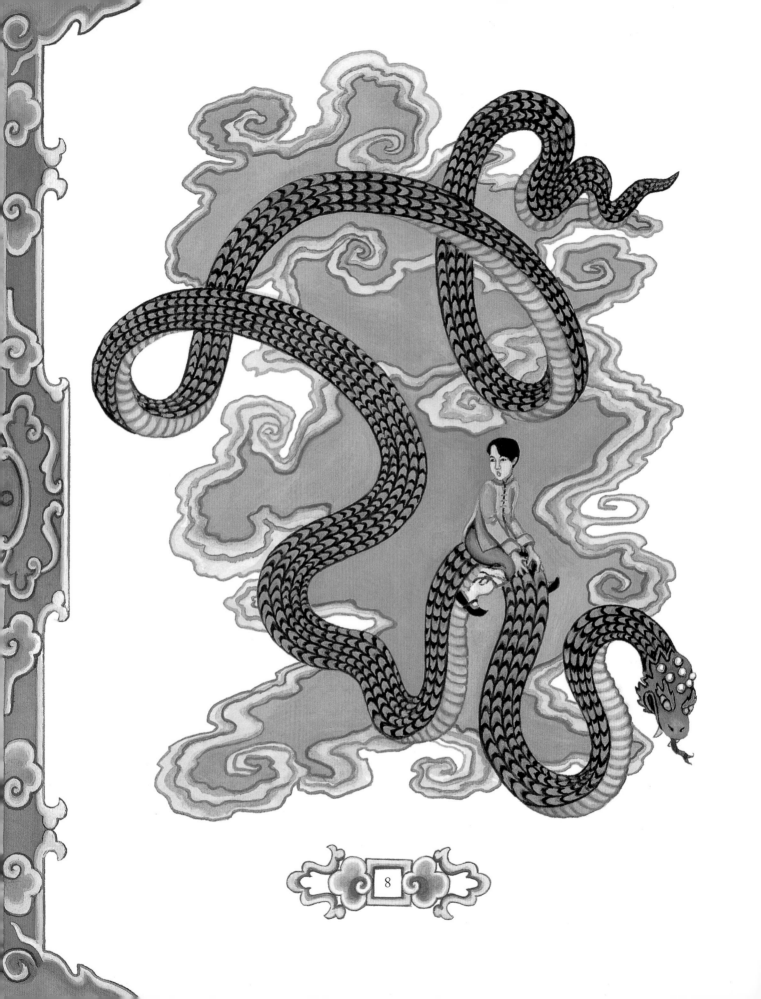

'Oh, I surely will!' said Po-wan nervously, hoping that the big reptile would continue to practise kindness and self-control and not eat him up in one gulp. 'That is, if I can get across this river. I'll never see Kuan Yin unless I can reach the other side, and at the moment I don't see how I can possibly do it.'

'Oh, that's no problem,' said the snake. 'Just jump on my back and I'll carry you across.'

So Po-wan climbed on to the snake's broad, scaly back and was soon safely across the river. He thanked the huge creature politely and said goodbye. Then he continued on his way towards the South Sea.

He walked a lot farther that day and was getting quite hungry when, luckily, he came to an inn where he was able to buy a bowl of rice. While waiting for his food, he had a chat with the innkeeper. He told him about the great snake who had taken him across the river and learnt that the creature was well known to the people of the region. He was called the Serpent of the Cliff and was well liked, too, because he kept bandits and other evildoers from crossing the river. As Po-wan was telling the innkeeper about his adventure, it came out that he was on his way to see the living Kuan Yin.

'Oh,' said the innkeeper. 'I would be so grateful if you would ask her a question for me. I have a daughter who is beautiful, good-hearted and clever. Yet she is now twenty years old and has never uttered a single word in her whole life. Could you please, please ask the goddess why she cannot talk?'

Po-wan could hardly refuse a request like this, so he told the innkeeper, 'Don't worry about a thing. I'll ask about your daughter for you, and I'm sure everything will turn out to be all right for her.' After all, Po-wan thought to himself, I am allowed three questions and I only need to ask one for myself.

Po-wan continued on his journey and, by nightfall, he was hungry again and quite tired, too. There was no inn to be found, so he knocked on the door of the

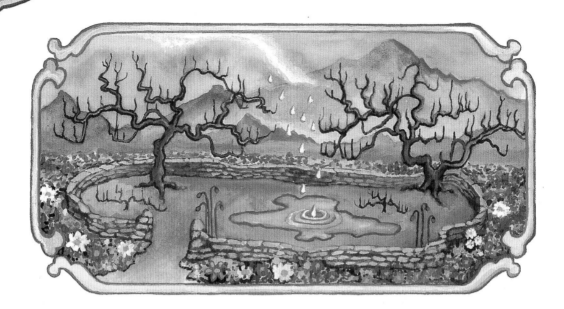

largest house he could find and asked to stay the night. The wealthy owner of the house welcomed him, gave him a good meal and something to drink, and then showed him to a lovely guest room. Po-wan woke up the next morning refreshed and ready to go. He thanked his host and said goodbye.

'Where will your journey take you?' his host asked.

'Oh, I am going to the South Sea,' replied Po-wan.

'Well, if you are going to the South Sea, perhaps you will see the living Kuan Yin and could ask her a question for me. I have been living in this house for twenty years and all that time I have taken the very best care of my garden. Yet no plant has ever borne flowers or fruit, which is bad enough; but what's more, because of that, the birds never come to my garden and sing, and there is no nectar for the bees to gather. My garden is such a sad place. I would be so grateful if you could ask the goddess why this is.'

'I shall be honoured to ask her your question,' said Po-wan and continued on his way. He did want to help the kind man with his garden and, besides, the living Kuan Yin allowed each person three questions, and he only had one of his own, one for the snake, one for the innkeeper and one for the man with the garden. 'Oh-oh...' Po-wan thought. He stopped and counted the questions on his fingers. Yes, he realised with a flutter of his heart, there was definitely one question too many.

What a predicament! He had four important questions to ask. One of them would have to go unanswered, but which one should it be? If he didn't ask his own question, his whole journey would be for nothing. But if he didn't ask the snake's question, or the innkeeper's, or the question of the man who had so kindly lodged and fed him, not only would one of them be very disappointed, but he would also be breaking a promise. As Po-wan walked, he turned the problem over and over in his mind.

Finally, he thought to himself, 'I made the promises, therefore I must keep them. Besides, even if I don't ask my own question, my journey won't be for nothing. At least those three people will have their problems solved.'

Happy with this decision, Po-wan came to the South Sea. He asked local people for directions and at last came into the presence of the living Kuan Yin. The goddess was so beautiful and radiated such kindness that Po-wan felt very meek and humble. He bowed to her and then quietly asked her his questions.

'The Serpent of the Cliff,' he began, 'has been practising kindness and self-control for a thousand years, but he has not yet become a dragon. Why is this?'

'On the serpent's head there are seven shining pearls. If six of them are taken away, he can become a dragon,' replied the goddess.

'Thank you, my lady,' said Po-wan. 'And now, here is my second question: there is a certain innkeeper whose daughter has reached the age of twenty without uttering a single word.

11

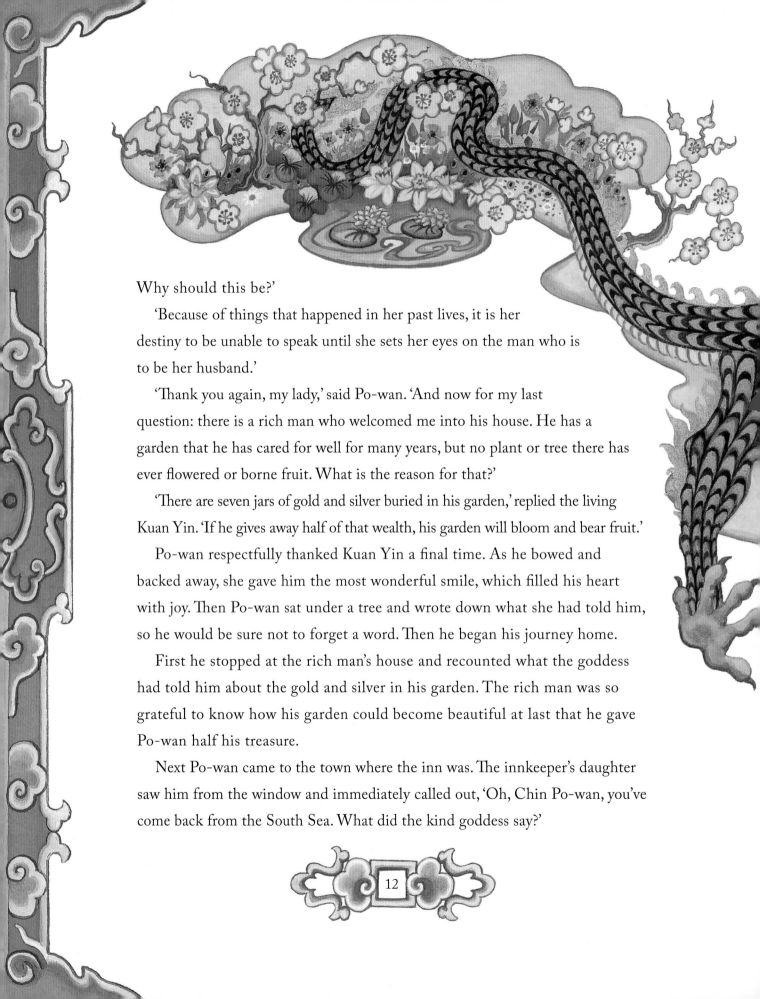

Why should this be?'

'Because of things that happened in her past lives, it is her destiny to be unable to speak until she sets her eyes on the man who is to be her husband.'

'Thank you again, my lady,' said Po-wan. 'And now for my last question: there is a rich man who welcomed me into his house. He has a garden that he has cared for well for many years, but no plant or tree there has ever flowered or borne fruit. What is the reason for that?'

'There are seven jars of gold and silver buried in his garden,' replied the living Kuan Yin. 'If he gives away half of that wealth, his garden will bloom and bear fruit.'

Po-wan respectfully thanked Kuan Yin a final time. As he bowed and backed away, she gave him the most wonderful smile, which filled his heart with joy. Then Po-wan sat under a tree and wrote down what she had told him, so he would be sure not to forget a word. Then he began his journey home.

First he stopped at the rich man's house and recounted what the goddess had told him about the gold and silver in his garden. The rich man was so grateful to know how his garden could become beautiful at last that he gave Po-wan half his treasure.

Next Po-wan came to the town where the inn was. The innkeeper's daughter saw him from the window and immediately called out, 'Oh, Chin Po-wan, you've come back from the South Sea. What did the kind goddess say?'

The innkeeper was filled with happiness at hearing his daughter speaking at last. The two young people had fallen in love at first sight, and the innkeeper insisted that they be married.

Then Po-wan went to the rushing river to give the snake the living Kuan Yin's message. The snake removed six of the pearls and gave them to Po-wan. Immediately he turned into a magnificent dragon, and the one remaining pearl in his forehead began to give out a powerful glow, which filled the countryside with a soft, gorgeous light.

That is how Chin Po-wan, through his kindness and generosity, married a beautiful wife and once again became as rich as his name.

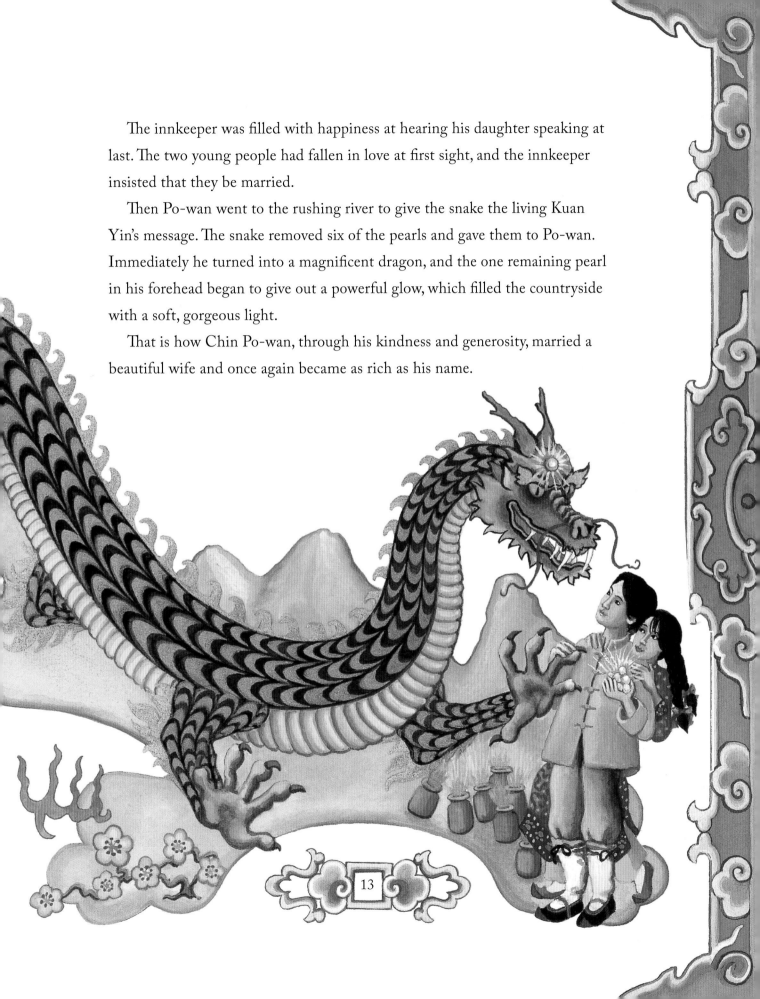

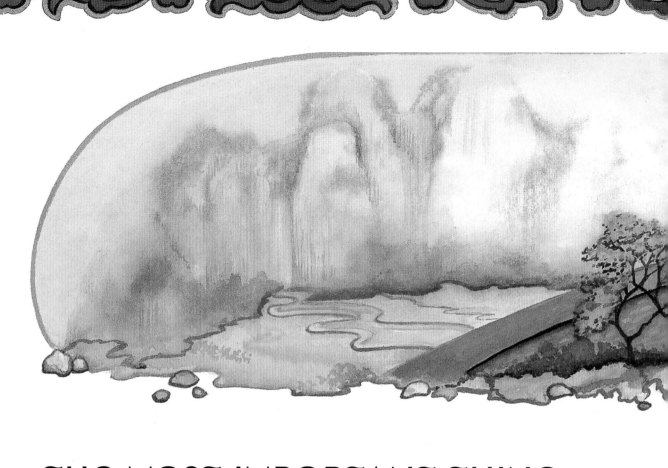

THE MOST IMPORTANT THING

Once a famous Chinese poet wanted to study the wisdom of the Buddha. He travelled a long distance to see a famous teacher and asked him, 'What is the most important thing in the Buddha's teaching?'

'Don't harm anyone and only do good,' replied the teacher.

'This is just too stupid!' exclaimed the poet. 'You are supposed to be a great teacher, so I travelled miles and miles to see you. And now is that all you can come up with? Even a three-year-old could say that!'

'Maybe a three-year-old could say it, but it is very hard to put into practice, even for a very old man like myself,' said the teacher.

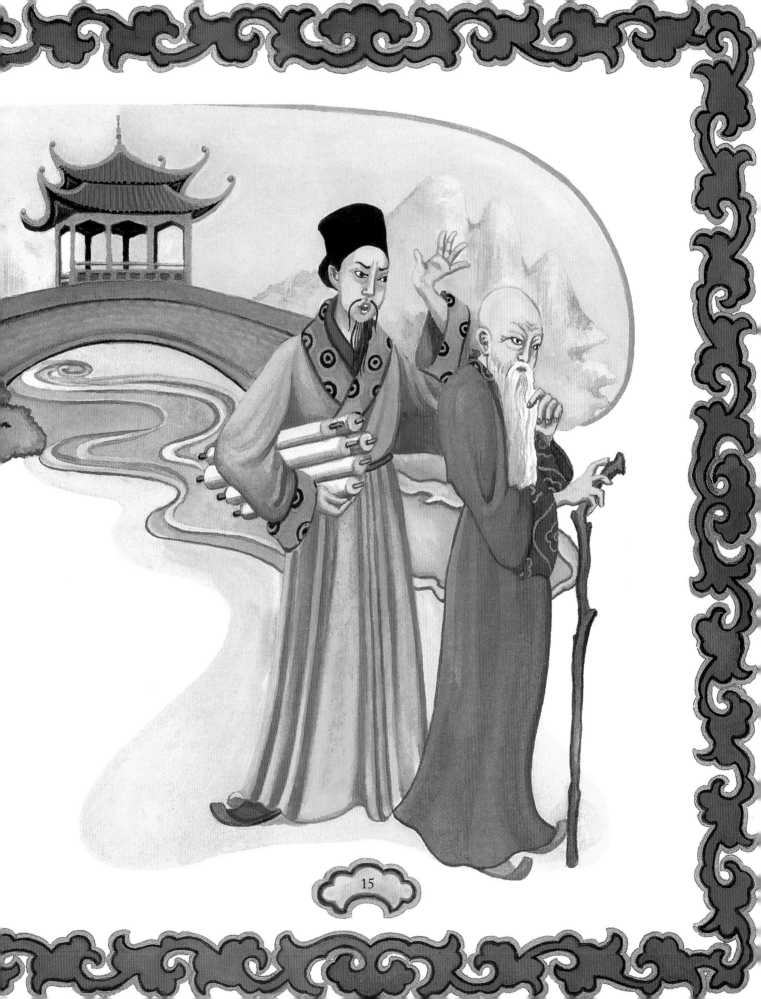

15

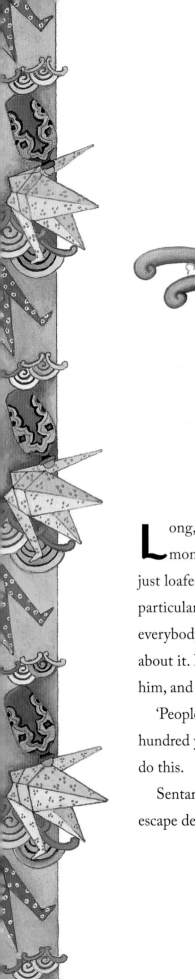

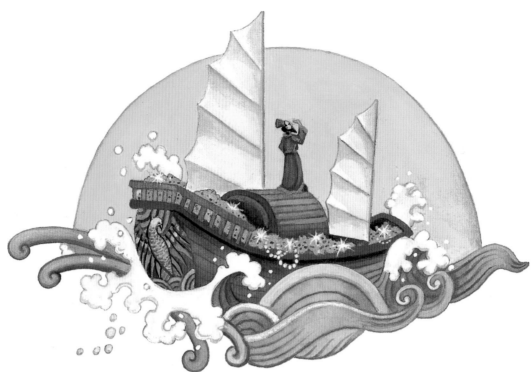

THE MAN WHO DIDN'T WANT TO DIE

Long, long ago, in Japan, there lived a man named Sentaro. He had inherited money from his father and had enough to live on, so he never worked. He just loafed through life until he was thirty-two years old. Then, one day, for no particular reason, he started thinking about sickness and death. He knew that everybody had to become sick and die some time, but he had never thought about it. Now he couldn't get rid of the idea that this was going to happen to him, and he started to feel very, very bad.

'People's lives are so short,' he thought. 'I would like to live at least five or six hundred years without getting ill.' And he began to wonder how he could actually do this.

Sentaro had heard the story of a Chinese emperor who had also wanted to escape death. The emperor was rich and powerful and could do whatever he

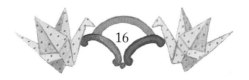

wanted, but, like everyone else, he still had to die. He felt sad about this, just as Sentaro did, and he wished for the same thing: to be able to live for a long, long time, or maybe even forever. This great emperor sent one of his trusted counsellors, a man named Jofoku, who until then had been able to accomplish anything he was told to accomplish, to find something called the elixir of life. According to stories they had heard, if you drank the elixir of life, you would live forever.

Jofoku set off across the sea to find the elixir of life, in a boat loaded with jewels and gold to pay for it. But he never returned. Sadly, without the elixir of life, the great emperor had to die just like everybody else.

But the story about Jofoku and the elixir of life lived on. According to what people told Sentaro now, Jofoku had gone to heaven and become a god, and the god Jofoku had become the special protector of hermits. Hermits were people who lived alone in the high mountains and spent their time meditating. People said that the hermits knew the secret of the elixir of life, and if Sentaro wanted to find it, he would have to ask them.

So Sentaro set off to get the elixir of life from the hermits. He wandered through all the high mountains of Japan, but he never found a single hermit. Bandits he found, in their hideouts in the mountains, but this didn't help him.

After he had spent a long time walking and climbing by himself in the mountains without success, he became very discouraged. But he didn't give up,

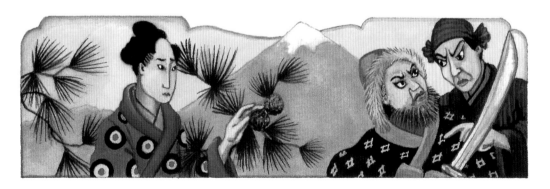

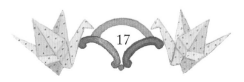

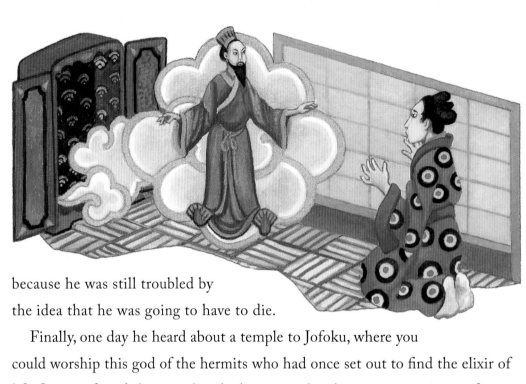

because he was still troubled by
the idea that he was going to have to die.

Finally, one day he heard about a temple to Jofoku, where you
could worship this god of the hermits who had once set out to find the elixir of
life. Sentaro found this temple, which was in a lonely spot in a mountain forest.
He went inside and began to pray. He prayed for seven days, begging Jofoku to
help him find a hermit who could fulfil his wish. At midnight on the seventh day,
a door on the little cabinet on top of the altar flew open, and Jofoku came out.
Hovering near Sentaro in the midst of a shining cloud, he spoke to him.

'To find the elixir of life, you would have to become a hermit yourself. A hermit's life
is too hard for you. A hermit has to eat only berries and the bark of trees. He has to stay
alone until his heart becomes as pure as gold and free from all desires. Finally, after a
long time, the hermit feels neither hunger nor heat nor cold. His body becomes so light
he can walk on water or ride on a bird. But you have been an idle man, used to comfort.
You could never do this. So I will answer your prayer in another way. I will send you to
the Land of Never-ending Life, where no one ever dies.'

With this, Jofoku put a tiny little crane, made of folded paper, into Sentaro's
hand and told him to sit on its back. At once, the crane began to grow, and
soon it was large enough for Sentaro to sit on it quite comfortably. It spread its
wings and rose high into the air. Together they soared over the mountains and
out across the ocean. For many days they flew over the waves, until at last they

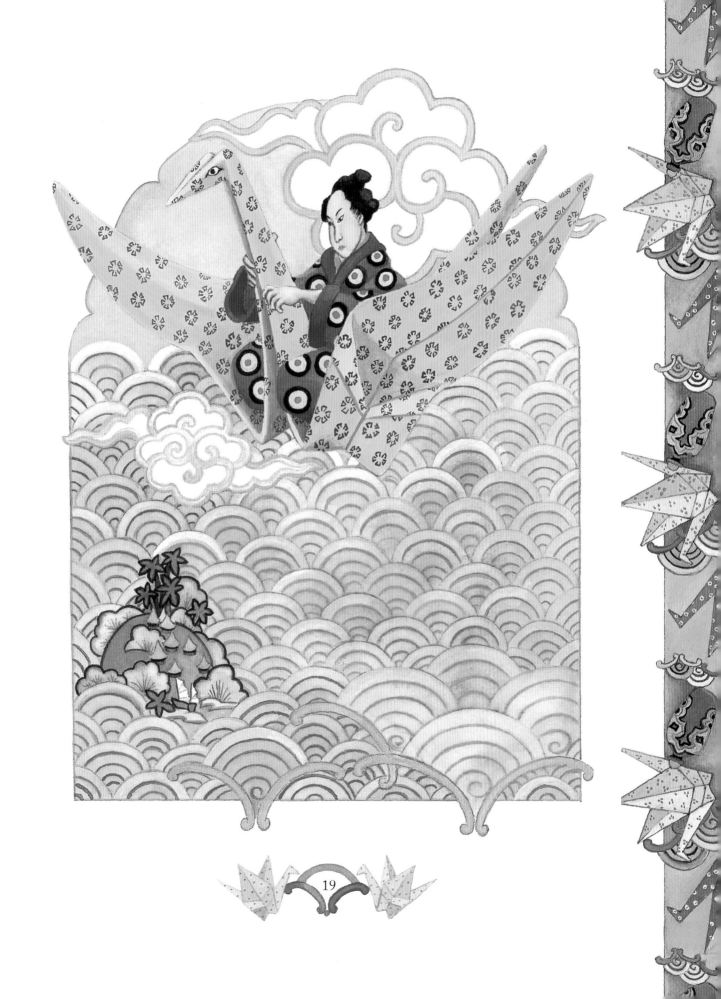

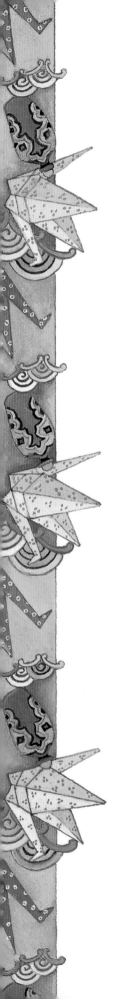

reached an island. The crane landed in the middle of the island, and as soon as Sentaro got off its back, it folded itself up and went into his pocket.

Sentaro was very curious about this Land of Never-ending Life. He walked around the country and then into the nearby town to talk to the people who lived there. Of course everything was very strange and very different from his own country. But the people seemed prosperous enough and there was plenty to eat, so he decided he should stay there.

At first he stayed at an inn. But when he told the innkeeper that he had come to the island for good, the innkeeper kindly found him a house and helped him to make all the arrangements necessary to stay there. So the Land of Never-ending Life became Sentaro's new home. He even set up a business for himself.

As time went on, Sentaro found out more about his island. The strangest thing of all, of course, was that no one could remember anyone ever dying or even getting ill. This made Sentaro very happy. He was very much looking forward to living forever, and he thought that the islanders must be the happiest people on earth. But this was not true at all. The people grew very bored and tired of their long, long, never-ending lives. Things kept being the same day after day, year after year. They wished very much to die, for it would be such an interesting change. On top of this, they had heard of a heaven or paradise, which you could enter only by dying.

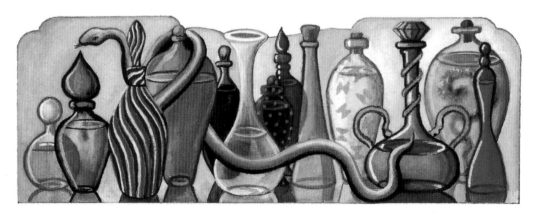

This sounded like something different and wonderful, and they were willing to try anything so they could die and go there. Whenever merchants came from distant lands, the islanders crowded around their booths trying to buy poisons. These they swallowed eagerly, but the poisons only made their health better. The most popular drink on the whole island was a potion that sometimes gave the drinker a few grey hairs and some stomach pains after he had drunk it every day for a hundred years. Poisonous snakes and fish were the islanders' favourite food, but still no one died. People didn't so much as get a cold.

Sentaro thought these people were strange, but for a long time he was happy in the Land of Never-ending Life. His business went well, and he always took pleasure in the idea that he would never die. But after many years, things began to change for Sentaro. He, too, became weary of an endless number of days, always the same. He started to have trouble with his business, and he was always getting into arguments with his neighbours. After about three hundred years, he was very tired and bored, and he began to be homesick. He wanted to get away from the Land of Never-ending Life and go to his old country again, where it was possible for people to die.

One day, Sentaro was trying to think of a way to get home, when suddenly he remembered Jofoku. He called out to Jofoku to help him, and as soon as the words were out of his mouth, the paper crane, which had been in the pocket of his old coat all this time, came flying to him and began to grow again to its full size. Sentaro climbed on to its back, and soon they were high in the air, flying over the ocean back towards Japan.

You'd think Sentaro would be happy, but no — not at all! Less than an hour had passed before he began to regret leaving all he had left behind on the island, and especially his never-ending life. He tried to turn the crane back, but it took no notice of him and continued to fly resolutely over the ocean towards Japan.

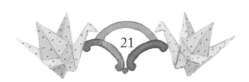

21

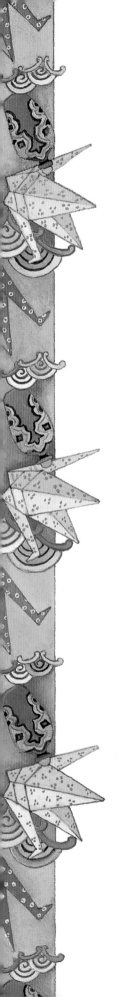

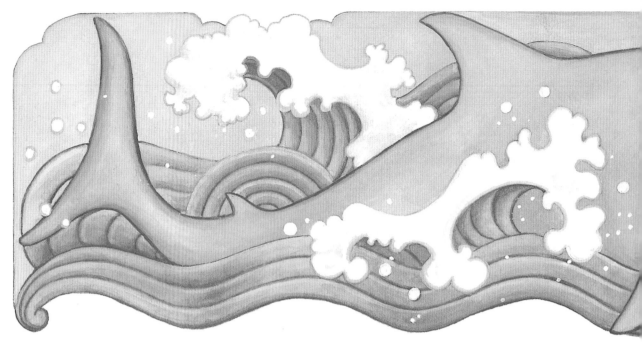

After a day or two of flying, storm clouds began to form and then rain fell in great sheets. The paper crane got wet, lost its shape and fell into the sea, Sentaro along with it!

Sentaro struggled to stay afloat. There was no ship in sight, and he was terribly frightened of drowning. As he looked around for help, what he saw instead was a huge shark coming towards him with a gaping mouth full of sharp teeth. Sentaro tried to cry for help, but he was so terrified that no sound would come from his mouth. When the shark was only a few inches away and he thought his end had come for sure, Sentaro finally managed to get out a huge scream, and he screamed as loud as he could for Jofoku to save him.

Sentaro woke up screaming and found he was on the floor in the lonely Jofoku temple on the mountainside. He had fallen asleep while praying, and all his adventures — the paper crane, the Land of Never-ending Life, the storm and the shark — had been nothing but a dream. A bright light came towards him, and in the light stood a messenger, holding a book.

This is what the messenger told Sentaro:

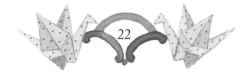

22

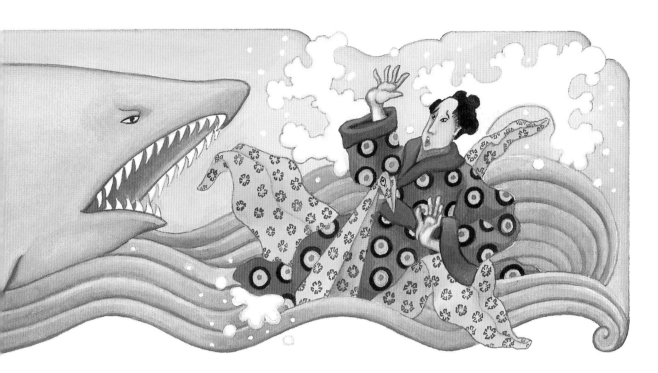

'In answer to your prayers, Jofoku sent you a dream so you could see the Land of Never-ending Life. But you grew weary of living there and begged to go back to your own country so you could die. Then Jofoku made you fall into the ocean and sent the shark, so you could die. But you didn't really want to die either, and you cried out for help. Then you woke up here.

'So you see, Sentaro, you don't want to live forever, and you are in no hurry to die either. So the best thing for you to do is to go back to your home and lead a good, normal life. Be good to your elders and be good to your children, and be a kind and generous friend, and you will find real happiness. Here is a book full of wisdom to show you how to lead the kind of life I have pointed out to you.'

Then the messenger disappeared. Taking the book, Sentaro went back to his old home. He studied the book and did his best to follow its wisdom. He gave up his desire to live forever and his desire to die. He gave up his selfishness and did his best to help other people. And he lived in contentment to a ripe, old age.

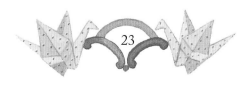

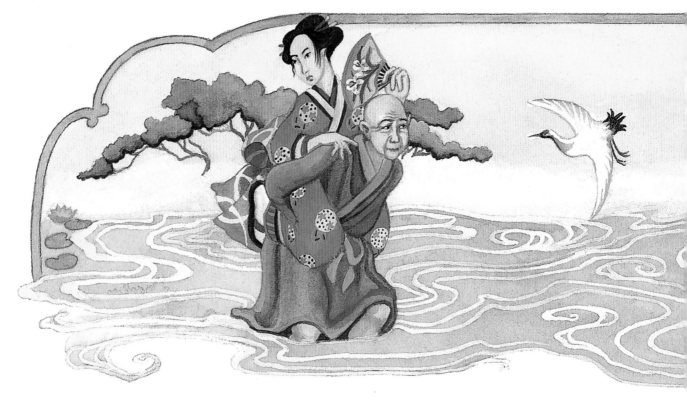

USELESS WORK

An old monk and a young monk were walking along the road when they came to a rushing stream. It was neither too wide nor too deep and they were about to wade across when a beautiful young woman, who had been waiting on the bank, approached them. She was elegantly dressed and she fluttered her fan and batted her eyelashes, smiling at them with big eyes.

'Oh,' she said, 'the current is so swift, the water is so cold, and if my kimono gets wet, it will spoil the silk. Won't one of you please carry me across the stream?' And she edged invitingly towards the young monk.

Now the young monk thought the woman's behaviour was disgusting. He thought she was spoilt and shameless and ought to be taught a lesson. On top of that, monks are not supposed to have anything to do with women. So

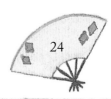

24

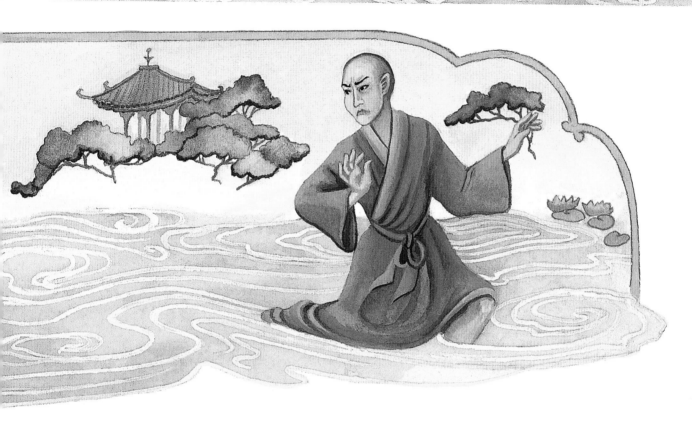

he ignored her completely and waded across the stream. But the old monk gave a shrug, picked up the young woman, carried her across the water and set her down on the other side. Then the two monks continued on their way down the road.

Though they walked in silence, the young monk was furious. He thought his companion had done entirely the wrong thing by indulging that spoilt young woman. And even worse, by touching her he had broken the monks' rule. He raved and ranted in his mind as they walked over hills and through fields. Finally, he could stand it no longer. Shouting loudly, he began scolding his companion for carrying the woman across the stream. He was beside himself with anger and completely red in the face.

'Oh, dear,' said the old monk. 'Are you still carrying that woman? I put her down an hour ago.' He gave a shrug and continued down the road.

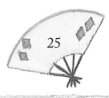

25

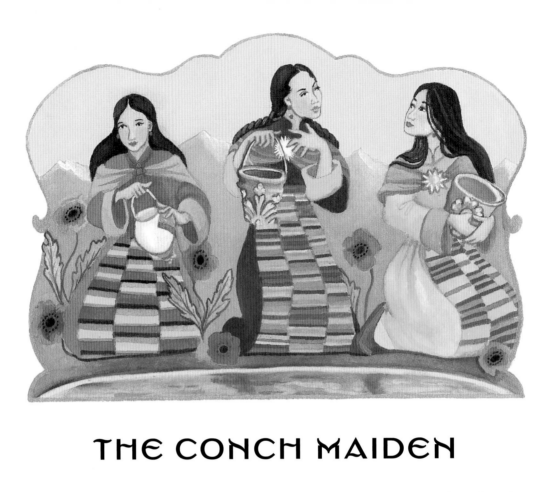

THE CONCH MAIDEN

Long, long ago, there lived three sisters in Tibet: the golden maiden, the silver maiden and the conch maiden. They were all very beautiful, and throughout the country there was not a young man that did not long to have one of them for his wife. But the golden and silver maidens were proud and fussy and thought only about how important and rich their suitors should be. Only the conch maiden wished for a husband with a good and kind heart.

One morning, the golden maiden took her golden bucket to go and fetch some water from the spring. When she opened the door, she found a beggar clothed in ugly, grubby rags lying in the dirt at the door of the house.

'What are you doing here, you filthy thing?!' screamed the golden maiden. 'Away with you! Out of my sight! Be gone!'

'All right, all right, I'm going,' said the beggar. 'But please help me to stand up, young miss. My old legs don't work so well.'

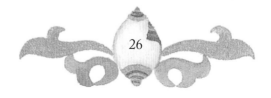

'Help yourself! Nobody told you to come here! You can leave the same way you came,' said the golden maiden. 'My father wants water to thin his beer. My mother needs water for her tea. I want water to wash my hair. So get moving! If you don't get out of my way, I'll step on your hand. I always do just what I want!'

No sooner said than done. She walked right over the beggar and in so doing trod on his hand. After she had passed, the beggar raised his head and looked after her with coals of fire burning in his black eyes. By the time the golden maiden came back from the spring, the beggar was gone.

The next morning, the silver maiden came out of the house carrying her silver bucket. The beggar was lying in front of the house again, and the maiden shrank back with disgust.

'How dare you lie in front of our house, you foul creature!' she cried. 'Get along with you! Out of my way!'

'It's not all that easy, lovely miss,' the beggar sighed. 'If you only knew how my old bones hurt. Please, won't you give me a hand to stand up?'

'Oh, isn't that a fine idea!' replied the maiden in a nasty mocking voice. 'My hand is the last thing you'll have! Now crawl away from here as fast as your hands and knees will carry you, or I'll step on you!'

Without waiting, she stepped over the beggar, but made sure that he got a good bang on the head from her silver bucket as

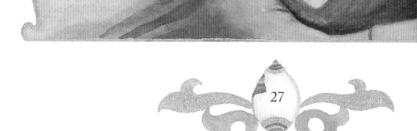

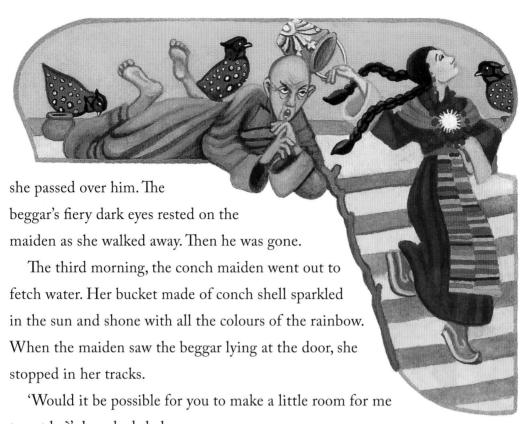

she passed over him. The beggar's fiery dark eyes rested on the maiden as she walked away. Then he was gone.

The third morning, the conch maiden went out to fetch water. Her bucket made of conch shell sparkled in the sun and shone with all the colours of the rainbow. When the maiden saw the beggar lying at the door, she stopped in her tracks.

'Would it be possible for you to make a little room for me to get by?' she asked shyly.

'I'd like to,' said the beggar, 'but my old bones hurt so much, I'll never be able to get up by myself.'

'Come on,' said the conch maiden. I'll help you.' And she gave the beggar her hand. He was so heavy, it was all she could do to get him up without falling down herself.

'I mustn't let him see how hard it is for me to lift him,' the maiden thought. 'Otherwise, he might think he's being a burden on me, and that might hurt his feelings.' So she smiled and chattered away in a kindly way: 'See there, upsy daisy, no problem at all. You're just a bit frozen from lying on the cold ground. Soon you'll be as good as ever.'

'How sweet and kind you are,' said the beggar. 'It's almost more than a man can believe. For your kindness, I wish you the richest husband in the land.'

'Let him be rich, let him be poor; the main thing is for him to have a good heart,' the maiden said, smiling again.

'That might be possible, too,' the beggar murmured half to himself, but with a gleam in his eye, and limped slowly behind the maiden. When she reached the spring, she knelt on the ground and began filling her bucket with water.

'Wait, let me help you,' said the beggar when she tried lifting the bucket into the sling on her back. But he was so clumsy about it, all the water spilled on to the ground.

The maiden laughed. 'Oh, don't bother about that. How many times I've done the same thing myself!'

They filled the bucket again, and the beggar lifted it so it could be slipped into the sling. But he held it too low for her to bend to get under it, so she said, 'If it isn't too hard for you, could you lift it just a little bit higher?'

'Gladly,' said the beggar. But now he lifted the bucket too high, so she still couldn't get it into the sling.

'Don't be angry with me,' said the conch maiden, 'but now you've got it too high for me.'

'No bother at all,' said the beggar. 'We'll just fix that.' But now when he lowered the bucket, he let it tip and the water spilled out all over the maiden's back.

'Oh, oh, I'm so clumsy!' the beggar cried.

'Not at all,' said the maiden. 'You're not clumsy. That could happen to anybody.'

The beggar gave the maiden a long, thoughtful look. Again they filled the bucket with water but as he lifted it, he made an awkward movement, and the bucket slipped from his grasp and crashed to the ground, shattering into a thousand pieces. At this, the conch maiden finally lost control of herself and began to cry bitterly.

'Oh, it's so sad, my beautiful bucket, my beautiful bucket!' she sobbed. But still through her tears, she said to the beggar, 'Don't blame yourself. You were doing the best you could. But, oh, my parents are going to be so angry with me!' She went on crying, 'A bucket made of conch is very hard to get.'

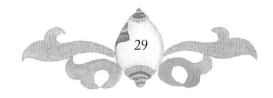

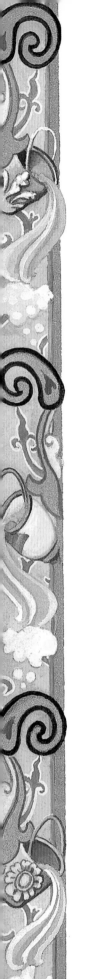

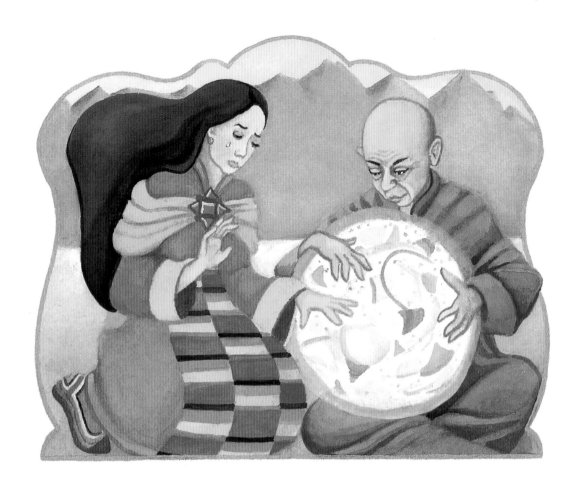

'Perhaps I can help you after all,' the beggar said softly with a little smile. Quickly and gracefully, he bent down and gathered all the shining pieces together into a little pile and began fitting them back together again. His hands moved very fast, then faster and faster. Finally, they were moving so fast that the maiden couldn't see them at all. Before she even had time to think, there before her eyes was her beautiful conch bucket all perfect and new, full of fresh, clean water from the spring. And the beggar showed no sign of clumsiness now when he lifted it on to her back. It seemed to slip into the sling almost all by itself. The conch maiden looked at the beggar with wonder.

'Can you do something for me?' the beggar then asked in a full, strong voice.

'Anything in my power,' the maiden cried. 'I'm so grateful to you for putting my bucket back together.'

'Then please ask your parents to let me spend the night in your kitchen.'

30

'Oh, I don't know if my mother would allow that,' said the conch maiden timidly. 'She doesn't like beggars. But I'll ask her anyway.'

'In exchange, she can keep what she finds at the bottom of the bucket,' said the beggar with a smile.

That aroused the maiden's curiosity. What could there be at the bottom of the bucket? There was something strange and special about all this. Somehow she knew the old man was no ordinary beggar. Despite herself, she thought there must be something wonderful about him.

She carried her bucket of water home and asked her mother to let the beggar spend the night in the kitchen.

'You're not talking about that awful beggar that has been hanging around the door for days now, are you?' she replied crossly. The conch maiden hung her head without replying and poured the water from her bucket into a big copper tub. To her surprise there was a clank as something hit the bottom of the tub, and when she looked in, there was a small object glittering in the water. The mother quickly stuck her hand into the water and came up with a heavy ring of gold. Then the conch maiden remembered what the beggar had told her.

'That's supposed to be payment for a night's lodging,' she quickly said.

'A beggar who pays in gold? That's a strange thing,' said the mother. 'All right, he can sleep in the kitchen.'

In the evening, the whole family gathered together as usual. The father drank tea with butter in it, the way people do in Tibet, the mother spun wool and the daughters sat together laughing and talking. After a while, they began talking about suitors.

'I want to marry the Prince of India at least,' declared the golden maiden. 'Otherwise, I won't marry at all.'

'Our own prince would be enough for me,' said the silver maiden.

31

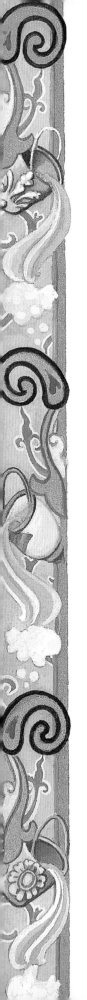

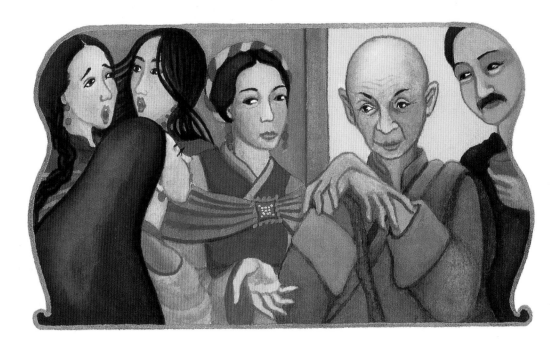

The conch maiden said nothing.

'And who would you like to marry?' the mother asked her.

Just then, the door opened and in came the beggar. 'I know the right husband for the conch maiden,' he said. 'The great Lord Mipham himself would count himself lucky to have such a kind-hearted and beautiful maiden as her for a wife!'

'Who is this Mipham?' the other two sisters immediately wanted to know. 'Is he as rich and powerful as the Prince of India?'

'Maybe richer and more powerful,' said the beggar mysteriously, and his dark eyes rested long on the conch maiden. 'He would be overjoyed to marry you, and you would be happy with him as with no other man. Do you think you would like to marry him, conch maiden?'

The conch maiden remembered how the beggar had miraculously repaired her broken bucket and quickly she nodded.

'Then follow the tracks of my crutches,' the beggar said. At once, he turned and hobbled out the door. The conch maiden didn't hesitate for a second, but jumped up from her chair and ran out of the door after him.

'Where are you going?' her mother screamed after her. 'Have you gone mad? A beggar will only lead you to another beggar.'

But it was too late. The maiden was already gone. Outside, she looked for the beggar, but all she could see was the trail of little holes in the ground made by his crutches. There was nothing for her to do but follow them, so off she ran over the hill into the darkness.

All through the night, the conch maiden followed the crutch tracks by the light of the moon, until the sky began to grow pale with dawn. Then she saw a big meadow ahead of her. On the meadow was a shepherd boy, watching over thousands of sheep.

'Did a beggar come by here?' asked the conch maiden.

'No, only Lord Mipham came by,' replied the boy. 'These sheep belong to him.'

The maiden ran on until she came to a huge herd of yaks. 'Did you see a beggar come this way?' she asked the man herding the yaks.

'No beggar,' said the yak herd, 'but Lord Mipham passed by a little while ago. These are his yaks.'

'Where could the beggar have gone?' the maiden thought. 'He himself might turn out to be this Lord Mipham, and then I'll end up married to a crippled old beggar.' But still she went on running until she came to large plain filled with horses.

'Have you seen a beggar?' she asked the man herding the horses.

'No, I only saw Lord Mipham, who came this way not long ago. All these horses are his.'

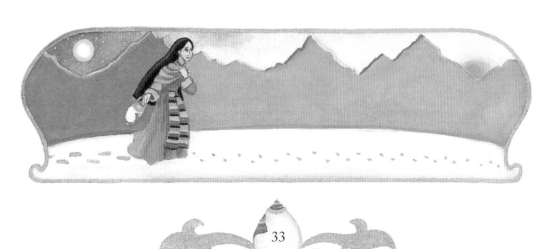

33

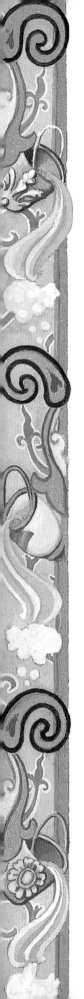

Just then, the sun came up over the horizon and in the morning light the maiden saw a sight that stopped her in her tracks. There before her was a golden castle, glinting and glittering in the first rays of the sun. At the castle door was an old man with white hair, who smiled at her.

'Is this the Buddha's temple?' the conch maiden asked the old man, for she could think of nothing else that could be so wonderful and magnificent as this.

'No, this is Lord Mipham's castle. Our master is waiting for you,' the old man told her.

The conch maiden gathered her courage and went forward. With every step she took towards the castle, fragrant flowers grew in her footprints. By the time she reached it, a carpet of blossoms lay behind her. A handsome youth met her at the door. His dark eyes sparkled with joy. He took her gently by the hand and said, 'I am Mipham. And I am the old beggar, too. Will you have me for your husband, as you said you would?' The conch maiden gazed at the handsome young man with rapture. Her heart was ready to burst with happiness. She nodded as though in a dream, and Mipham led her into the castle.

There, his servants dressed the conch maiden in a white gown that shone with all the colours of the rainbow when she moved, and adorned her with corals and glittering gems. Then she took her seat on a golden throne next to Mipham. Together they picked a date for their wedding, which took place very soon indeed. And since Mipham and the conch maiden both had kind and good hearts, they lived happily ever after.

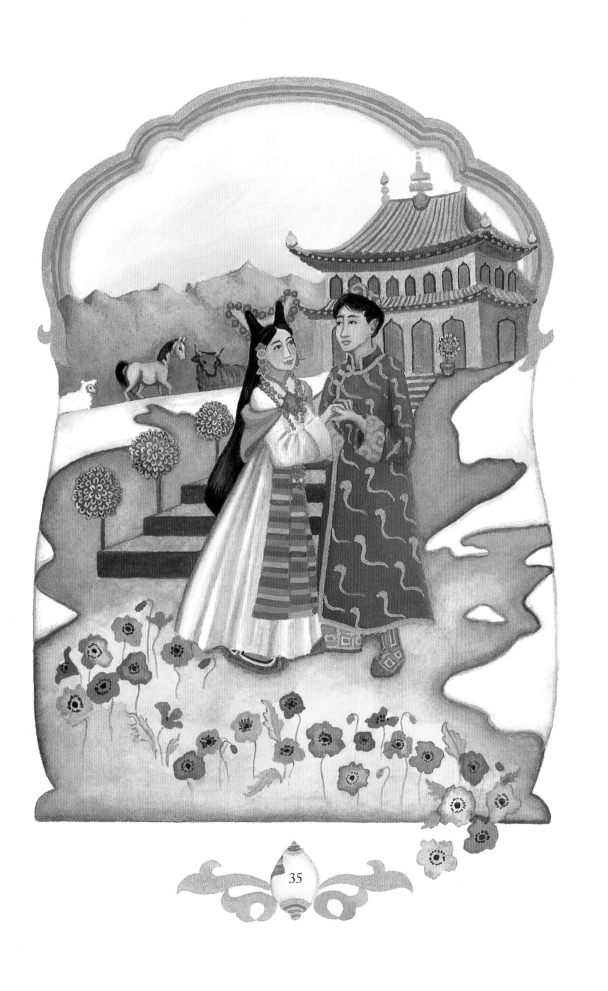

35

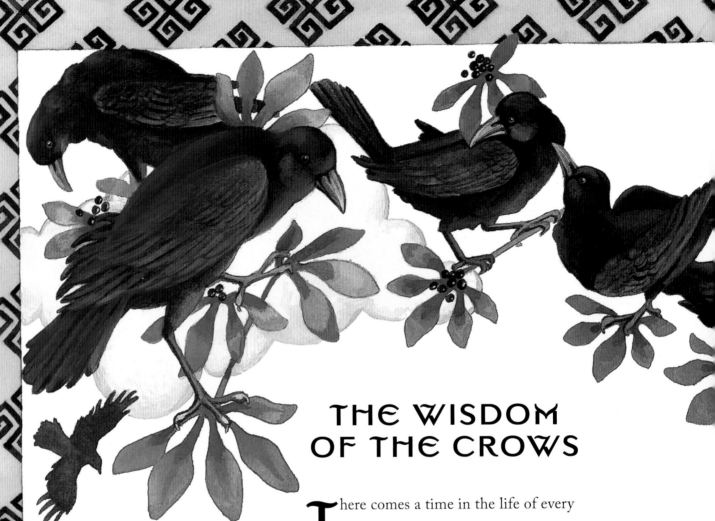

THE WISDOM
OF THE CROWS

There comes a time in the life of every kind of creature when they have to go out on their own and join the company of their elders. Crows are no exception.

It happened one day that the elder crows were testing three young ones to see if they had reached the age where they had the wit and maturity to fly with their elders. To the first of the young ones, the leader of the crows put the following question: 'In this whole world, what do you think crows should fear the most?'

The young crow thought a moment and then answered, 'The most fearsome thing is an arrow, for it can kill a crow with one strike.'

When the elder crows heard this, they thought it was a very clever answer. They flapped their wings and cawed with approval. 'You speak the truth,' said the leader. 'We welcome you into the flock.'

Then she asked the second young crow, 'What do you think we should most fear?'

'I think a skilled archer is more to be feared than an arrow,' the young one said, 'for only the archer can aim and shoot the arrow. Without the archer, the arrow is no more than a stick, like the twig I am perching on.'

The crows thought this was one of the most intelligent comments they had ever heard. The parents of the second young crow croaked with pride and beamed at their brilliant child. The leader said, 'You speak with great intelligence. We are pleased to have you as a member of the flock.' Then she asked the third young crow, 'And what do you think is the thing most to be feared in the world?'

'Neither of the things mentioned already,' responded the young bird. 'The thing in the world most to be feared is an unskilful archer.'

Here was a strange answer! The bewildered crows stood about silent and embarrassed. Many thought the third young crow was simply not bright enough to understand the question. 'Why do you say a thing like that?' the leader of the flock finally asked.

'The second of my companions is right. Without the archer, there is nothing to fear from an arrow. But a skilled archer's arrow will fly where it is aimed. So when you hear the twang of the bowstring, you only have to fly to one side or the other, and his arrow will miss you for sure. But with an unskilled archer, you never know where his arrow will go. If you try to get away, you may fly right into its path. You never can know whether to move or stay still.' When the birds heard this, they knew that the third young crow had real wisdom, which sees beyond the surface of things. They spoke of him with admiration and respect. Not long afterwards, they asked him to become the leader of the flock.

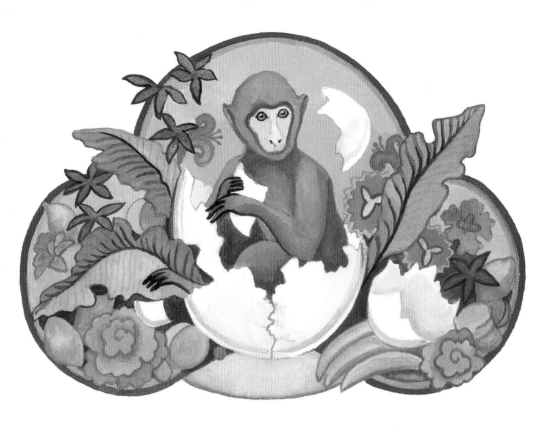

THE STONE APE

Many years ago, in a time long past, there was a beautiful island, which lay right in the middle of the Great Eastern Sea. The name of the island was Mountain of Flowers and Fruits, and on it was a large rock.

Since the beginning of the world, this rock had absorbed all the secret powers of heaven and earth and sun and moon, so by the time this story begins, it was full of magic.

One day, the rock split open, and out came a stone egg. After a while, the egg hatched, and out of it jumped a little stone ape. He bowed to the four corners of the earth — east, south, west and north — and then ran off bursting with energy and joy.

The stone ape grew up wilful and strong. When he played with the other apes of the island, he was always in charge of the games and adventures. One day, he led the whole tribe to swim and bathe in a clear, blue pool. As they approached the pool, they heard a great roaring sound. They looked up and saw that the sound

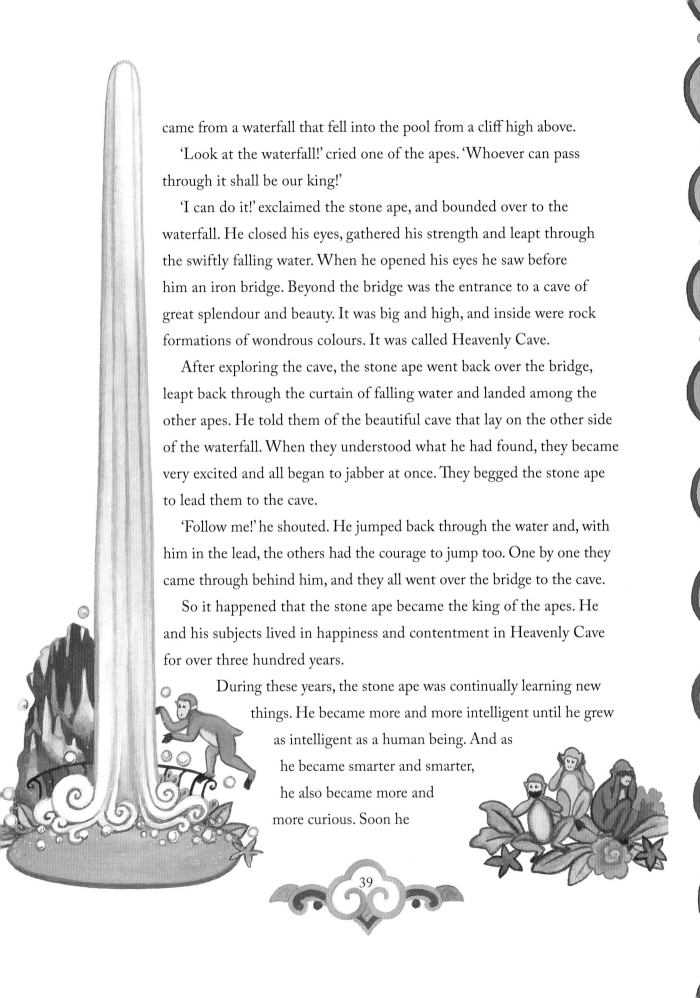

came from a waterfall that fell into the pool from a cliff high above.

'Look at the waterfall!' cried one of the apes. 'Whoever can pass through it shall be our king!'

'I can do it!' exclaimed the stone ape, and bounded over to the waterfall. He closed his eyes, gathered his strength and leapt through the swiftly falling water. When he opened his eyes he saw before him an iron bridge. Beyond the bridge was the entrance to a cave of great splendour and beauty. It was big and high, and inside were rock formations of wondrous colours. It was called Heavenly Cave.

After exploring the cave, the stone ape went back over the bridge, leapt back through the curtain of falling water and landed among the other apes. He told them of the beautiful cave that lay on the other side of the waterfall. When they understood what he had found, they became very excited and all began to jabber at once. They begged the stone ape to lead them to the cave.

'Follow me!' he shouted. He jumped back through the water and, with him in the lead, the others had the courage to jump too. One by one they came through behind him, and they all went over the bridge to the cave.

So it happened that the stone ape became the king of the apes. He and his subjects lived in happiness and contentment in Heavenly Cave for over three hundred years.

During these years, the stone ape was continually learning new things. He became more and more intelligent until he grew as intelligent as a human being. And as he became smarter and smarter, he also became more and more curious. Soon he

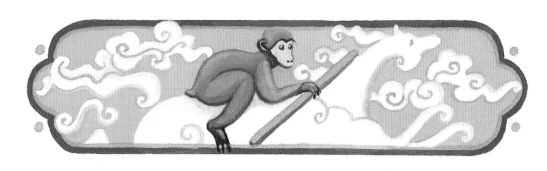

began to learn unusual things, and he became the master of seventy-two different kinds of miraculous powers. He could take the shape of anything he wished — human, plant, animal or mineral; he could ride clouds as if they were horses; and he was not afraid of any being or thing.

This was all very well and good, except that the stone ape used his powers only for his own amusement and glory and didn't seem to care how much trouble he made for others.

Now the stone ape had a magic iron rod, which he had stolen from the palace of the dragon king under the sea, and this rod was a very powerful weapon. He used it to fight his way into the underworld, the realm of the dead. There he forced the ten princes of the dead to give him the book of life and death. This book held the names of every creature and the number of years each had to live. He looked through the book until he found the page where his own name was written. He tore the page out and crumpled it in his hand. Now the stone ape would never die.

Just to make sure of this, he stole into the Western Heaven, where the sage Lao-tzu lived, who brewed the elixir of eternal life. As wise as Lao-tzu was, it took him a long time to make just a little of this elixir, and just one drop was enough to make a being live forever.

The stone ape found five gourds filled with the elixir and drained them all to the bottom. 'Now I will surely live forever!' he shouted with joy. Then to escape the wrath of the gods, he made himself invisible and crept out of the west gate of that heaven. 'Now I'll go back to earth and rule as king,' said the stone ape to himself.

Another time, he stole the peaches of Hei-wang-mu, the mother of the fairies. These were no ordinary peaches. They grew only in the fairy mother's orchard,

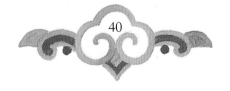

and only once every three thousand years. And once every three thousand years, when the trees were laden down with fruit, the fairy mother would invite all the gods and fairies to her orchard to feast on the magical peaches.

Now on the very day of the fairy mother's peach party, before the guests arrived, the stone ape stole into the orchard and stuffed himself with all the peaches he could possibly eat. By the time he had finished, he was so full and heavy that he just had to lie down to sleep. He thought to himself, 'If the fairy mother and her guests should come, I won't be able to run away!' So he turned himself into a tiny little peach worm, crawled under the bark of one of the trees and fell asleep. When the gods and fairies came and found their feast spoilt, they looked high and low for the thief, but nobody suspected the little peach worm, asleep in the tree.

Now the Lord of Heaven had been watching the stone ape and saw all the trouble he was causing. 'This must stop,' he thought. But as the stone ape was so wily and clever and had so many miraculous powers, it was very difficult to control him. 'Only the Lord Buddha can tame him now,' the Lord of Heaven concluded. So he sent a messenger to the Buddha and respectfully requested him to do something to keep the stone ape from wreaking havoc in heaven and on earth.

The Lord Buddha came out of the West. When he saw him, the stone ape shouted at him, 'Who are you that dares to disturb me?!' The Buddha looked at him calmly. 'I am the Buddha,' he said, 'and I am here to tame you.'

'Do you know to whom you are speaking?' said the stone ape, full of pride and defiance. 'I am the stone ape. I am a king. I hold the hidden knowledge. I am master of seventy-two different kinds of miraculous powers and the holder of eternal life! I am afraid of no one, certainly not you!'

The Buddha smiled. 'I've heard that you can somersault over the clouds and that each somersault takes you a thousand miles. Can you really do that? If you can, show me.'

41

'I can do anything!' shouted the stone ape. And off he went, somersaulting through the sky. He went head over heels so fast and so many times, he became like a whirlwind, high up beyond the clouds. He continued for a long, long time, covering an immense distance with every turn. Finally, he came to what seemed like the edge of the sky, where he saw five huge, reddish pillars. They were very tall and disappeared into the sky above. 'My goodness!' he thought. 'I must have reached the end of the world!' He was very proud of himself. To show he had been there, he somersaulted up to the middle pillar and made his mark on it. Then he somersaulted back to where he had started. The Buddha was waiting for him.

'Well, not only can I somersault a thousand miles at a time, but I have somersaulted to the end of the world!' he boasted. 'If you don't believe me, go and have a look for yourself. I left my mark on one of the pillars.'

'Perhaps you should have a look at this,' said the Buddha and held up his hand. On the Buddha's middle finger the stone ape saw the mark he had made on the pillar at the end of the world. He was stunned and afraid. The whole time he was somersaulting, he was in the palm of the Buddha's hand!

The stone ape realised he had met his master and he tried to escape. But the Buddha put his hand down over him. Then he made a magic mountain out of the basic elements of the world — water, fire, wood, earth and metal — and put it over the stone ape. Try as he would, using all his miraculous powers, the stone ape was unable to escape from beneath the magic mountain. At last earth and heaven were safe from his mischief.

The apes say that after a thousand years beneath the magic mountain, the stone ape reappeared on the island. They say that time brought about in him a change of heart, and nowadays, though he still has lots of fun, he uses his intelligence and powers to help others.

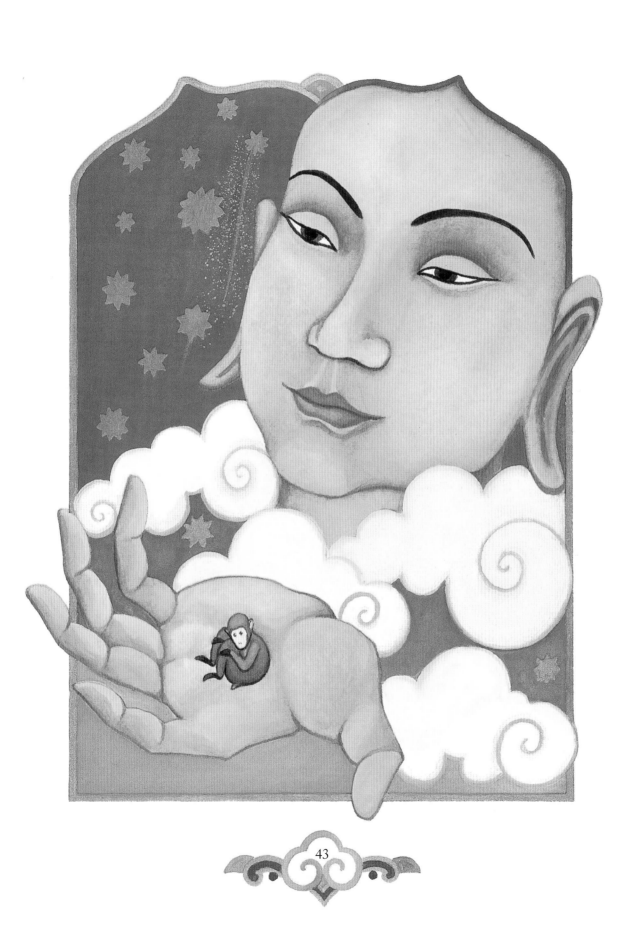

43

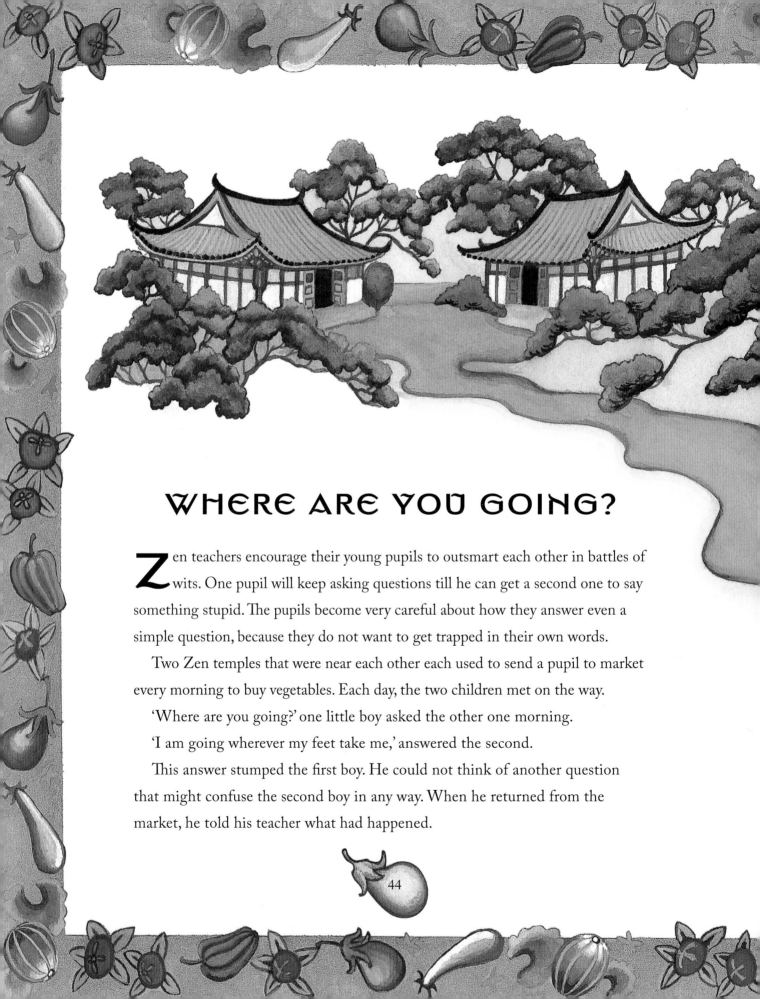

WHERE ARE YOU GOING?

Zen teachers encourage their young pupils to outsmart each other in battles of wits. One pupil will keep asking questions till he can get a second one to say something stupid. The pupils become very careful about how they answer even a simple question, because they do not want to get trapped in their own words.

Two Zen temples that were near each other each used to send a pupil to market every morning to buy vegetables. Each day, the two children met on the way.

'Where are you going?' one little boy asked the other one morning.

'I am going wherever my feet take me,' answered the second.

This answer stumped the first boy. He could not think of another question that might confuse the second boy in any way. When he returned from the market, he told his teacher what had happened.

44

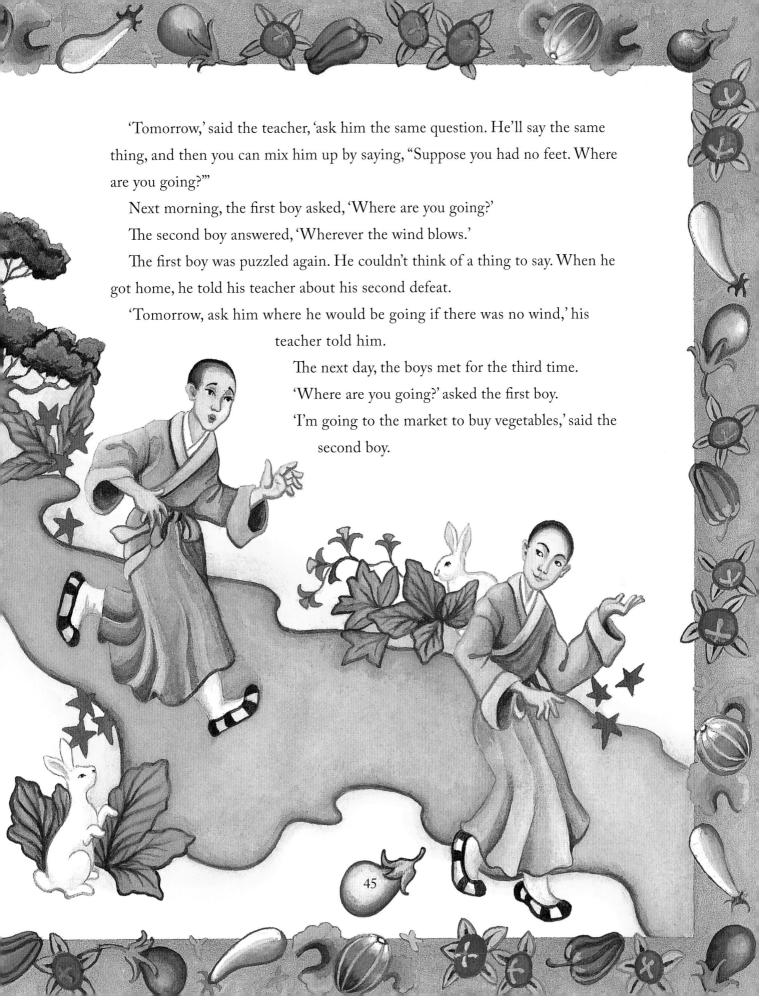

'Tomorrow,' said the teacher, 'ask him the same question. He'll say the same thing, and then you can mix him up by saying, "Suppose you had no feet. Where are you going?"'

Next morning, the first boy asked, 'Where are you going?'

The second boy answered, 'Wherever the wind blows.'

The first boy was puzzled again. He couldn't think of a thing to say. When he got home, he told his teacher about his second defeat.

'Tomorrow, ask him where he would be going if there was no wind,' his teacher told him.

The next day, the boys met for the third time.

'Where are you going?' asked the first boy.

'I'm going to the market to buy vegetables,' said the second boy.

45

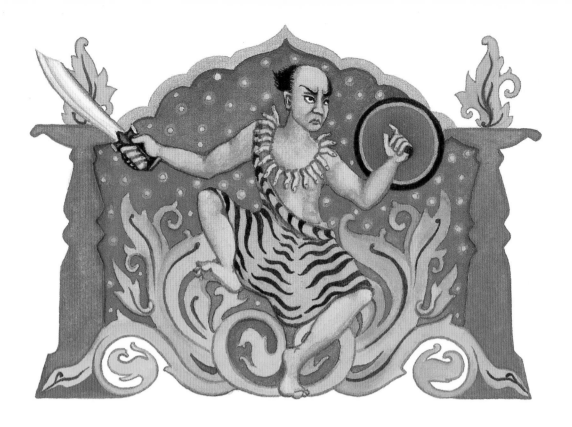

ANGULIMALA THE BRIGAND

Thousands of years ago, in the land of India, there was a prosperous kingdom called Kosala. The king's name was Prasenajit and his palace was in the glittering city of Shravasti, which was full of splendid shops, beautiful parks and magnificent mansions.

All was well and happy in the kingdom of Kosala until a terrible blight fell upon it. It was not the usual kind of catastrophe — a flood, famine, plague or war. Rather, it was all caused by one man — a fearsome brigand, whose name was Angulimala, which means 'finger necklace'. This is because he had made a vow to kill a thousand people, and to keep count, he saved a finger from each of his victims and wore it on a cord around his neck.

No one could stop Angulimala. The king's men could never catch him because he could run faster than the fastest horse and he was tremendously strong and very clever. Once a party of forty men on horseback went out to

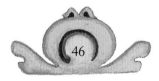

catch him, and he killed them all and strung their fingers on his necklace. Whole villages in the countryside became empty as all the people took refuge in the city out of fear of Angulimala. No one went out of doors at night for fear of Angulimala, and even during the day people stayed far, far away from the part of the country where he lived.

Now, at that time, it so happened that the great teacher called the Buddha, whose name means 'the awakened one', was also living in Kosala near the city of Shravasti. He was called 'the awakened one' because he had awakened from all the hopes and fears that torment human beings and keep them lost in a kind of dream. When they are happy, they hope to be happier and are afraid to lose the happiness they have. When they are unhappy, they fear they will remain that way. They blame other people for their problems and somehow hope to get out of them that way. But the Buddha had awakened from all that. He was content to be just as he was.

The Buddha lived as a monk, without any money or possessions. Every morning, after he had spent some time sitting calmly and peacefully without thinking about anything (which is called meditating), he would walk into the city of Shravasti to beg for his morning meal — his only meal of the day. He would start at the end of a street and go around to the back of each house, to the kitchen door, and stand there with his begging bowl without saying anything. India is a very hot country, so people kept their kitchen doors open. They would see the monk standing at the door, and if they had any extra food they would put some in his bowl. Everyone knew the Buddha was an awakened person, so when people saw him they felt honoured that he had come to their house, and he usually didn't have much trouble collecting a bowlful of food.

47

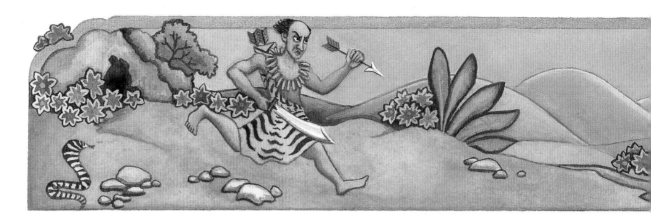

One particular morning, as he was on his begging round in Shravasti, he heard people complaining bitterly about Angulimala. They said that a great number of people were going to King Prasenajit's palace to demand that the king take his army and go out and catch the fearsome, invincible brigand. After hearing this, the Buddha carried his bowl of food back to his sleeping place, ate quietly and put his things in order. Then he set out along the road that led to where Angulimala lived.

As he walked along, the Buddha met people coming in the other direction. 'Do not go that way, monk,' they told him. 'Angulimala lives down there. Anybody who goes in that direction is sure to get killed!'

The Buddha listened politely to what they said, but then continued on his way in silence. At first, there were quite a few passers-by going in the opposite direction who gave the Buddha this warning. But the closer he got to Angulimala's lair, the fewer people were on the road. At last, except for him, the road was completely deserted. The Buddha continued walking quietly along.

Up on the hill in the forest, Angulimala saw the Buddha coming. 'How amazing!' thought the brigand. 'He can't have heard of me. People don't dare come this close even in groups of a hundred armed men — and here comes this unarmed monk all by himself. Wonderful! In a few minutes, I shall have another finger for my necklace, and with hardly any trouble at all!'

So saying, the brigand picked up his bow and arrows and buckled on his

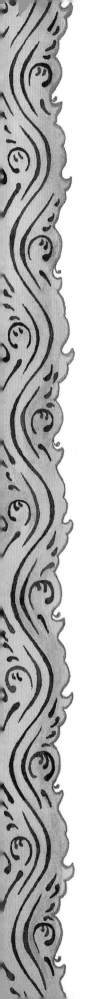

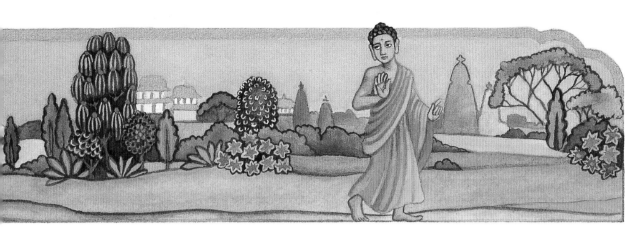

sword. Swiftly and nimbly, he ran down through the trees. Without making a sound, he came out on to the road a short distance behind the Buddha.

Then a strange thing happened. Angulimala couldn't catch up with the Buddha. As we know, Angulimala was a very fast runner, faster than a horse or a deer, but no matter how fast and long he ran, the Buddha was always just out of his reach. And the strangest thing was that the Buddha himself was not running at all. He was just walking along at his normal pace.

Angulimala could not understand this, and he became more and more furious at being unable to get his hands on the Buddha. He ran and ran, panting and sweating, panting and sweating. He ran until at last he could run no more. Then he stopped in his tracks and shouted at the Buddha, 'Stop, monk, stop, stop!'

The Buddha kept walking quietly along, but now the amazing thing was that although the brigand had stopped completely, the distance between them grew no greater.

'I have stopped,' said the Buddha, turning his head to look the brigand in the eye. 'Now, you should stop too.'

'What do you mean by that?!' shouted the infuriated brigand, who thought things were just the other way around.

'I've stopped living in dreams of hope and fear and so I have stopped hating and harming others. So instead of being stuck as you are, I can move just as I please. Now, listen, Angulimala: if you want to be able to go as you like, as I can, you should stop too.'

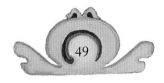

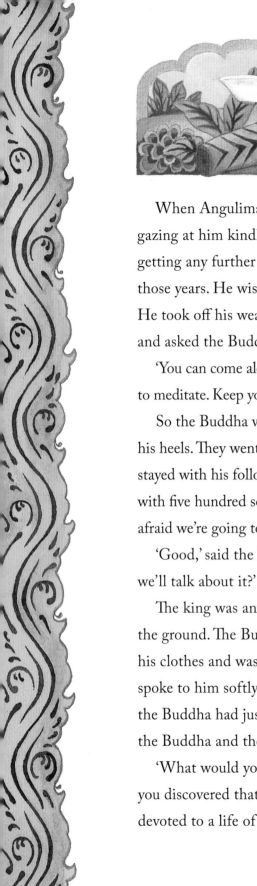

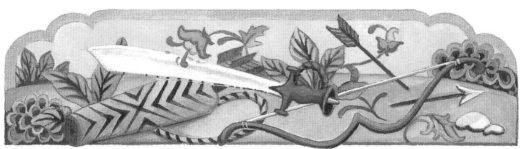

When Angulimala heard these words and looked at the Buddha, who was gazing at him kindly from just beyond his reach, walking calmly along without getting any further away, suddenly he realised how stupidly wrong he'd been all those years. He wished with all his heart that he'd never done harm to anyone. He took off his weapons and threw them in the ditch. Then he fell on his knees and asked the Buddha to help him.

'You can come along with me and be a monk,' said the Buddha. 'I'll teach you how to meditate. Keep your heart open the way it is now, and everything will be just fine.'

So the Buddha walked back into Shravasti with Angulimala walking humbly at his heels. They went to the Jeta Grove, a park in the city where the Buddha often stayed with his followers. Not long after they got there, King Prasenajit arrived with five hundred soldiers. 'We're going after Angulimala,' said the king. 'But I'm afraid we're going to have a difficult time, so I have come to ask your advice.'

'Good,' said the Buddha. 'Why don't you sit down and have a cup of tea and we'll talk about it?'

The king was anxious to seek the Buddha's help, so he sat down near him on the ground. The Buddha beckoned to Angulimala, who had by now changed his clothes and was wearing a simple monk's robe. He took him to one side and spoke to him softly. And so, when the water was ready, following the instructions the Buddha had just given him, the once fearsome brigand, Angulimala, served the Buddha and the king tea.

'What would you do,' said the Buddha to the king as they sipped their tea, 'if you discovered that Angulimala had become a simple monk, without possessions, devoted to a life of meditation and doing good for others?'

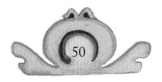

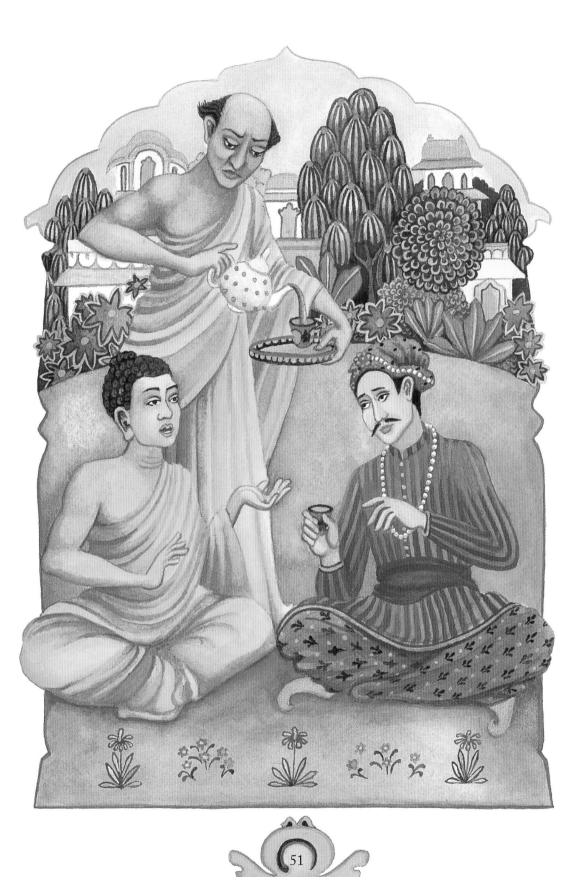

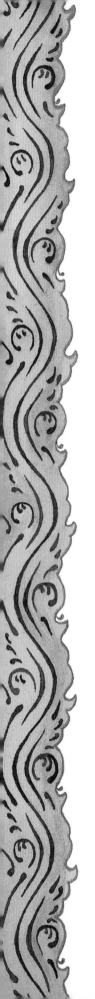

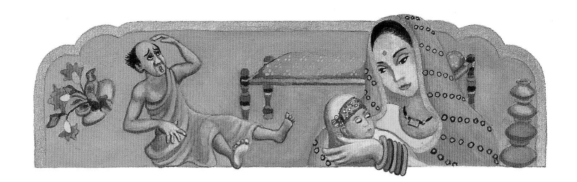

'To begin with, I'd be really amazed,' said the king. 'But if it really happened, I suppose I would pardon him and treat him with the respect due to a monk.'

'Good,' said the Buddha, 'because that is Angulimala who has served you tea.'

The king jumped up, white with fear and anger. But the Buddha soothed him, explaining that Angulimala had really changed and no one need be afraid of him anymore. After he had had a few minutes to get used to the new situation, the king let go of his bad feelings and began to feel really quite pleased. Then he took leave of the Buddha, explaining that he had other things to do, and he and his army all went home.

Angulimala became a very eager follower of the Buddha and spent a lot of time in the forest meditating according to his master's instructions. As sometimes happens to people who meditate a lot, after a while he began to develop special abilities which he used to help other people. Angulimala seemed to have a special talent for helping mothers give birth to their children. Whenever there was a problem with a birth, Angulimala was always called. It seemed he only had to be there for everything to go smoothly. So although many people remembered his bad deeds of earlier days and turned away from him when he was on his begging rounds, there were always enough grateful mothers or mothers-to-be, and Angulimala usually received enough to eat, so he could go back to the forest and meditate.

But when anyone has done as much evil as Angulimala had, killing all those people, there are bound to be bad results. After a few years, when the former brigand went to the city to beg, he began to have accidents. If a flowerpot fell off

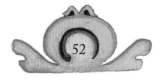

a windowsill, it would hit Angulimala. If anywhere near him someone was beating an animal, somehow the blows all landed on Angulimala. If someone threw a stone at someone else in anger, it hit Angulimala. Any time one person used a weapon on another, instead of hitting the intended person it hit Angulimala.

And it got worse and worse.

Finally, bruised and broken and only half alive, Angulimala dragged himself to the Buddha and begged him for help and advice.

The Buddha told him: 'Young man, gather your courage and hold out for a while longer. Though you may not think so, this is the very best thing that could be happening. All those murders you committed had to be paid for. If you had not changed your ways, you would have been reborn again and again and experienced terrible punishments in all your future lives. But since you have worked so hard to make your heart pure and have done so much to help other people, all your bad deeds are ripening now. If you can stand it just a little longer, it will be over. Your debt will be paid.'

So Angulimala took heart and he endured the painful accidents a while longer. Gradually, they happened less and less and finally stopped altogether. Angulimala went on meditating in the forest and giving his help whenever it was needed to mothers in childbirth. He lived a long time and came to be admired and even loved by the very people who once hated and feared him. Gradually, like the Buddha, he awoke entirely from his dream of hope and fear and became completely fearless and wholly contented.

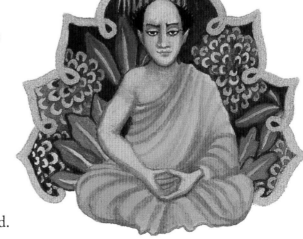

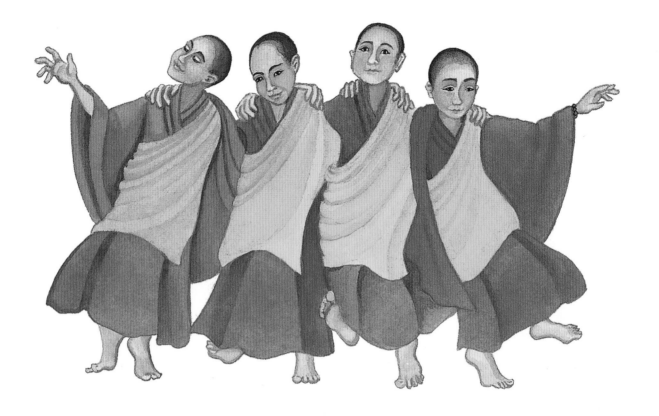

LEARNING TO BE SILENT

A group of four friends were all studying meditation. They decided, in order to clear their minds, to take a vow of silence and not talk for seven days. The first day, they meditated all day without saying a word. But when night fell and the oil lamps in the meditation hall grew dim, one of the friends whispered to a servant, 'Take care of those lamps.'

One of the others, shocked to hear his friend speaking, said, 'You are not supposed to be talking!'

The third one was overcome with irritation. 'You idiots!' he said. 'Why did you talk?'

'I am the only one who hasn't talked,' said the fourth friend, smiling proudly.

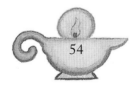

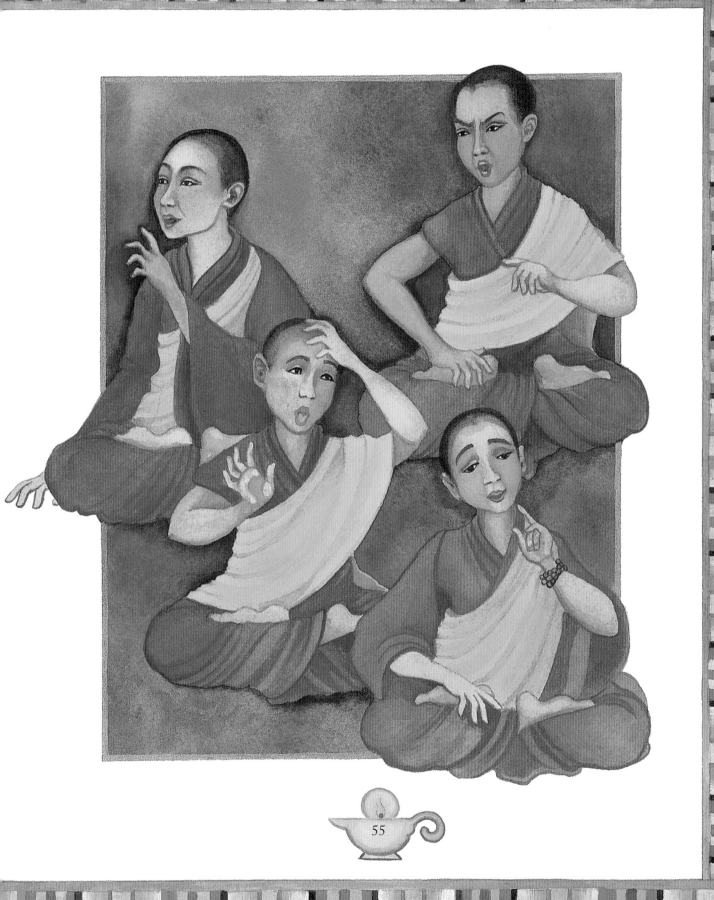

55

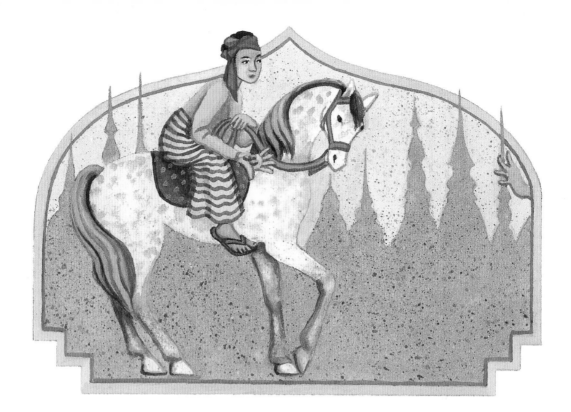

GOODHEART AND THE GODDESS OF THE FOREST

Once there lived a rich merchant who had three sons. The elder two sons had already long ago brought home well-to-do brides; only the youngest didn't seem to want to think about marriage. He spent all his time hanging around the town being friendly to the poor and giving them money. That is why everybody called him Goodheart.

But his two elder brothers and their wives were not happy about Goodheart's behaviour, because he was giving away the family money. One day, the brothers went to their father and said, 'Don't you see how carelessly our brother is giving away our money? Soon our entire fortune will be gone. You should throw him out of the house.' The father agreed and sent for his youngest son.

'Your brothers have been complaining about you,' he said. 'You've been giving our money thoughtlessly to the poor, and soon we'll all be beggars

ourselves. What you need is to go out into the world and learn how hard it is to earn a living. On top of that, it's high time you found a wife and got married.' Then he gave the youth a horse, three gold coins and his blessing to send him on his way. Goodheart thanked his father, said goodbye to his brothers and rode out of the town towards the south.

He wandered for days and weeks. Before long he gave his gold coins away. Then he sold his horse. He ate whatever he found or kind people gave him, and he slept wherever he was at the end of the day, mostly on the ground under the stars. He passed through many towns, always going south. One day he came to a part of the country where there were no more people or houses. He walked the whole day without meeting a single person or getting anything to eat. It grew dark, and he could not see a light in any direction. He seemed to have become lost in a very empty place, and he was afraid.

All at once, out of nowhere, an old man with white hair appeared in front of him. 'Good evening,' said Goodheart and bowed to the old man. 'Are you from this place? I'm lost and I'm looking for somewhere to spend the night.'

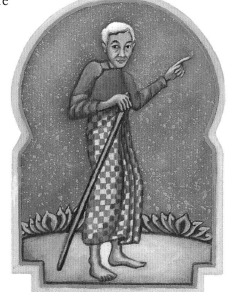

'I have come to give you a piece of advice,' said the old man and smiled mysteriously. 'Stop travelling south. Go north. Go north until you come to the edge of a forest. There you will find a fir tree with a slender trunk. Sit down under it and wait. When evening comes, it will begin to shiver and sigh, and then it will turn into a beautiful goddess. Then don't hesitate for an instant, but take hold of her by the hem of her dress and ask her to be your wife.'

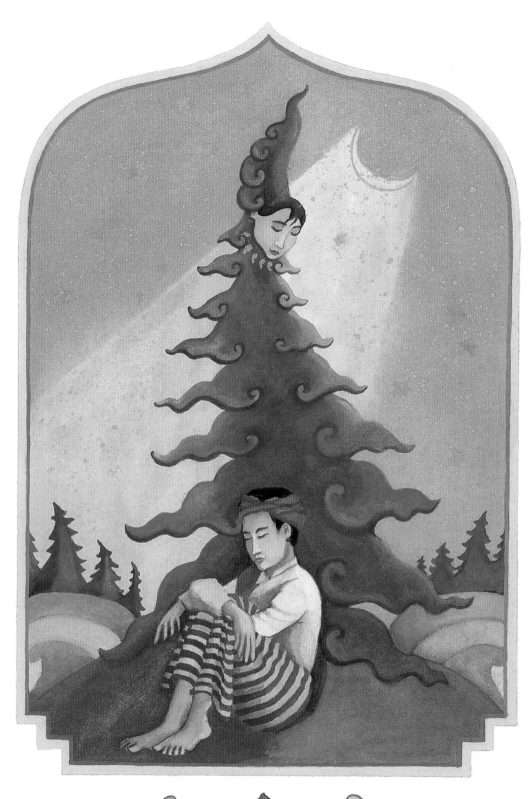

Then the old man disappeared as suddenly as if he had been swallowed by the earth. Goodheart lay down and went to sleep. The next day, he began walking north. He walked until he came to the edge of the forest and found a place where there was a fir tree with a slender trunk. He sat down and leant his head against it and waited. Night fell and the moon began to rise. As moonlight touched the forest, the trunk shivered and the tree gave a deep sigh. Before Goodheart's eyes, it turned into a beautiful goddess, who looked at him and smiled.

Goodheart fell in love with the goddess as soon as his eyes met hers. He took hold of the hem of her dress and said, 'O beautiful woman, please don't ever leave me. Please stay with me always and be my wife.'

'You ask much,' said the goddess, 'yet so it is to be.' And she gave him her hand.

'I am poor,' said the youth. 'I have nothing but my hands, but I will do everything to make us happy.'

'Let that be my worry too,' laughed the goddess. She unknotted her green headcloth and tossed it back over the top of her head. In an instant in front of them stood a lovely, snug little hut with the table already set in front of the hearth. Oh, how happy the young couple were!

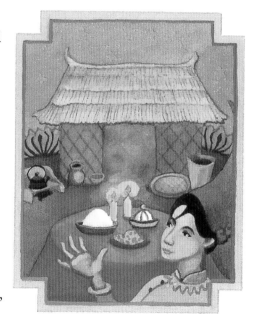

But after they had eaten, the goddess said, 'We can't stay here longer than three days. Whatever shall we do then?'

Before Goodheart could utter a word in reply, a messenger arrived and announced, 'The goddess's father commands Goodheart to come immediately and split wood for him.'

The goddess took the youth by the hand and whispered to him, 'That's what I was afraid of. My father is the forest giant. He wants to test you. He has three huge piles of firewood lying in his yard, but no mortal man can chop that wood. Take this axe and swing it three times over each heap.'

Goodheart took the axe and went to the giant's yard, and there he found three huge heaps of wood that were as hard as stone. Goodheart swung the axe over each heap three times, and an invisible hand chopped the wood into little pieces. In no more than an instant, the wood was split and neatly piled.

'Oh-ho,' said the giant, 'you're not a bad fellow. But you won't win my daughter that easily. Tomorrow her mother wants to see you.'

Goodheart went home to the goddess and told her everything.

'Oh, that's awful!' said the goddess. 'My mother is the forest witch. A visit to her can only end badly.

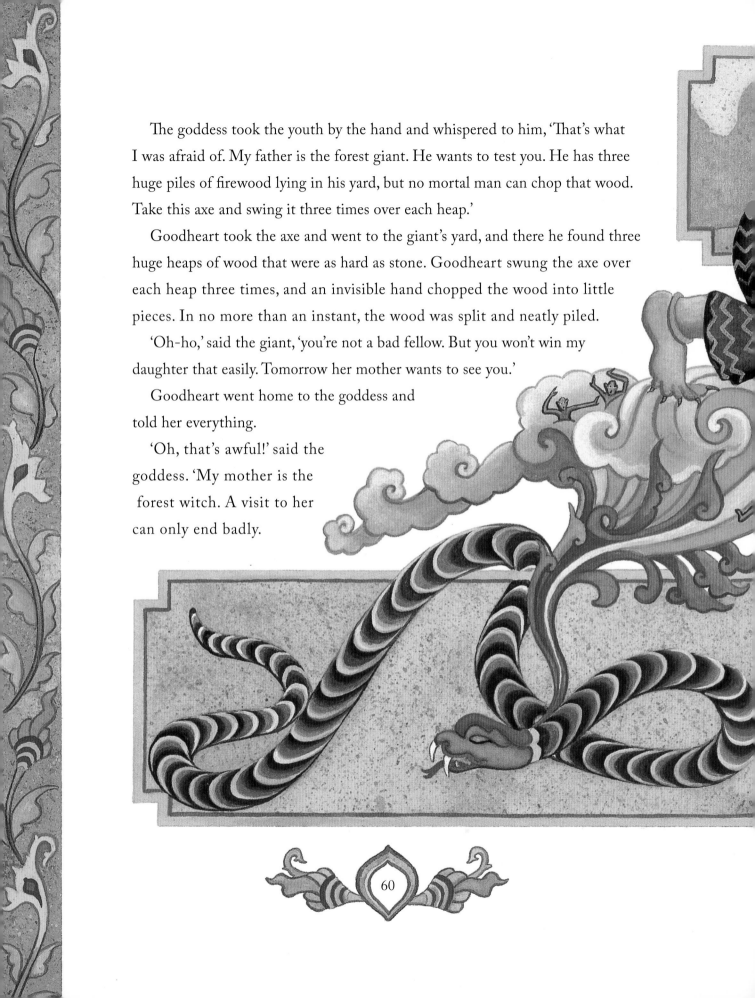

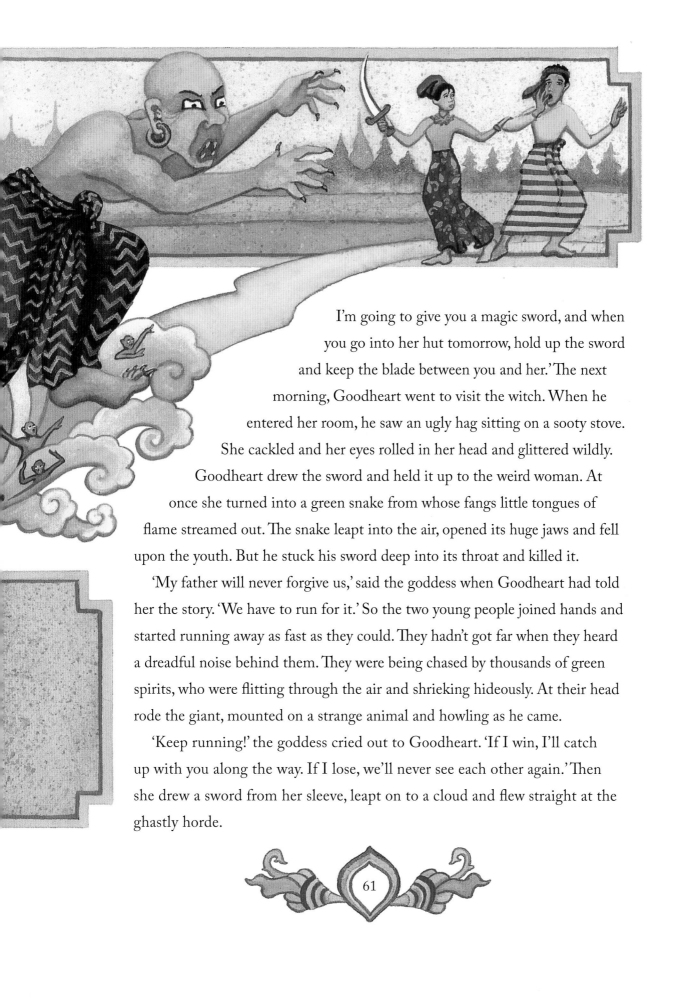

I'm going to give you a magic sword, and when
you go into her hut tomorrow, hold up the sword
and keep the blade between you and her.' The next
morning, Goodheart went to visit the witch. When he
entered her room, he saw an ugly hag sitting on a sooty stove.
She cackled and her eyes rolled in her head and glittered wildly.
Goodheart drew the sword and held it up to the weird woman. At
once she turned into a green snake from whose fangs little tongues of
flame streamed out. The snake leapt into the air, opened its huge jaws and fell
upon the youth. But he stuck his sword deep into its throat and killed it.

'My father will never forgive us,' said the goddess when Goodheart had told
her the story. 'We have to run for it.' So the two young people joined hands and
started running away as fast as they could. They hadn't got far when they heard
a dreadful noise behind them. They were being chased by thousands of green
spirits, who were flitting through the air and shrieking hideously. At their head
rode the giant, mounted on a strange animal and howling as he came.

'Keep running!' the goddess cried out to Goodheart. 'If I win, I'll catch
up with you along the way. If I lose, we'll never see each other again.' Then
she drew a sword from her sleeve, leapt on to a cloud and flew straight at the
ghastly horde.

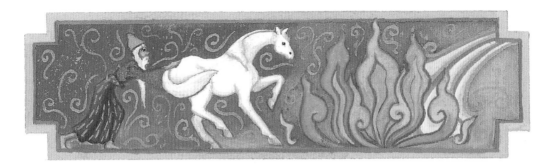

'Miserable creature! You've bound yourself to a mortal and destroyed your own mother. You'll be sorry!' the voice of the giant thundered out of the cloud.

There was a fierce battle. Sword clattered on sword and there were many screams and cries. The goddess fought with deadly courage and finally she put the horde of green spirits to flight. As the noise of the battle died away, the sky cleared. There was just one white cloud in the sky, which was sailing gently down to earth. The goddess jumped from the cloud, unknotted her green headcloth and tossed it back over the top of her head. In an instant, she changed into a white stallion and galloped away after Goodheart.

When the stallion appeared next to the youth, he grabbed it by the tail, swung himself up on its back and trotted into the nearby town. There he met a magician who was disguised as a merchant. The magician had only to glance at the beautiful white stallion to know it was no ordinary horse. He told Goodheart he was a horse dealer and offered him another horse, complete with saddle, for the stallion and a bag of gold coins into the bargain.

'That's a deal!' said Goodheart and gave the stallion to the magician.

'And now let's see what this horse really is,' said the magician when he got home. He fired up his stove, and when it was so hot that flames were licking out of the chimney top, he pushed the horse into the oven. But as soon as he closed the oven door, it popped open again and out flew a little bird.

'Wait till I catch you!' shouted the magician in a rage. He turned himself into a hawk and flew after the little bird. He was just about to catch the little creature, when it changed into a golden ring and fell to the ground in the midst of a crowd of playing children.

'That's a pretty ring!' cried a boy and ran home with it to put it in his special box.

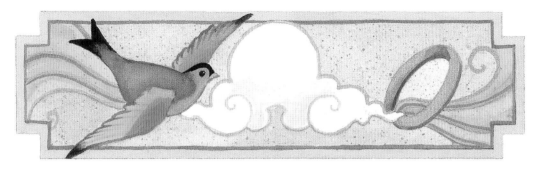

But the magician got there first and met him at the door. 'Give that ring to me!' he snapped.

'No, it's mine!' said the child.

'No, it's mine! I lost it. It's got my sign on it.' Then he snatched the ring out of the child's hand.

'Now you won't get away,' gloated the magician, looking down at the ring in his hand. But at the same moment it slipped from his grasp and fell to the ground. The magician got down on his hands and knees and looked everywhere, but no matter how hard he looked, he couldn't find it.

'Look all you like, you'll never find me!' called a voice above his head. The magician looked up in time to see a white cloud sailing away with the forest goddess on it, laughing at him.

Now the goddess raced like the wind after Goodheart. When she caught up with him, she jumped from the cloud and said, 'So I was to be your wife, but I changed myself into a white stallion so I could become your wife; then you went and sold me to a magician which almost cost me my life!'

'Don't be angry, darling goddess,' said Goodheart. 'I didn't know it was you.' He took her by the hand and they went home together. What a joy it was when the youngest son returned home with his beautiful bride! They immediately invited all their family and friends to their wedding. The two elder brothers came, and there was also an old uncle, who had one hen eye and one all-seeing cock eye. The uncle looked the wives of the two older brothers over with approval, but he couldn't take his gaze off Goodheart's beautiful bride. Something seemed to him not quite right about her.

The wives of the elder brothers could only carry one bowl at a time when it came to serving the guests, but Goodheart's bride always brought several. In the kitchen, she was a marvel. The food seemed to turn into wonderfully cooked meals all by itself.

'There's something strange here,' thought the uncle. He shut his hen eye tight and looked at her piercingly with his cock eye. After a while, he said to himself, 'She's not from this world.' He took Goodheart's father aside and said, 'Look, brother, this is none of my business, but there's something I don't like about the bride. It wouldn't do to have an evil spirit in the family. You'd better throw her out of the house before it's too late.'

'What are you saying?!' Goodheart cried when his father told him of his uncle's suspicions. 'Do you have any idea how hard and rare it is to win such a bride? I will never be parted from her.'

The uncle said no more. Then the time came for his own only daughter to be married. He invited the wives of the three brothers and gave them the task of making a hundred dresses for the bride. All the dresses had to be ready in three days. The wives of the two older brothers went straight to work. But Goodheart's wife lay about the house, singing to herself and not lifting a finger. At the end of two days, the elder brothers' wives had made only five dresses each. Desperately they stared at all the bolts of cloth that still had to be made into dresses.

'Give them here,' said Goodheart's wife and carried all the cloth into her room. 'Tonight, I'll do some sewing,' she said.

That night, the goddess took nine candles, set them up in a row and lit them one after the other. From the flames of the burning candles, nine pillars of smoke arose. They found their way out the windows and rose higher and higher until they reached all the way up into the sky. Then nine maidens came down the pillars of smoke and set to work making dresses. First they measured and cut the

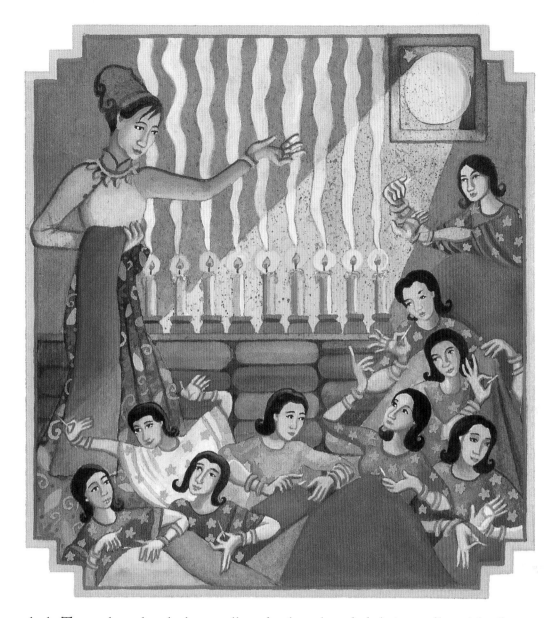

cloth. Then when the cloth was all ready, they threaded their needles with silver moonbeams and sewed the dresses with such fine stitches that no seams could be found. Before long, stacks of gorgeous dresses lay all about the room. When the last dress was done, the candles went out and the maidens disappeared.

In the morning, the uncle came and said, 'So, now, ladies, have you finished your work?'

Said the older brothers' wives, 'We worked as hard as we could, but we were only able to make five dresses apiece. Goodheart's wife took all the rest of the cloth.'

65

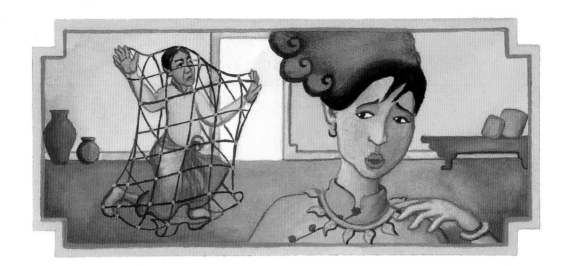

'And how many dresses did you make?' he asked Goodheart's wife.

She pointed at the dresses all piled up in her room. 'Here are ninety dresses,' she said. The uncle shut his hen eye tight and, winking his cock eye very quickly once for each dress, he counted up the dresses. Now he was sure there was no mistake. This wife of Goodheart's was not from this world. But he still said not a word.

One day when the goddess was alone in the house, there came a loud banging on the door. When she opened it, the uncle pushed his way into the room with a net of the kind that is used to catch spirits. The goddess knew right away what the uncle was up to, and before he could even try to catch her, he was all tangled up in his own spirit net. Then the goddess ran to Goodheart and said, 'You know I come from no earthly race. I have no choice now but to leave this place. Come with me if you want. Otherwise, we must separate forever.'

'A man and a wife should face together whatever good or evil comes to them,' declared Goodheart. 'I will never leave you.'

'Then close your eyes and give me your hand,' said the goddess. Goodheart closed his eyes, gave her his hand and at once began to feel himself flying through the air. A long time passed before he felt firm ground under his feet. As he opened his eyes, he saw the goddess unknot her green cloth and toss it back over her head. In an instant, a small but very cosy little hut stood before them,

and there they lived, happy and contented. Before a year had passed, the goddess gave birth to a beautiful son.

At the time that the little boy was taking his first steps, it happened that the imperial army was passing through the region. The soldiers saw the young woman and how beautiful she was, and they tried to carry her off as a gift to the emperor. But once again she threw her green cloth over her head. At that very instant, a white cloud floated down from the sky, took the goddess, her son and Goodheart, and flew away as the soldiers looked on in amazement.

Higher and higher and higher flew the cloud, into the depths of the sky, where it finally stopped. Since that time, the goddess and her husband and her son have lived in the sky. And whoever does not believe it has only to look up at the stars at night. If you're lucky, you'll see three lights — two big ones and a small one — that never, never grow apart.

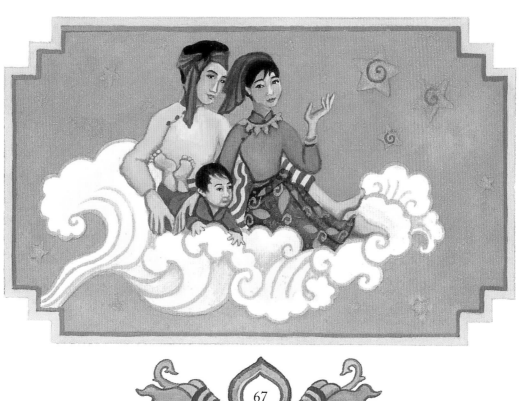

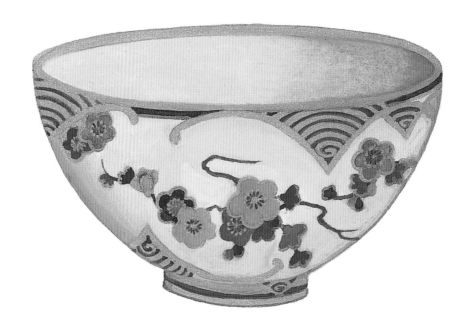

THE DEATH OF A TEACUP

There was once a great teacher of Zen, a school of the Buddha's teaching that is very down to earth about how the things in life really are. This great teacher's name was Ikkyu. Even as a young boy he was very clever and always found a way of getting himself out of trouble.

One day as he was playing, Ikkyu knocked over a teacup, which fell to the floor and shattered into pieces. Now the teacup belonged to his teacher, and it was very old and precious, and his teacher valued it greatly. As Ikkyu was worrying about this accident, he heard his teacher coming and quickly hid the pieces of the cup behind his back. When his teacher appeared, Ikkyu asked him, 'Why do people die?'

'That is just natural,' his teacher replied. 'Everything only has so long to live, and then it must die.'

At these words, Ikkyu showed his teacher the pieces of the broken teacup.

68

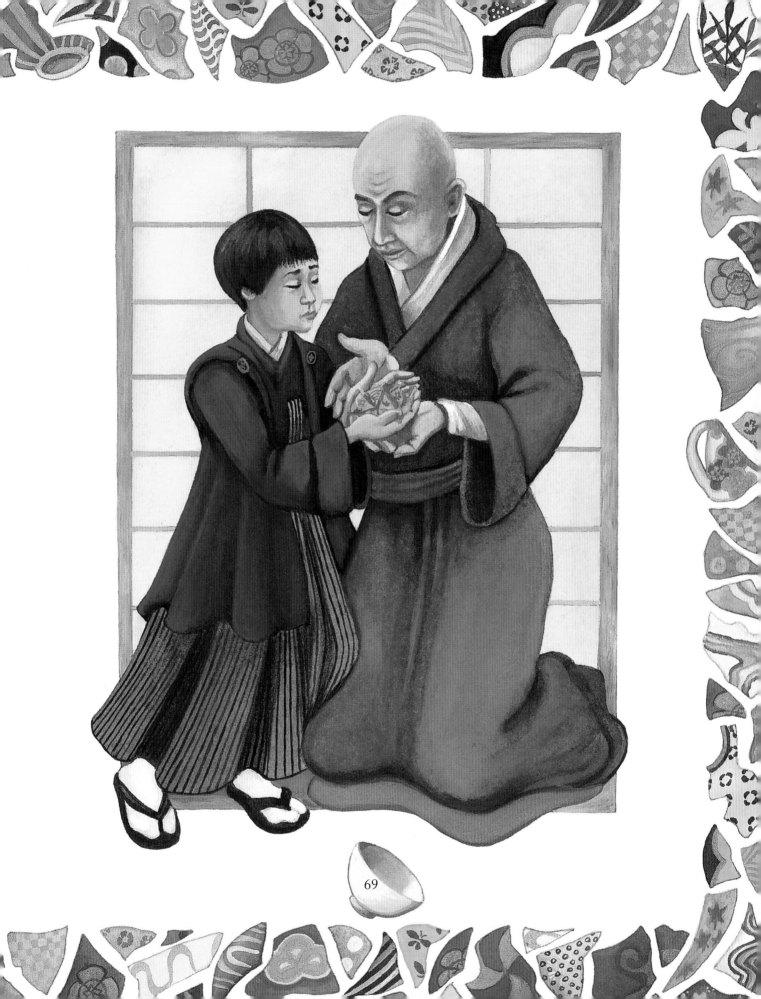

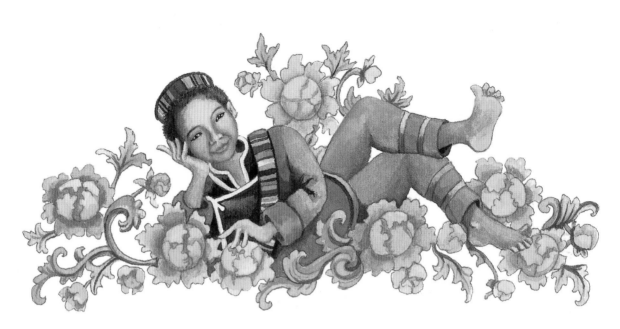

THE FOOLISH BOY

There was once a boy who lived with his poor mother in a small cottage. As the boy grew up, he was found to be rather weak-minded. He was continually getting into trouble because he was so simple. The other children made fun of him by getting him to believe the most outrageous stories.

One day, he went for a walk in a field full of yellow spring flowers — barefoot, of course, since he had no shoes. He was sitting among the flowers when another boy passed and called to him, 'Hey, do you know that the soles of your feet have turned all yellow? That's a sure sign you're going to die right away.'

The poor foolish boy was very frightened, but he thought to himself, 'If I am going to die, then I'll need a grave.' So he began digging. Pretty soon he had made a shallow hole. He lay down in it and began waiting to die.

Just then, one of the king's servants came by carrying a big earthenware jar full of oil for the king. He saw the boy lying in the hole and asked him what he was doing.

'The soles of my feet have turned yellow, and as you know, that's a sure sign I'm about to die. So I've made myself a little grave and I'm waiting.'

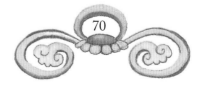

'That's ridiculous!' said the king's servant. 'You couldn't talk to me like that if you were dying. Why don't you get out of that hole and do something useful? Look, help me carry this jar of oil to the king, and in return I'll give you a hen.'

So the foolish boy climbed out of the hole, lifted the big jar of oil on to his back and started off for the palace with the king's servant. As they went along, the boy thought about what he would do with the hen he was going to get.

'When the hen lays eggs, I'll let her hatch them,' he thought. 'I should end up with quite a few chicks. When the chicks grow up into cocks and hens, I'll sell them at the market. Then I'll take the money and buy a cow. Then the cow will have a calf, and I'll sell both the cow and the calf and buy a nice little house. Once I have a house, I'll be able to get married. Then my wife and I will have a baby. When the child grows up, I'll have to make sure it behaves properly. If it's good and does what it's told, I'll be very kind to it. But if it's disobedient, I shall be very firm with it and stamp my foot, just like this!'

And the boy stamped his foot so hard that the jar slipped off his back and smashed to bits on the ground. When the king's servant saw the broken jar and the spilled oil, he lost his temper.

'What do you mean by stamping your foot like that and spilling the king's oil?!' he screamed. The boy felt he could explain everything, but when he tried, the servant lost patience, took him by the ear and dragged him off to the king.

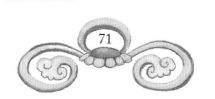

71

'Your Majesty, I tried to get this boy to help carry your oil. But as we were walking along, suddenly he started stamping his foot like a maniac. The jar slipped off his back and broke into a hundred pieces!'

The king asked the boy to explain his behaviour.

'Well, your Majesty,' he replied, 'your servant offered me a hen in payment for carrying the oil. Since I knew I was going to get a hen, it was only natural for me to plan what I would do with it. I quickly figured that by selling the chickens I could buy a cow, and then the cow would have a calf, and by selling the cow and calf, I could buy a house. Then I could get married and have a child. I had to plan how to raise the child properly. I resolved that if it was disobedient, I would have to be firm with it and stamp my foot to show it I meant business.'

When the king had heard this ridiculous story, he was quite amused. He had a good laugh, gave the boy a gold coin and told him to go home to his mother.

When the boy reached his house, he saw a strange dog sneaking out of the front door with a purse full of money in his mouth. He became extremely excited and began shouting to his mother that a dog was running off with her purse. When the mother saw what was happening, she was afraid the boy would attract other people with his cries and somebody else would chase the dog and get the money. So she ran up on to the roof of the house and sprinkled sugar all over it. Then she called to the boy to come up as quickly as he could.

'Look!' she said. 'It's been raining sugar on the roof!'

The boy loved sugar and immediately set to work gathering it all up. With her son busy in this way, the mother slipped out of the house, quickly found the dog and got her purse back.

Some time later, the boy's mother arranged to marry the boy into a rich family who lived far enough away that they hadn't heard of the youth's simple-mindedness. The custom was for the man to go to live with the bride's family.

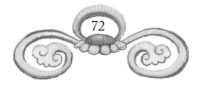

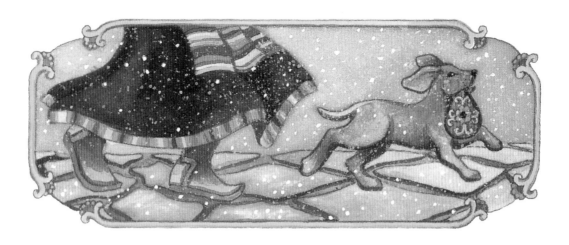

First the men of the bride's family came to the groom's house for a feast, and then they were to take the groom back home with them. The boy dressed in his best clothes, but when the feast was over, he asked the men from his bride's family to go on ahead, since he wanted to take some time to say goodbye to his mother.

At nightfall, he rode off alone by moonlight. As he went, he could see his shadow moving along beside him. He could not see it exactly, but he was afraid it was a ghost or demon, so he kicked his horse into a gallop to get away. But the faster he went, the faster his shadow went too. He saw he was not going to escape, so he grabbed his hat and threw it hard at the shadow to try to frighten it. That didn't work, so he threw his coat at it too, then his shirt, then his trousers and so on, until he didn't have a stitch left on his body. But the shadow was not frightened and continued to follow him closely. Thinking he might slip away, he jumped off his horse and began running along the road on foot. He ran till he reached the shade of a big tree that grew by the side of the road.

Once under the tree, he was overjoyed to find that the shadow had disappeared. But as soon as he peeped out from the shadow of the tree, no matter in which direction, the shadow appeared again. This was very upsetting. Finally the foolish boy decided the safest thing was to stay in the shade of the tree, so he climbed up into the branches and soon was fast asleep.

Some travellers came along the same way some time later. As they approached, they were surprised to find articles of clothing scattered along the

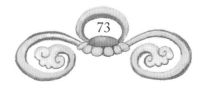

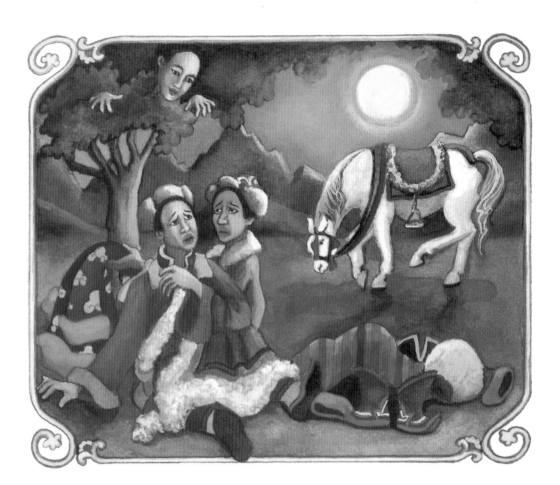

road. They gathered them up one by one, and when they found a horse grazing by the roadside, they took that too. They came to the big tree and sat down beneath it to divide up what they had found. Just then the boy woke up and saw what was going on below. So he cried out, 'What about me! I want my share too!'

Hearing a loud voice coming out of the tree, the travellers were frightened out of their wits. Thinking that it must be a demon demanding his share, they ran as fast as they could, leaving the clothes and the horse behind. The boy climbed out of the tree, put on his clothes, mounted the horse and rode off to his bride's house.

When he got there, he found he wasn't so very late. The bride's parents led him to a big room where family, friends and neighbours were waiting to begin the wedding feast. Everyone started to celebrate. There was laughing and singing and lots to eat and drink. The boy was having quite a good time, but he also found he missed his mother. He thought the least he could do was save her

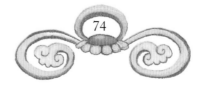

some of this excellent food. He found a copper vase with a small mouth and hid it in his lap. As he ate, he kept dropping choice bits into the vase for his mother. He was putting a little cake in the vase very carefully, when his hand went in too far and got stuck. He couldn't get it out! This was quite awkward. With his hand stuck in the vase, he couldn't eat. Everybody noticed he wasn't eating and pressed him to have more. But he just sat there with his hand in his lap saying he'd had enough, though he was still very hungry.

Hours later, the guests left and the boy was left alone with his bride. She asked him what was the matter with him and why he was acting so strangely. At first, he was too shy to say anything, but finally he had to tell her the story and show her his hand stuck in the vase.

'Oh, that's not such a big problem,' she said sweetly. 'There's a big white stone at the foot of the stairs. Just beat the vase against the stone and it's bound to break or come off.'

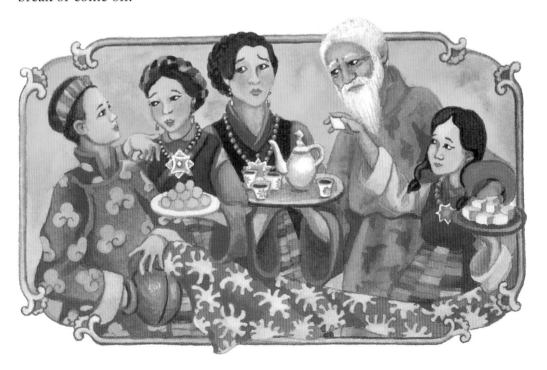

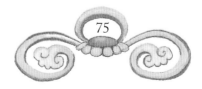

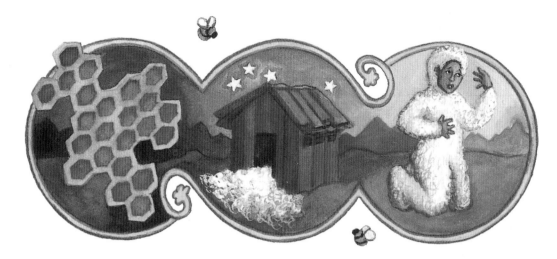

So the young fellow stole down the stairs in the dark and came to what looked like a big white stone near the bottom of the steps. He crept up to it, raised his arm and brought down the copper vase with all his might on the round white object. The vase broke and came off his hand, but to his horror instead of the clank he expected, he heard an awful groan. Looking closer, he found that what he had hit wasn't a stone at all. It was his white-haired father-in-law to whom he had given a violent blow on the head. The poor man had drunk too much beer at the feast and fallen asleep at the foot of the stairs.

Terrified and sure that he had killed him, the boy ran out of the house into the night. After a while, he came to a farm. A large honeycomb had been left in a corner of the farmyard. Not knowing what it was, the boy lay down on it and fell asleep. He was soon smeared all over with honey. In the middle of the night, he grew cold and crawled into a shed where wool was stored. He lay down on that and slept until dawn.

When he awoke, he saw in the morning light that he was all white and woolly. 'Oh, no!' thought the poor, simple boy. 'As a punishment for killing my father-in-law, I've been turned into a sheep!' He was very unhappy, but he ran out of the courtyard and joined a flock of sheep grazing on a nearby hillside. He spent the whole day wandering around with the sheep, trying his best to learn the customs and habits of his new companions. At night, he went with them into the enclosure where they slept.

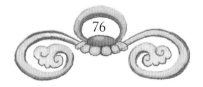

At midnight, some robbers came. They felt around among the sheep, trying to get hold of a nice plump one. The boy was the most meaty, so one of them hoisted him up on his back and they carried him off to their hideout. They laid him on the ground and were getting ready to cut him up for their dinner when the boy became so frightened, he forgot he was supposed to be a sheep. He shouted loudly, 'Please don't kill me, kind robbers!'

Hearing a sheep with human speech, the robbers went white with fear and took to their heels. The boy was hungry and exhausted from his adventures as a sheep, so he went back to his bride's house. There he found out that the bride's father was not dead but had only been hurt. When the whole story came out, the poor youth was completely forgiven, and he settled down to live happily with his wife.

After some years, he thought he would like to make a bit of money as a trader, so he gathered some things to sell and set off for India. One night on the way, he stopped at a large inn. The innkeeper made the young man comfortable and invited him to his table for dinner. As they ate, the innkeeper told him all sorts of strange stories. Finally, the young man had to blurt out that he didn't believe him.

'To prove I'm telling the truth, tonight I'll show you something stranger than anything I've told you. I'll bet you when dark falls tonight, a cat will carry a lantern into this room.'

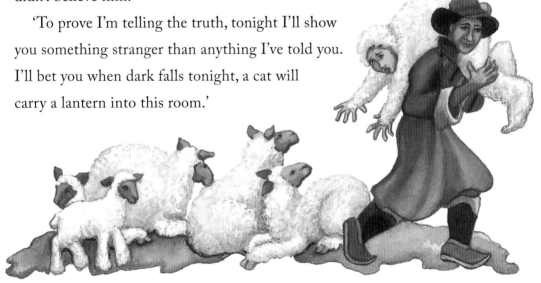

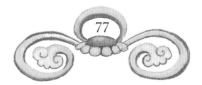

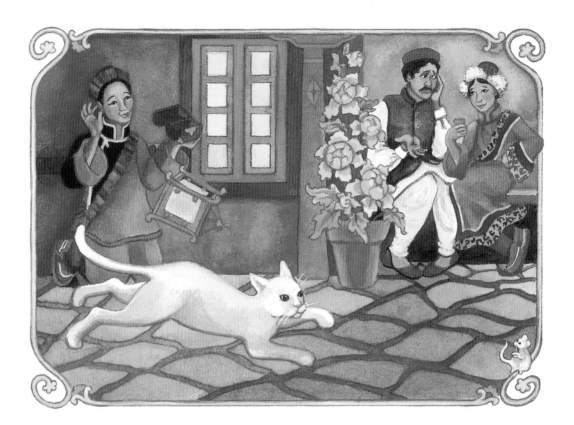

The young man thought his host's boasting was quite silly, so he said, 'All right, I'll bet you anything you like.'

'Very well,' said the innkeeper, 'I'll bet everything I have, my house and all, against everything you have, all of your possessions.'

'Fine,' said the young man, quite pleased with himself. 'The bet is on.'

Sure enough, that evening just at twilight, a large white cat walked into the room carrying a lantern in its mouth. It seems that the innkeeper had spent a long time training it to do this, so he could trick people who stayed at his inn. So the young man had to give everything he had to the innkeeper. He had no choice but to remain at the inn as a servant.

After some months, the young man's wife became worried about him. Knowing him as she did, she was afraid he'd got himself into some kind of trouble. She decided to go and see for herself. Disguising herself as a merchant, she took a few loads of wool to sell and set out to follow her husband.

Some days later, she arrived at the inn where he was living as a servant. They

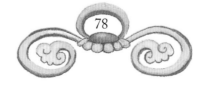

were very happy to see one another, and the young man told her everything that had happened. She told him to say nothing to the innkeeper and went inside and took a room for the night. As he usually did with his guests, the innkeeper invited her to dinner, and during dinner he managed to make the same bet with her as he'd made with her husband. If a cat came in with a lantern when night fell the next evening, the innkeeper was to have all her possessions, and if not, she was to have all of his.

The following day, the wife gave her husband a little box with three mice in it and some special instructions. Then she went to sit with the innkeeper to wait for the cat. Just at twilight, the big white cat started across the courtyard with the lantern in its mouth. The husband did what his wife had told him. He let out one of the mice, which ran right in front of the cat. The cat jumped in the air and almost ran after the mouse. But it had been so well trained, it regained control of itself and continued across the courtyard with the lantern. The husband let out another mouse, which also scampered right in front of the cat. The cat was so tempted that it stopped and turned around in a circle three times, but still its training held, and it continued towards the doorway with the lantern. When it was just about to open the door, the husband released the last mouse. This time the temptation was too much for the cat. It dropped the lantern and ran off after the mouse.

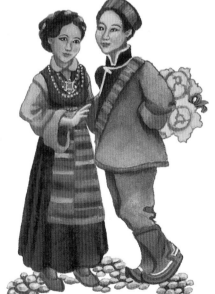

Darkness fell and the cat never appeared with the lantern. The innkeeper finally had to admit that he had lost his bet. He handed over to the disguised wife not only his own property but also everything he had won from her husband. The young man and his wife, taking all these possessions with them, returned to their own house, and they lived happily ever after.

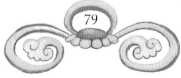

79

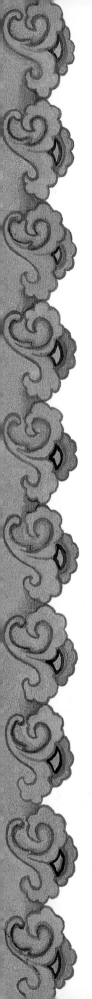

SOURCES

'**The Living Kuan Yin**': Carol Kendall and Yao-wen Li. *Sweet and Sour: Tales from China.* New York: Seabury Press, 1978.

'**The Most Important Thing**': Seikan Hasegawa. *The Cave of Poison Grass: Essays on the Hannya Sutra.* Arlington, VA: Great Ocean Publishers, 1975.

'**The Man Who Didn't Want to Die**': Yei Theodora Ozaki. *Japanese Fairy Book.* Tokyo: Charles E. Tuttle, 1970.

'**Useless Work**': This story comes from an oral tradition. It has been told for centuries, and the source is unknown.

'**The Conch Maiden**' and '**Goodheart and the Goddess of the Forest**': D. and M. Stovickova. *Tibetische Märchen: Märchen, Mythen und Legenden aus Tibet und anderen Ländern des Ferne Osfens.* Hanau, Germany: Verlag Werner Dausien, 1974.

'**The Wisdom of the Crows**': Post Wheeler. *Tales from the Japanese Storytellers.* Toyko: Charles E. Tuttle Company, 1964.

'**The Stone Ape**': Lim Sian-tek. *Folk Tales from China.* New York: John Day Company, 1944.

'**Where Are You Going?**', '**Learning to be Silent**' and '**The Death of a Teacup**': Paul Reps. *Zen Flesh, Zen Bones.* Garden City, NY: Anchor Books / Doubleday & Company, n.d.

'**Angulimala the Brigand**': Sherab Chödzin Kohn. *The Awakened One: A Life of the Buddha.* Boston: Shambhala Publications, 1994.

'**The Foolish Boy**': Captain W. F. O'Connor. *Folk-Tales from Tibet.* London: Hurst and Blackett, 1906.

The tales gathered in this collection are all traditional ones and may also have appeared elsewhere than in the sources given above.

Barefoot Books, 294 Banbury Road, Oxford, OX2 7ED

ISBN 978–1–84686–823–8

British Cataloguing-in-Publication Data: a catalogue record for this book is available from the British Library

1 3 5 7 9 8 6 4 2

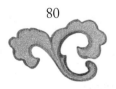

The Barefoot Book of
BUDDHIST
TALES

RETOLD BY Sherab Chödzin & Alexandra Kohn
ILLUSTRATED BY Marie Cameron

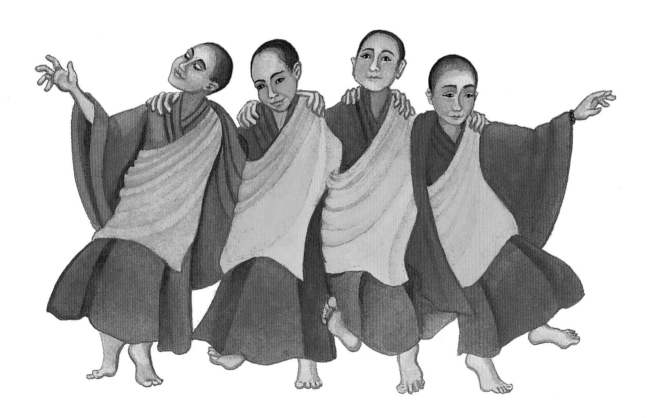

Barefoot Books

CONTENTS

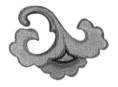
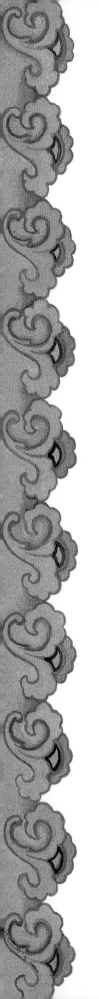